Designing a More Inclusive World

Springer
London
Berlin
Heidelberg
New York
Hong Kong
Milan
Paris
Tokyo

Simeon Keates, John Clarkson,
Patrick Langdon and Peter Robinson (Eds)

Designing a More Inclusive World

With 84 Figures

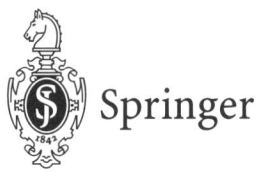 Springer

Simeon Keates, MA, PhD
John Clarkson, MA, PhD, MIEE, CEng
Patrick Langdon, BA, PhD
Engineering Design Centre, Department of Engineering, University of
Cambridge, Trumpington Street, Cambridge, CB2 1PZ, UK

Peter Robinson, MA, PhD, CEng
Computer Laboratory, University of Cambridge, William Gates Building,
JJ Thomson Avenue, Cambridge, CB3 0FD, UK

British Library Cataloguing in Publication Data
Cambridge Workshop on UA and AT (2nd : 2004 : Fitzwilliam
    College, Cambridge)
    Designing a more inclusive world
    1. Self-help devices for people with disabilities –
    Congresses 2. People with disabilities – Rehabilitation –
    Technological innovations - Congresses 3. User interfaces
    (Computer systems) – Congresses
    I. Title II. Keates, Simeon
    617'.03
ISBN 1852338199

Library of Congress Cataloging-in-Publication Data
A catalog record for this book is available from the Library of Congress

ISBN 1-85233-819-9 Springer-Verlag London Berlin Heidelberg
Springer-Verlag is part of Springer Science+Business Media
springeronline.com

Typesetting: Electronic text files prepared by author
Printed and bound at The Cromwell Press, Trowbridge, Wiltshire
69/3830-543210 Printed on acid-free paper SPIN 10948057

Preface

The second Cambridge Workshop on Universal Access and Assistive Technology (CWUAAT) was held at Fitzwilliam College, Cambridge, in March 2004.

CWUAAT '04 represents the continuation a new series of workshops that are held every two years and encourage discussion of a broad range of interests. There is a general focus on product/solution development. Hence the principal requirements for the successful design of assistive technology are addressed and these range from the identification and capture of the needs of the users, through to the development and evaluation of truly usable and accessible systems for users with special needs.

The best submissions received for CWUAAT '04 are contained in this book; the contributors are all leading researchers in the fields of Universal Access and Assistive Technology and represent a large part of the international research community. They include, though not exclusively, computer scientists, designers, engineers, industrial representatives, ergonomists and sociologists.

Universal Access and Assistive Technology have increasingly important roles to play in the future as the global population grows older and many more people exhibit some degree of functional impairment. Hence, there is a need to encourage wide-ranging discussion, co-operation and collaboration within and between the Universal Access and Assistive Technology research communities. One of the principal aims of the first CWUAAT and this book is to promote such discussion.

This book is divided into three sections.

Part I – Design Issues for Universal Access and Assistive Technology – focuses on helping designers to adopt inclusive design into their mainstream design practice.

Part II – Enabling Computer Access and New Technologies – looks at methods for making computer access as inclusive as possible. This section also includes four chapters focusing on the issues of social acceptability, in other words designing not just for functional performance, but also trying to enhance 'softer' properties such as aesthetic values.

Part III – Assistive Technology and Rehabilitation Robotics – looks at the latest state-of-the-art in purpose-built assistance for users with more severe impairments.

In summary, the book provides a snapshot of the best current thinking on Universal Access and Assistive Technology, with contributors from academic, public and commercial institutions spread across four continents.

Finally, our thanks must go to all those who contributed to the success of CWUAAT and to the compilation of this book. Many thanks are due to all the contributors who, with the assistance of the Programme Committee, were responsible for setting the high standards of reporting seen in this book. Particular thanks are also due to Christa Croghan who, with the staff at Fitzwilliam College, so enthusiastically helped to organise and host the workshop.

Simeon Keates and John Clarkson
On behalf of the CWUAAT Organising Committee
University of Cambridge
March 2004

Contents

Part II Enabling Computer Access and New Technologies

Part III Assistive Technology and Rehabilitation Robotics

List of Contributors

Adams R., School of Computing Science, Middlesex University, London, UK

Adlam T., Bath Institute of Medical Engineering, University of Bath, Wolfson Centre, Royal United Hospital, Bath, UK

Allen J.L., Department of Design, Monash University, Melbourne, Australia

Arnott J., Division of Applied Computing, Dundee University, Dundee, UK

Astbrink G., School of Medicine, University of Tasmania, Hobart, Tasmania, Australia

Baxter G.D., Department of Psychology, University of York, Heslington, York, UK

Beomonte Zobel P., Department of Energetica, University of L'Aquila, Roio Poggio, Italy

Billard A., Adaptive Systems Research Group, Department of Computer Science, The University of Hertfordshire, Hatfield, Hertfordshire, UK

Black K., ACE Centre Advisory Trust, Headington, Oxford, UK

Blythe M., Department of Psychology, University of York, Heslington, York, UK

Brown S.S., Computer Laboratory, University of Cambridge, Cambridge, UK

Cardoso C., Engineering Design Centre, Department of Engineering, University of Cambridge, Cambridge, UK

Cassim J., Helen Hamlyn Research Centre, Royal College of Art, London, UK

Clarkson P.J., Engineering Design Centre, Department of Engineering, University of Cambridge, Cambridge, UK

D'Amico A.M., Istituto di Psicologia, Viale Marx 15, Rome, Italy

D'souza N., School of Architecture and Urban Planning, University of Wisconsin, Milwaukee, Wisconsin, USA

Dautenhahn K., Adaptive Systems Research Group, Department of Computer Science, The University of Hertfordshire, Hatfield, Hertfordshire, UK

Dewsbury G., Department of Computer Science, University of Lancaster, Lancaster, UK

Dickinson, A., Division of Applied Computing, University of Dundee, Dundee, UK

Dodds G., Virtual Engineering Centre, Queen's University of Belfast, Belfast, UK

Donahue S.J., North Carolina State University, Raleigh, NC, USA

Doughty K., Department of Psychology, University of York, Heslington, York, UK

Driessen B.J.F., TNO Institute of Applied Physics, Stieltjesweg 1, Delft, The Netherlands

Durante F., Department of Energetica, University of L'Aquila, Roio Poggio, Italy

El Kaliouby R., Computer Laboratory, University of Cambridge, Cambridge, UK

Faulkner R., Bath Institute of Medical Engineering, University of Bath, Wolfson Centre, Royal United Hospital, Bath, UK

Ferguson S., Virtual Engineering Centre, Queen's University of Belfast, Belfast, UK

Fornara F., Istituto di Psicologia, Viale Marx 15, Rome, Italy

Gelderblom G.J., IRV, Institute for Rehabilitation Research, Zandbergseweg 111, Hoensbroek, The Netherlands

Gheerawo R.R., Helen Hamlyn Research Centre, Royal College of Art, London, UK

Gibbs C., Bath Institute of Medical Engineering, University of Bath, Wolfson Centre, Royal United Hospital, Bath, UK

Giuliani M.V., Istituto di Psicologia, Viale Marx, 15, Rome, Italy

Goggin, G., School of Medicine, University of Tasmania, Hobart, Tasmania, Australia

Goodman, J., Department of Computing Science, University of Glasgow, Glasgow, UK

Hekstra D., Handicom, Oranjelaan 29, Harderwijk, The Netherlands

Hine N., Division of Applied Computing, Dundee University, Dundee, UK

Hwang F., Engineering Design Centre, Department of Engineering, University of Cambridge, Cambridge, UK

Joel S., Division of Applied Computing, Dundee University, Dundee, UK

Judson A., Division of Applied Computing, Dundee University, Dundee, UK

Keates S., IBM TJ Watson Research Center, Hawthorne, NY, USA

Langdon P.M., Engineering Design Centre, Department of Engineering, University of Cambridge, Cambridge, UK

Lysley A., ACE Centre Advisory Trust, Headington, Oxford, UK

McCreadie C., Institute of Gerontology, King's College London, London, UK

McStay J., Virtual Engineering Centre, Queen's University of Belfast, Belfast, UK

Meegahawatte D., Bath Institute of Medical Engineering, University of Bath, Wolfson Centre, Royal United Hospital, Bath, UK

Monk A.F., Department of Psychology, University of York, Heslington, York, UK

Newell, C., School of Medicine, University of Tasmania, Hobart, Tasmania, Australia

Nicolle C., Ergonomics and Safety Research Institute, Loughborough University, Loughborough, Leicestershire, UK

Orpwood R., Bath Institute of Medical Engineering, University of Bath, Wolfson Centre, Royal United Hospital, Bath, UK

Poulson D., Ergonomics and Safety Research Institute, Loughborough University, Loughborough, Leicestershire, UK

Raiche H., School of Medicine, University of Tasmania, Hobart, Tasmania, Australia

Raparelli T., Department of Mechanics, Technical School of Turin, Italy

Rentoul R., Division of Applied Computing, Dundee University, Dundee, UK

Robins B., Adaptive Systems Research Group, Department of Computer Science, The University of Hertfordshire, Hatfield, Hertfordshire, UK

Robinson P., Computer Laboratory, University of Cambridge, Cambridge, UK

Schofield S., Division of Applied Computing, Dundee University, Dundee, UK

Scopelliti M., Istituto di Psicologia, Viale Marx, 15, Rome, Italy

Shikler T.S., Computer Laboratory, University of Cambridge, Cambridge, UK

Sobecki J., Wroclaw University of Technology, Wybrzeze Wyspianskiego 27, Wroclaw, Poland

Syme A., Division of Applied Computing, University of Dundee, Dundee, UK

te Boekhorst R., Adaptive Systems Research Group, Department of Computer Science, The University of Hertfordshire, Hatfield, Hertfordshire, UK

ten Kate T.T., TNO Institute of Applied Physics, Stieltjesweg 1, Delft, The Netherlands

van Woerden J.A., TNO Institute of Applied Physics, Stieltjesweg 1, Delft, The Netherlands

Versluis, A.H.G., TNO Institute of Applied Physics, Stieltjesweg 1, Delft, The Netherlands

Weihberg M., Wroclaw University of Technology, Wybrzeze Wyspianskiego 27, Wroclaw, Poland

Yu W., Virtual Engineering Centre, Queen's University of Belfast, Belfast, UK

Part I

Design Issues for Universal Access and Assistive Technology

Chapter 1

Is Universal Design a Critical Theory?

N. D'souza

1.1. Introduction

Universal design is a term that was first used in the United States by Ron Mace (1985) although forms of it were quite prevalent in Europe long before. For the purpose of this chapter Universal Design is defined as 'the design of all products and environments to be usable by people of all ages and abilities to the greatest extent possible (Story, 2001, p.10.3). Universal design in recent years has assumed growing importance as a new paradigm that aims at a holistic approach ranging in scale from product design (Balaram, 2001) to architecture (Mace, 1985), and urban design (Steinfeld, 2001) on one hand and systems of media (Goldberg, 2001) and information technology (Brewer, 2001) on the other.

Given the popularity, Universal design still remains largely atheoretical i..e. the researchers of Universal design do not explicitly affiliate themselves to any form of theoretical paradigm. One of the reason is perhaps because Universal design is a melting point between cross paradigms. By paradigms I mean basic orientations to theory and research (Newman, 1997, p.62). In this sense Universal design can come under functionalist paradigm (because it caters to utility), pragmatic (because it is instrumental in nature), positivistic (because it strives for universal principles), normative (because it prescribes certain rules) and critical theorist paradigms (because it gives voice to the oppressed).

Conventionally the word *universal* is synonymous to *general* and refers to a set of principles that are stable, timeless and value free. In this sense universal design could be interpreted as deriving from a positivist paradigm. However, given its history and perspective, and with the universal design examples I provide, I will demonstrate several instances where the universals do change, are time bound and value laden. In this sense I argue that Universal design follows a critical theory paradigm in its conception and knowledge generation. By conception I mean how universal design came into being as a body of concepts and by knowledge generation I mean how the concepts pervade and are shared by the community of researchers.

1.2 Universal Design as a Critical Theory in its Conceptualisation

1.2.1 Social Emancipation

Social emancipation is to help people change conditions and build better world for themselves. Critical researchers conduct research to critique and transform social relationships by revealing the underlying sources of such relationships and empowering people, especially less powerful. Such an emancipatory role is demonstrated in universal design concept as the researchers argue for the importance of making through design, so-called weak component in the society as strong as every other part (Balaram, 2001).

Social emancipation is to help people change conditions and build better world for themselves. Critical researchers conduct research to critique and transform social relationships by revealing the underlying sources of such relationships and empowering people, especially less powerful. Such an emancipatory role is demonstrated in universal design concept as the researchers argue for the importance of making through design, so-called weak component in the society as strong as every other part (Balaram, 2001).

Mullick and Steinfield (1997) argue that in the beginning years of universal design in United States, the concept sprang up from the new thinking of the era dominated by the famed Brown v/s Board of education case of 1954. In this case the Supreme Court ruled that separate educational facilities are inherently unequal. The decision forced the desegregation of public schools in 21 states. The axiom *separate is not equal* inspired the beginning days of the universal design concept.

This reformation was not unlike the social changes that occurred in other European countries such as Sweden. For example, Universal design emerged when Karl Grunewald of the Swedish Social Sciences Department and his team started to translate the normalisation principle into the built environment (Sandhu, 2001, p.3.5). The normalisation principle was originally created to normalise the way in which one perceived and portrayed people who are disadvantaged and to establish people with a handicap in socially valued roles so far as their capabilities allow. Hence the roots of universal design can be attributed to emancipatory attitudes reflected in that era.

1.2.2 Social Inclusion

Critical theory argues for social inclusion. By social inclusion one means that social reality consists of multiple layers and includes several segments of society. By probing into these layers the critical researcher can identify and provide voice to the oppressed. While, the beginnings of Universal design catered to the special groups of people, i.e. people with diminished abilities such as physical impairment, retardation, advanced age, pregnancy, and so on, the current trend provides for the needs of the majority. According to Lawton (2001) this is demonstrated in the ADA (American with Disabilities Act) venture that has extended the boundaries of design for everyone by translating special-user design to mainstream designs. This is done by enhancing the aesthetics and the commonplace look of products and give it as much attention as the function. In this way equality and inclusiveness is conveyed socially.

1.2.3 Social Reality as Probabilistic

For the critical researcher reality is seen as constantly shaped by social, political, and cultural factors. The critical science approach considers that people have a great deal of unrealised potential, are creative, changeable and adaptive In this sense critical theory is probabilistic.

A similar outlook can be seen in Universal design. Lawton (2001) defines Universal design as the best approximation of an environmental facet to the needs of the maximum possible number of users. In recognition of this, Lawton argues that personal need motivates affordances (where affordances are what the environment offers, provides, furnishes, and invites).

Lawton lists a variety of probable affordances that the environment could offer for a variety of needs. Some of them include physical privacy, proper orientation of features, social opportunity and so on. The probabilistic view is also expressed in the principles of universal design which allow for 'flexibility of use' (Story, 2001, p.10.1-10.8). Flexibility means to provide choices in methods of use, accommodate right or left hand access, provide adaptability to the user and facilitate the user's precision. In this sense Universal design is probabilistic in its conceptualisation rather than deterministic.

1.2.4 Social Reality as not Value Free

Critical theory is based on belief that facts require an interpretation from within a framework of values, theory and meaning. Theories are based on beliefs and assumptions about what the world is like and on a set of moral-political values. In order to interpret facts, one must understand history, adopt a set of values, and know where to look for underlying structures. Hence, different versions of critical science offer different value structures (e.g. Marxism v/s feminism). Although the word universal could be attributed as value neutral, in the recent times, Universal design researchers have embraced cultural differences as an integral part of social reality.

Balaram (2001) for example, argues that in the non-industrialised majority world, where there is overwhelming diversity in language and customs, disability refers to issues beyond physical disabilities, and is essentially a social construct. He argues that in Asia it is an extremely unsociable act to send their disabled or elderly relative to institutional care. Hence he advocates an Universal design which can work with the relevant value system. He proposes interventions such as changing societal attitudes, educating for the future, positive thinking, welfare networking and so on.

The idea of value laden universal design is also reflected in two of the seven principles of universal design: 'simple / intuitive' and 'perceptible information' (Story, 2001, p.10.7-10.8) Both these principles refer to environmental legibility in diverse settings that accommodate wide range of literacy and language skills.

1.2.5 Critical Theory as a Third Way in the Subject-Object Debate

On one hand critical theory considers that the subjective ideas are important. On the other hand it assumes an objective world in which there is unequal control of resources and the power in which subjective opinions are based. This paradox is aptly demonstrated in the many examples of universal design in the dichotomy between universality and subjective needs.

Lawton (2002) has argued to bridge this gap by catering to several individual issues such as self-actualisation, systematic consideration of each need for every prospective user, systematic assessment of individuals on the characteristics of representation members of each group, assessment of environment in terms of affordances and a participatory design process. As needs and competencies are assessed environmental design affordances are matched to the personal characteristics. Hence the individual and subjective attributes are considered important to what is ultimately defined universal.

1.3. Universal Design as a Critical Theory in its Knowledge Generation

1.3.1 Critical Theory as a Provision of Resources

According to Newman (1997), critical theory seeks to provide people with a resource that will help them understand and change their world. Once people discover the resources they can use them to alter social relations, and to improve how things are done. Hence, a critical theory grows and interacts with the world it seeks to explain. Such knowledge generation is also seen in universal design.

Story et al. (2001) has used several versions (almost four versions in a period between 1994-1997) to formulate the seven principles of universal design. In her paper she charts out how these seven principles evolved from its fuzzy beginnings and how different studies suggested new changes in the principles. Hence, the seven principles of universal design emerged from a variety of sources which were made available to the society.

Subsequently, the principles themselves became a resource for others to make use of. For example, Manley (2001) uses the seven principles to create an accessible public realm in England where she argues for an universal approach to street design. She argues for street spaces which provide freedom to walk without interruption in city streets. Similarly Calkin et al. (2001) use Universal design principles for a comparative study with the design guidelines of Dementia care nursing home. Hence knowledge generation occurs through the resources being made public and constantly deliberated.

1.3.2 Replication of Facts in Critical Theory

Unlike positive science where facts are neutral and agreeable, according to critical theory facts are set within the framework of values. Researchers in different countries consider universal design principles as a loose body of concepts which could be reinterpreted to their own settings. Hence the replication of facts has to adhere to the respective value systems.

For example, in Japan Universal design has to include factors to tackle earthquake disasters (Takahashi, 2002). In Israel there exists a great sensitivity to provide universal design to injured soldiers (Ramot, 2002).

In Switzerland, universal design has inspired a new place types such as care apartment complex in Switzerland (Hurlimann, 2002). Care apartments were created so that it fosters more social relationship than the convention hotel-like care of the nursing homes. The care apartments are integrated into regular housing without standing out or causing social stigma. Hence the replication of facts in universal design is not deterministic or based merely on facts but takes the prevailing social attitudes into consideration.

1.3.3 Knowledge Accumulation

In critical theory knowledge is accumulated by the consequence of action. Universal design also strives to accumulate knowledge through design action. In the environmental behaviour research it is generally believed that environment causes people to behave in a certain way. Calkins *et al.*, (2001), for example, assumes that specific interventions in the environment of Dementia patients cause improvement in their stress levels.

Among the several interventions mentioned, one of them amounts to reducing negative stimulation. Negative stimulation is done by reducing scale of the environment, controlling ambient conditions such as auditory and visual backgrounds, limiting unnecessary choices and providing a place for retreat. Hence by catering to specific interventions in the environment, it is assumed that relevant changes occur in behaviour.

Similarly, Lawton uses several environmental indicator examples to demonstrate how certain environmental affordances can be accomplished by intervention. For example to fulfil an affordance called preference he uses an environmental indicator such as toilets near activity spaces.

The core of Lawton's model is, therefore, a set of human needs, and a parallel set of affordances, that can be fulfilled through relevant environmental interventions. Hence the knowledge accumulation is universal design comes from interventions and the consequences.

1.3.4 Testability and Modification and Change in Critical Theory

A researcher tests critical theory by describing accurately the conditions that are generated by underlying structures and then by applying that knowledge to change social relation. Hence critical theory informs practical action or suggests what to do, but the theory is also modified on the basis of its use. The testability and modification in universal design has been proposed by the Post Occupancy evaluation (POE) (Preiser, 2001). According to Preiser universal design performance can be measured by defining the degree of fit between people and their environment, testing the human activity support systems, measuring the adverse effects of products and understanding how designs cater to multiple uses. Hence, the performance is based on the seven universal design principles laid down by Story (2001). Changes for increased performance are then prescribed based on the outcomes. Hence knowledge grows by an ongoing process of eroding ignorances and enlarging insights through action.

1.4. Prologue

Much of the information on Universal design is fragmented and hence its' theory has not been adequately developed. However, as demonstrated in this study, Universal design can be seen in the paradigm of critical theory in terms of conceptualisation and knowledge generation. In application, perhaps, it is closer to a normative paradigm. Some have called critical theory follow an universal pragmatic logic as against universal reductionist logic of positive science (Habermas, 1972) i.e. an universality that takes into account pragmatic conflicts of society and not an universality that is devoid of everyday life of people. While Universal design does not fit neatly into such the mainstream critical thought (such as Marxism and feminism), it consists many facets of a critical theory that may perhaps indicate that it operates as an universal pragmatic system.

1.5. References

Balaram S (2001) Universal Design and the Majority world. In: Universal Design Handbook, McGraw-Hill

Brewer J (2001) Access to the World Wide Web: Technical policy and perspectives. In: Universal Design Handbook, McGraw-Hill

Calkins M, Sanford JA, Proffitt MA (2001) Design for Dementia: Challenges and Lessons for Universal Design. In: Universal Design Handbook, McGraw-Hill

Goldberg L (2001) Universal design in film and media. In: Universal Design Handbook, McGraw-Hill

Habermas J (1972) A postscript to knowledge and human interests. In: Philosophy of the Social Sciences, Beacon Press, Boston

Hurlemann M (2001) The Care Apartment Concept in Switzerland. In: Universal Design Handbook, McGraw-Hill

Lawton P (2001) Designing by degree: Assessing and Incorporating Individual Accessibility needs. In: Universal Design Handbook, McGraw-Hill

Mace R (1985) Universal Design, Barrier free environments for everyone. Designers West, Los Angeles, CA

Manley S (2001) Creating an Accessible Public Realm. In: Universal Design Handbook, McGraw-Hill

Mullick A, Steinfield E (1997) Universal Design: What it is and what it isn't. Innovation, the Quarterly Journal of the Industrial Designer Society of America, 16(1): 14-24

Newman (1997) The meanings of methodology. In: Social Research methods: Qualitative and Quantitative Approaches, Third edition, Allyn and Bacon, Boston, pp 73-84

Ostroff E (2001) Universal Design as practiced in the United States. In: Universal Design Handbook, McGraw-Hill

Preiser WFE, Ostroff E (eds.) (2001) Universal Design Handbook, McGraw-Hill

Preiser WFE (2001) Towards Universal Design evaluation. In: Universal Design Handbook, McGraw-Hill

Ramot A (2001) Israel: A Country on the Way to Universal Design. In: Universal Design Handbook, McGraw-Hill

Sandhu J (2001) An Integrated Approach to Universal design: Towards Inclusion of all ages, Cultures and Diversity. In: Universal Design Handbook, McGraw-Hill

Steinfield E (2001) Universal Design in Mass transportation. In: Universal Design Handbook, McGraw-Hill

Story MF (2001) Principles of Universal Design. In: Universal Design Handbook, McGraw-Hill

Takahashi G (2001) From Accessibility for Disabled People to Universal Design: Challenges in Japan. In: Universal Design Handbook, McGraw-Hill

Chapter 2

Cross-market Product and Service Innovation – the DBA Challenge Example

J. Cassim

2.1 Introduction

The DBA Design Challenge is an annual competition run by the Small Business Programme of the Helen Hamlyn Research Centre (HHRC) at the Royal College of Art (RCA) in collaboration with the Design Business Association (DBA), the UK's official trade body for design consultancies. Leading design firms are challenged to work with young disabled consumers to develop inclusive design prototypes in a concentrated period of three months.

Now in its fourth year and with twenty projects undertaken to date, the event builds on existing initiatives at the HHRC – the Design for our Future Selves Awards and the Helen Hamlyn Research Associates Programme. These match RCA design students and new graduates respectively with marginalised groups, placing end-users at the centre of the design process from inception to end to encourage more socially responsive design.

The DBA Design Challenge aims to capture the interest of the professional design community in these objectives, not just the student or postgraduate community at the RCA. This external focus meant that it was important for the HHRC to form an alliance with a professional body with its own established network of design firms to whom the Challenge could be addressed.

It turned again to the Design Business Association, reviving a partnership and replicating a mechanism first used with great success in the early days of the DesignAge action research programme at the RCA – a programme, which subsequently evolved into the Helen Hamlyn Research Centre in 1999. The only major difference was that where its DesignAge namesake focused on the design needs of ageing populations, the new DBA Design Challenge and the Small Business Programme, of which it is part, centre on partnerships with young disabled users.

This chapter discusses the rationale behind this and some of the mechanisms employed to achieve the objectives of both.

2.2 Perceptions of Disabled and Older Users

The inauguration of the Small Business Programme in 2000 coincided with the publication of three reports by the Audit Commission (Audit Commission, 2000), Needs Must (Frazer and Glick, 2000) and the United Kingdom Department of Trade and Industry (DTI 2000). The latter outlined the impact on older and disabled people of the poor ergonomic design of such everyday consumer products as kettles, refrigerators and generic packaging types and its relation to accidents in the home.

By identifying the nature of problems in five areas (manipulation, grip, lifting, reach and transport), it sought to determine the characteristics and capabilities that should be measured to provide designers with information that would result in safer products.

The Needs Must and Audit Commission reports described the financial impact of inadequate provision in the UK's social services programmes and National Health Service (NHS) equipment respectively.

Absent from all three was any discussion of the psychological impact of 'special needs' design on disabled or older consumers – the emphasis was on function, efficacy or the financial cost of failure. The Audit Commission Report, for example, stated that the services were a 'gateway to independence' that could 'make or break' the quality of life of the 4 million disabled people and the 1.7 million informal carers who used them in the UK.

It further stated that 'the right equipment can make the difference between an enriched, independent life or a miserable, isolated existence'. The Audit Commission Report acknowledged that much NHS issue equipment was of 'dubious quality' but provided no design guidelines even for such standard items of equipment as crutches or hearing aids, nor did it single out existing examples of good design.

Absent too was any comparison between the lifestyles, aspirations or consumer patterns of older people with the multiple minor disabilities of age and younger people with more severe congenital or acquired disabilities. They were seen as a single homogeneous group, united in their desire for functional products and accessible services but with no distinction made between their actual tastes or consumer behaviour.

Their primary profile was a combined medical one of age and/or disability and while both groups were seen as aspiring to good design, what each meant by that expression was not explored aesthetically or otherwise. Their respective roles as consumers whom mainstream market forces might target by virtue of their significant market share was also ignored (Employers Forum on Disability, 2001). Instead, they were viewed as passive NHS clients and not consumers in the usual sense.

Another aspect absent from these reports was any discussion of their potential role as advisors to the design process, one which went beyond their usual limited status as test subjects who could highlight the ergonomic failure of products.

2.3 Yo-Yo's, WOOF's and Rainbow Youth

Marketing agencies have traditionally focussed on the aspirations of young people in the development of new products with 35 seen as the cut-off age of interest in them as consumers (Compton *et al.,* 2003).

With falling birth-rates, the impending pensions crisis and the ageing of the 'Woodstock Generation', there is, growing recognition that post-war baby boomers – the so-called Yo-Yo (Young-Old) (Taylor, 2002), WOOF (Well Off Older Folks) or 'Rainbow Youth' (Stevenson, 2003)– are a lucrative market of consumers who cannot be defined by age alone in their buying patterns (Scales *et al.*, 2000).

As product and technology literate as their children and grandchildren, they use the same work or leisure-related consumer products yet require enhanced functionality. They desire a form of inclusivity by stealth - one that takes into consideration their declining physical, sensory even cognitive capabilities but lacks the aesthetic stigma so common to special needs products that would single them out as old or disabled, for they view themselves as neither.

2.4 Young Disabled Users as Crossover Consumers

Recognition of this scenario has brought into focus the important role that young disabled consumers can play in the product and service development process. They simultaneously embody the aspirations and lifestyles of youth but the limitations imposed by their disability demand a flexible, alternative and non-stigmatising design response that is cross-market and mainstream in appeal.

This reasoning underpinned the decision to strategically position the DBA Design Challenge around the aspirations of younger disabled consumers and frame it as a creative response to their need for mainstream consumer design. It ensured that emphasis was placed equally on aesthetics and function, thereby promoting the idea that inclusive products and services of this kind had the ability to span generations. Other considerations came into play as described in the following sections.

2.5 Empathy between Contemporaries

Matching designers with their disabled contemporaries was seen as a means to facilitate empathy and dialogue between two groups with broadly similar tastes and lifestyles but radically different ways of achieving the same ends. Efforts have been made to match the designers with disabled users from the creative industries or professions directly related to the project in question.

For example, the lead (graphic) designer for Coley Porter Bell's 'c' system, which won the DBA Design Challenge Inclusive Design Award in 2002, consulted extensively with Rebecca Harris, a congenitally blind artist and her exact contemporary in age. The proposed 'c' system consists of a labelling system for clothing using a tactile language of shapes representing colour and size to be used on the swing tag and silk label of the garment. The system enables visually impaired users to identify over 60 colours by learning 16 core tactile shapes. A bar code reader gives additional product information relating to style, material, pattern, care instructions and the whole system has applications for other products where colour selection or co-ordination is important (Cassim and Dong, 2003).

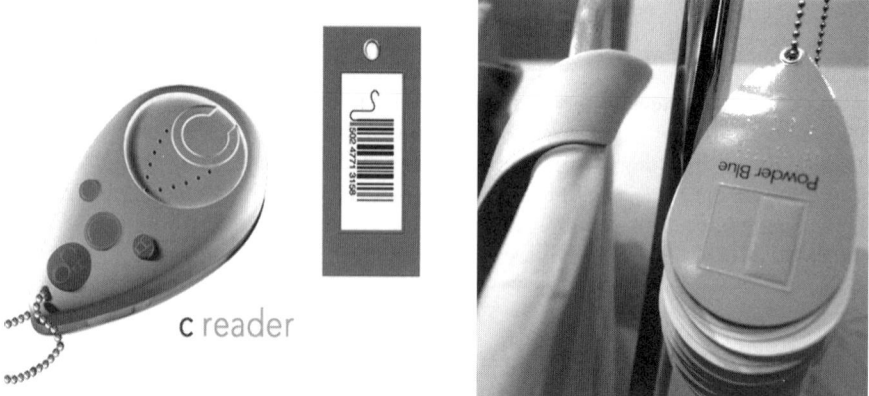

Figure 2.1. 'c' system bar code reader and tag itself

For this project, the lead designer and Harris went on shopping trips together, developing an open-ended relationship that took place outside of the academic or test framework common to user research involving severely disabled people.

Experiences such as these tend to concretely reinforce the practical considerations and psychological reality of the context in which the final design must exist. In the case of the 'c' system, this had been outlined anecdotally by the other visually impaired participants in the user forum and formally in the mentoring session held by the author at an initial stage of the project.

2.6 Innovation Triggers

Severely disabled young people were targeted in preference to older users with minor disabilities for the user forums that are an integral element of the competition. It was felt that the former could offer complex scenarios of everyday situations informed by the lateral, creative coping strategies they adopted individually in response to the deficiencies of design or service provision.

It was hoped that these would act as triggers for new concepts or for innovative features in the final design. Secondly, it was a mechanism to ensure that those design teams wishing to rethink such standard items as kettles, saucepans, milk cartons etc would return to first principles in product and service concepts and not merely re-style them cosmetically.

A further rationale behind this decision to prefer youth over age and severe disability over minor impairment was that the young users were likely to display higher degrees of competence and understanding of mobile communications technology and interfaces (Cassim and Dong, 2003).

Where the project involved their use, it was essential that those who advised the designers were not 'technophobes,' had an understanding of the technology under discussion and could discuss such issues on a basis of equality, shared expertise and contextual relevance. Many such users were members of the British Computer Association of the Blind (BCAB) or the Foundation for Assistive Technology (FAST) and had volunteered their services in response to calls circulated through their email networks by the author.

There was sufficient informal evidence from the first two Design Challenges to indicate that these assumptions regarding the difference in response between older users with minor disabilities to young users with severe disabilities (i.e. critical users) were accurate. However, in order to test them, two older users from the University of the Third Age were invited to participate in the forum held for Fitch: London's 'i-connect' project in 2002. This looked at ways to redesign such complex transport interchanges as Waterloo Station through environmental design measures that harnessed the service potential of Bluetooth technology (Cassim, 2003a).

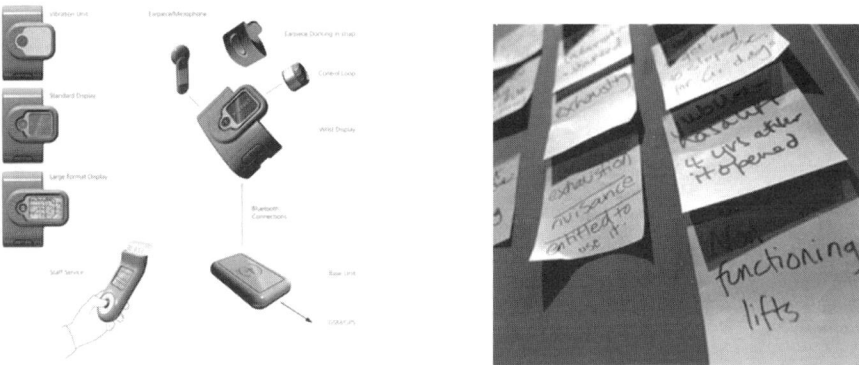

Figure 2.2. i-connect wearable device and storyboard for the project

Frequent users of public transport with physical and sensory disabilities participated in the user forum, which took the form of a complex question and answer session. Each stage of their individual journey was mapped and analysed. The disabled users described in detail their coping strategies and offered logistical and technological solutions to the kind of impasse in which they routinely found themselves.

In contrast, the two able-bodied older users, one in her late sixties, the other in his early eighties could describe such general issues as the tiring nature of stairs or the difficulty of reading signage but offered few coping strategies beyond the commonplace. Neither possessed mobile phones nor were they familiar with the principles and possibilities of Bluetooth which was central to the design team's proposals.

2.7 Creation of the End-User Network

Each DBA Design Challenge depends upon a network of 'critical users' of the type described above. Appeals are made through email networks and online discussion forums to members of such organisations as the Computer Association of the Blind and the Foundation for Assistive Technology (FAST). Many are computer engineers or software developers who can introduce designers to relevant developments and new technologies that would assist them in realising their 'blue-sky' product concepts. Not all projects are 'blue-sky' concepts or involve the use of complex technology.

To ensure that issues relating to motor, visual and cognitive skills are comprehensively covered in user forums which relate to the design of such well-established products as kettles –KettleSense by Alloy in 2001 (Cassim, 2002), drinks containers – Milkman by Factory Design in 2000 (Cassim, 2000) and packaging – SiebertHead in 2001 & 2002 (Cassim, 2002) similar appeals are made to members of such charities as Arthritis Care, Different Strokes and the Parkinson's Disease and Multiple Sclerosis Societies. As a result, a significant network of individual expert end-users has been created with new volunteers being added each year.

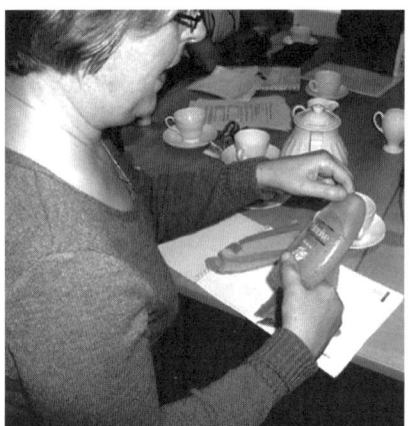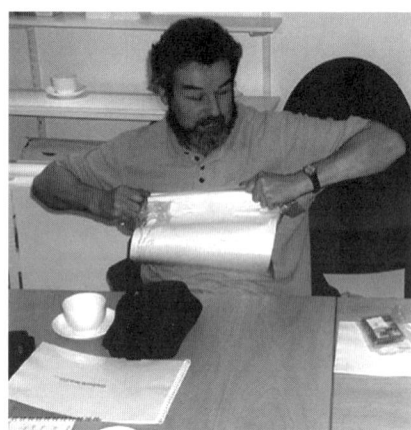

Figure 2.3. User Forums for the DBA Design Challenge

2.8 New Areas of Innovation

An overriding aim of the DBA Design Challenge is to convince design firms and small businesses, that the inclusive design process and partnerships with their young disabled contemporaries in particular can be a fertile source of ideas for new product and service innovation in areas that they may not have considered. This being so, great emphasis is placed on the business and creative case for engagement with disabled people, in the briefs and initial presentations held to encourage DBA members to participate. In 2002 and 2003, the new area of 'smart wearables' (Cassim, 2003b) was delineated resulting in Pearlfisher's project of the same name in 2002 and a rise in entries centred on wearable or embedded forms of technology (Cassim, 2002). Pearlfisher a branding and futures company worked with a fashion designer to develop a range of clothing using Outlast™ a temperature regulating fabric developed by NASA. It has since gone on to market a clothing range for young children as a result of their experience of participating in the DBA Design Challenge in 2002 and the new product ideas that the process generated.

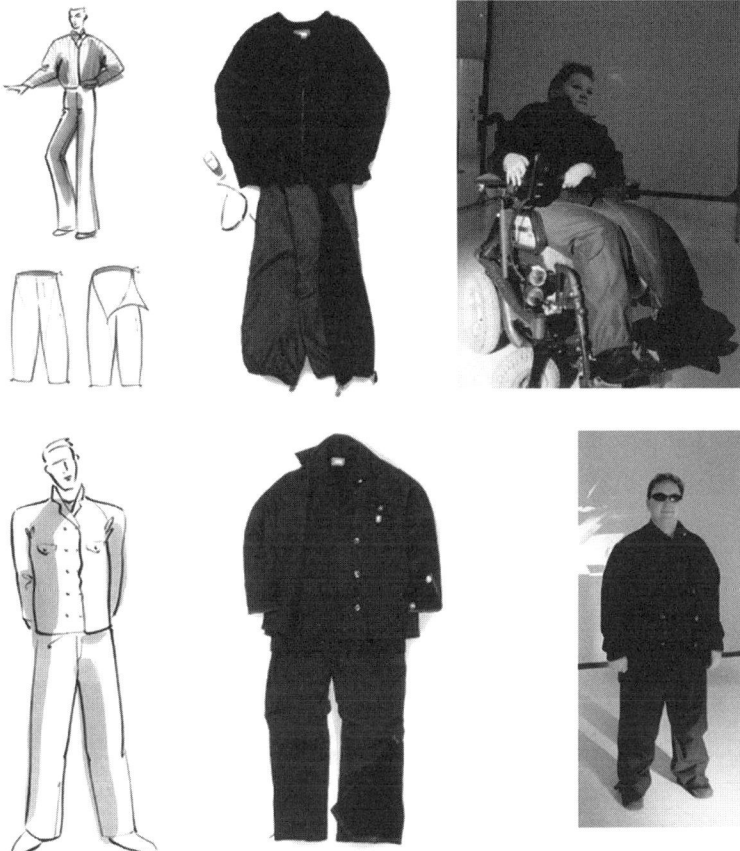

Figure 2.4. Part of Pearlfisher's clothing range for DBA Design Challenge 2002

The participating design teams range in age from their early twenties to early forties providing a typical cross section of the design community. There is evidence to suggest that firms submitting entries are using the opportunity for various reasons. Some cite its importance as a means of building teamwork in-house and a way of challenging and stimulating them creatively with projects that they would normally encounter.

There is recognition, too, of its role as a training exercise to enable staff to gain new skills in an area of increasing importance to their clients in light of the ratification of the Disability Discrimination Act (DDA) in October 2004 in the UK. The final presentation, be it in PowerPoint or movie formats, is restricted to six minutes with the latter medium encouraged. The rationale offered to firms by the HHRC is that it can serve as a portrait of best practice and their own company culture and processes – caring, creative, responsive and so on – which can be used by them when pitching to new clients or for more general public relations purposes. Many commercial projects they undertake are bound by client confidentiality and cannot be described in detail for these reasons. No such restrictions apply to their Design Challenge projects, hence its value as a promotional tool.

Interestingly, although the Challenge was first structured as a simple invitation to designers to participate in the inclusive design process, it was changed to a competition in the second year at the request of the DBA. This strong competitive element has meant that it is not viewed as an altruistic training exercise alone but as an event on par with other professional design competitions. Accordingly, the quality and quantity of entries has grown each year along with its profile as one of the major events of the design calendar.

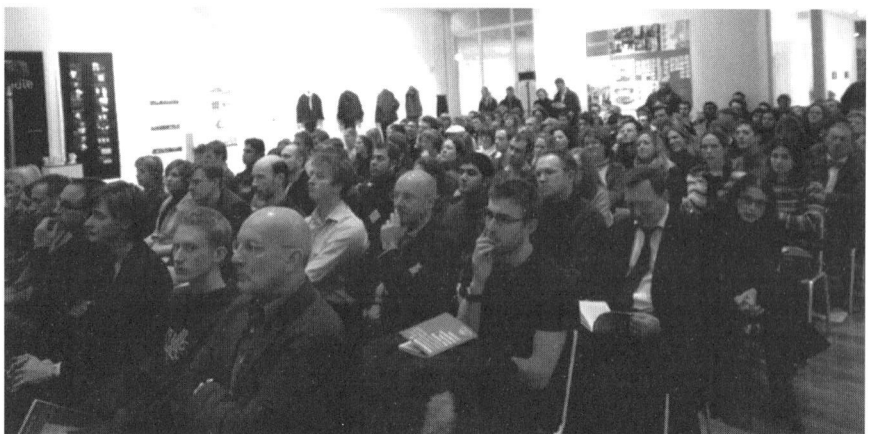

Figure 2.5. The audience at the DBA Design Challenge 2002

Importantly, it has yielded a varied cross-section of concrete exemplars of mainstream inclusive design practice of relevance to the constituencies it seeks to serve – the business, academic, healthcare, design and disabled communities – the five key players vital to the improvement of industry standards in the healthcare sector.

2.9 References

Design for our Future Selves Competition. Available at:
  www.hhrc.rca.ac.uk/programmes/cp/competition/index.html
Employers Forum on Disability. Available at:
  www.employers-forum.co.uk/www/csr/sttn/sfacts/sfacts1.htm
HHRC Research Associates Programme. Available at:
  www.hhrc.rca.ac.uk/programmes/ra/index.html
DBA Design Challenge. Available at: www.hhrc.rca.ac.uk/events/DBAChallenge
Audit Commission (2000) Fully Equipped – the provision of equipment to older or disabled
  people. Audit Commission, London
Cassim J, Dong H (2003) Critical Users in Design Innovation. In: Inclusive Design – design
  for the whole population, Springer Verlag, London, UK
Cassim J (2000) Innovate 1: how 4 design teams faced the user challenge. Helen Hamlyn
  Research Centre, Royal College of Art, London, UK
Cassim J (2001) Innovate 2: the business case for inclusive design. Helen Hamlyn Research
  Centre, Royal College of Art, London, UK
Cassim J (2002) Innovate 3: how a human focus on human needs can generate great ideas.
  Helen Hamlyn Research Centre, Royal College of Art, London, UK
Cassim J (2003a) Innovate 5: can insights on disability help to design better products?
  London, Helen Hamlyn Research Centre, Royal College of Art, London, UK
Cassim J (2003b) Smart Wearables – a new frontier for inclusive design innovation. In:
  Include 2003, RCA, London, UK
Compton N P, Chenecy S (2003) Boomer Brands. In: Viewpoint 13, London, UK
DTI (2000) A study of the difficulties disabled people have when using everyday consumer
  products. Department of Trade and Industry, London, UK
Frazer R, Glick G (2000) Out of services – A survey of social services provision for elderly
  and disabled people in England. Needs Must, London, UK
Rainbow Youth – designing, marketing & retailing to Europe's new old. In: Viewpoint 13,
  (2003) London, UK
Scales J, Scase R (2000) Fit & Fifty? Report prepared for the Economic & Social Research
  Council EPSRC, Swindon, UK
Stevenson T (2003) Datamonitor marketing survey cited in Glad to be Grey. The Observer
  Magazine, 5 October, UK
Taylor J (2002) Bringing originality and delight into communication with older people.
  Helen Hamlyn Research Associates Programme, Royal College of Art, London, UK

Chapter 3

Introducing User-Centred Design Methods into Design Education

R.R. Gheerawo and S. J. Donahue

3.1 Introduction

A crucial part of the practical application of inclusive design lies in working with user groups and involving them at all key stages within the design process. It is therefore increasingly important to introduce inclusive design principles into mainstream design education so that they can diffuse outwards into industry. This chapter looks at how design students and educators can be encouraged to work with user groups and it evaluates some of the practical methodologies that can be used to involve users within the design process.

The chapter also gives case studies and examples of how this can be implemented, citing work from postgraduate design students at the Royal College of Art (RCA) and from undergraduate design students at the College of Design, North Carolina State University (NCSU).

3.2 Background and Context

The Department of Trade and Industry (DTI Foresight, 2000) defines inclusive design as a process whereby 'designers ensure that their products and services address the needs of the widest possible audience'. Designers are therefore centrally placed to effect this change, but whilst there is Government recognition of the need for professional designers to work inclusively, there is little legislation, or even encouragement, for design educators to teach design students about inclusive design processes, methods or benefits.

It is crucial to introduce inclusivity into design education and this needs to take place at two levels. The first is to drive a socially inclusive agenda into the heart of a design college or university through the teachers, tutors and professors, the people who are the core of design education and management. The second is to work directly with the design students themselves to engender a more inclusive approach in their personal design practice.

However, there are a number of challenges. Relatively few design courses teach inclusive design as a distinct unit and an introduction to the subject is often left to one or two seminars or lectures (Nicolle, 2003).

Even those courses where user-centred approaches are favoured, timetable demands mean that little time can be spent exploring the core benefits and wider practice of inclusive design.

> *'In a marketplace driven by features, style, cost and time to market, the elements of problem solving are often small and the compression of timescales precludes a truly rigorous comprehensive design process. ...Inclusivity therefore offers ... a catalytic design environment for enhanced creativity and provide(s) the opportunity for more creative solutions than had initially been conceived for a 'received product type'*

(Warbuton, 2003)

Design is a time-pressured profession and design education is no less demanding. Teaching both the creative and the constructive elements of a design course can fill most of the available studio time.

As design is a subject that requires the constant development of both personal taste and expression, a large amount of individual time and focus is required for each student designer to discover and explore their specific potential. There are therefore relatively few opportunities to get inclusive thinking into an already packed curriculum. Where this is impossible, other ways of attracting the interest of students are needed.

3.2.1 Work at the Royal College of Art (RCA)

At the Helen Hamlyn Research Centre (HHRC) based at the RCA, the key mechanism for addressing these issues is an annual competition for graduating MA design students. The award scheme gives students a platform for creative interaction with social trends and key user groups.

The competition in 2003 had five briefs, each addressing a social issue and all looking for an innovative approach rather than mundane problem solving. Two briefs addressed the socially invisible groups of older people and young disabled people; two investigated the major social challenges of balancing work and life and urban mobility and transport; and the last brief made any particular social issue more visible through communication design.

Responding to this mix of issues is central to the concept of design inclusion (Coleman, 94). By using each brief to highlight one social issue, the students could immediately engage with potential user groups and set their creative thinking against the background of a "real world" issue or problem. This, in turn, allowed them to experience the value and benefit of an inclusive approach without detracting from their studio work.

3.2.2 Work at North Carolina State University

Vehicles for addressing these issues at North Carolina State University (NCSU) were initiated by Sean Donahue. While functioning as the Designer in Residence in the Spring of 2003, Donahue worked on methods to rethink design studio education. The foundation of his work was to establish methods for engaging inclusive design as a vehicle for re-evaluating the use, role, and context of mainstream design. The approach aimed to:

- address the specific requirements of undergraduate design education within a general studio environment;
- to avoid segmenting inclusive design practices to secondary courses but to incorporate them into traditional classroom contexts;
- to allow the notions of inclusive design to provide valuable insight into issues of context and appropriateness for application in mainstream communication design;
- by integrating methods of investigation that move the designer outside of the studio in order to expand their understanding of audience, user and appropriateness.

These issues were of particular value because they allowed students to take these methods of inclusive investigation into any mode of practice they embark on upon gradation. The aim was to infuse all design thinking and not simply relegate 'inclusivity' to a particular type of specialised design practice.

3.3 Working with Users

Inclusive design theory was successfully introduced into studio practice at an educational level in the following two ways. The first was to involve design students with users, encouraging them to understand their needs and involve them in the design process as a way of 'seeding' innovation. The second was to challenge students to address the powerful social changes that surround them. Both of these worked well together; the students were attracted to the process by the chance to creatively problem-solve for a 'real life' situation, and the key to doing this successfully was demonstrated through meaningful interaction with users.

'Design processes work when they build on natural human behaviour'

(Beyer and Holtzblatt, 1998)

This was the core principle made clear to the students. By talking to one person other than themselves, designers can effectively increase the number of people who can use their product or service by a significant factor. By selecting a few key users with some reduced ability (such as older or disabled people) this consumer base can massively increase as the design becomes easier for everyone to use (Nussbaum, 2001).

3.3.1 Methodology

Working with users and involving them in the design process does not have to be a hugely involved and time-consuming process. Students were encouraged to use simple and effective methods that did not add much 'lead time' to their design development but which gave design insights into both user need and market effectiveness. The key was for each student to empathise with the user, even if only for a short while. Objective observation had to be maintained throughout the experience. All this had to then be filtered and fed back into the design brief without losing any design value or impact. Knowing how to turn user feedback into useful material for the design brief was found to be a crucial part of inclusive design education.

3.3.2 Research Methods

The research methods that were used maximised the amount of information of design value, whilst minimising the time spent collecting. Direct observation of people 'in situ' yielded potent design clues as to how users actually behaved. Questionnaires revealed a host of lifestyle information as well as detailed preference of prototypes tested. User diaries documented difficulties with current designs and helped to evaluate prototypes over a period of time.

Interviews, conducted in either a formal or semi-formal structure, contributed valuable insights into lifestyle preferences as well as product needs. Focus groups, convened for between two to four hours, elicited responses on everything from frustration with current designs to detailed prototype testing and alternative coping strategies.

3.3.3 Evaluation of Research Methods

The methods that were of most immediate use were those that allowed the design student to get close to the user and understand their needs, preferences, aspirations and lifestyle. Questionnaires and observation of people were found to be only really useful at the beginning of the project when the brief was being developed or the project direction established. The type of dry data generated by these two methods meant that the important human element necessary wasn't there, and therefore these methods were of limited use in design development. Focus groups, interviews and diaries, on the other hand, could be modified for use throughout the process and were found to be of greater benefit.

For example, groups of up to six users focussing on the project brief could be approached later in the project to comment on potential designs (see Figure 3.1). In some cases, users were asked to keep project diaries throughout the project to help the designer record the effectiveness of the brief, the development and the final proposal.

3.3.4 Critical Users

Rather than canvass the opinion of a large number of people, the guiding principle was to team up students with a number of key users, selected on a project-by-project basis, who would drive the students to think beyond the standard boundaries of design solutions. This developed into the idea of 'critical users', groups of users who subjected the design ideas to the strongest challenges because of their capabilities – for example people with arthritis working on packaging design solutions.

> *'In practice, though, for successful inclusive design, the definition of users needs to move ... to embrace users with different functional capabilities.'*

> (Keates and Clarkson, 2003)

These types of users were found to drive students towards more innovative solutions by challenging their proposals and showing them life from another point of view. The students who successfully engaged with the process and empathised with their critical users found the experience stimulating and thought provoking. The users also welcomed this type of approach, with many feeling that they made both a valid and valued contribution to the project.

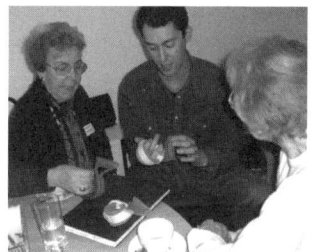   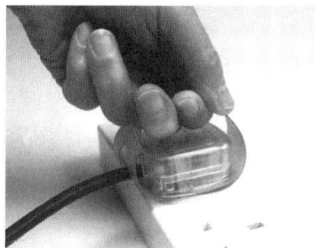

Figure 3.1. A focus group of older users   **Figure 3.2.** Pull the Plug'

3.4 Case Studies

3.4.1 Royal College of Art Case Studies

Over the last five years, many projects focused on very specific problems experienced by people, but did so in ways that were both practical and life enhancing. These case studies demonstrate the design innovation and commercial potential of student work that was developed with groups of 'critical' users.

Martin Bloomfield's 'pull the plug' (RCA Industrial Design Engineering 1999 - Figure 3.2) is a low-cost plastic strip which makes a UK power plug easy to remove from wall sockets. The coloured strip also allows for easy identification of plugs when a number of appliances are in use. Bloomfield worked with focus groups of older people with limited dexterity to develop the usability of his design.

This group of 'critical' users was then expanded to include younger people and was site-tested at offices and in the domestic environment.

Hugo Glover's 'pill pusher' (RCA Design Products 2002 – Figure 3.3) greatly aids the dispensing and taking of pills, especially for users with extreme physical conditions caused by arthritis or sciatica, or those with reduced dexterity and eyesight.

The required tablet is positioned over a small, circular depression that 'catches' the tablet as it is pressed through with a finger or thumb from the blister pack. The tablet can be then easily tipped into the hand or directly into the mouth. As the product needed to be developed with such a specific type of user, Glover focussed on one individual who fulfilled the above criteria and who was also a regular pill taker.

He worked closely with this person and immersed himself in their daily regime. Prototypes were tested over weeks and he spent mornings and afternoons filming both vocal feedback and contextual use of his prototypes. He then supplemented this user research with interviews and product testing with a wider selection of users. The combined methodology allowed him to iteratively work up his ideas into a product that met real user need and is at present, being further developed to market.

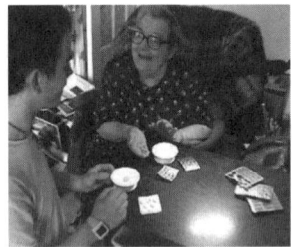

Figure 3.3. Working with a key user on the 'Pill Pusher'

Ben Wilson's 'hand driven trike' (RCA Design Products 2001 – Figure 3.4) was designed for an active eight-year old end user with lower body paralysis and a desire for a machine styled like the mountain bikes of his able-bodied friends. The overall concept, however, is for riders of all ages and abilities and can be easily customised for either hand propulsion or pedal power.

Ready-made high tech components and 'street-cred' styling ensure the trike's place in mainstream bike design. Wilson's main user drove the development and design of the bike from brief-writing stage through to final design. Although working with just one main user, Wilson went deep into his lifestyle, combining informal interviews with more immersive techniques to empathise with his needs and aspirations over a two-year period.

This resulted in key insights that resulted in a unique mechanism in the saddle area that allows the rider to corner and steer the vehicle by moving their upper body from side to side. Working with a user who had a 'critical' set of needs pushed the design boundaries, driving the student to innovate. The success of the design can be measured by the fact that the user refused to return the working prototype and his health has considerably improved from using it.

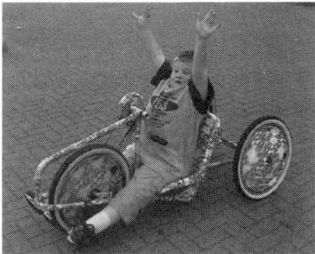

Figure 3.4. Eight year old key user on the prototype trike

Disability is something that can affect us all at any time in our life, and often does so for limited periods of time. William Welch's adaptable cutlery (RCA Goldsmithing, Silversmithing, Metalwork and Jewellery 2001 – Figure 3.5) is designed for people with poor grip or restricted hand movement.

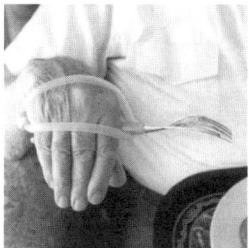

Figure 3.5. Cutlery with assistive strap for users with limited dexterity

The oversized handle is filled with a smart material that moulds itself to the individual user's hands while the head bends sideways to optimise hand-to-mouth co-ordination. A looped strap fits over the hand and slots into the suction pad at the base of the handle. Its mainstream design aesthetic, however, makes it an attractive rather than stigmatising product, and the designer has posted do-it-yourself instructions on his web-site for making a similar but temporary product from readily available materials for those whose need for the cutlery is not permanent. Welch worked with groups of older people, and people with arthritis or strokes to iteratively develop the design. The mainstream aesthetic and looped strap was a direct result from user consultation, and focus groups helped to confirm the designs developed with his main users. As well as creating an innovative product through addressing user need, Welch discovered that his work carried enough demand to be commercially developed. He has since set up a company to produce, develop and market the cutlery.

3.4.2 North Carolina State University Case Study

The projects that are assigned and the resulting artefacts that are created in design education establish a student's preconception of what design is, how it is used and who it is applicable to. This is particularly true in undergraduate education. It can also be said that these define and shape what a student understands their future professional practice to entail.

The argument therefore becomes very persuasive for establishing methods of design education that move away from limiting the contribution of design methods to the resultant artefacts. Relying on these artefacts to define a course permits the student and future professional to limit what they may contribute or make, based on pre-existing notions of existing design. Instead, by focusing on the process of establishing social context, a contribution can be formulated that addresses the specifics of user research findings, with the ultimate goal of expanding the design question and the contextual base for the project.

The foundation project for this was rethinking the designer's approach to a logo. It began by reposing the design question for the students. Instead of assigning a project to redesign a logo for company X, the project was positioned in a way that allowed students to integrate inclusive design methods of investigation in order to develop a communication system that spoke to a potentially broader user group.

The project was entitled 'Designing communication systems that build brand recognition'. This was a very traditional undergraduate studio project that repositioned the design issue away from being defined by preconceptions of artefacts conjured by using the word "logo", towards an understanding of the design project based on recognising the goals of the communication in terms of its user groups. This encouraged the students to create a communication system that provided opportunities for brand recognition to include a wider audience. This redefinition of the design issue provided room for a dialogue that opened up the discussion to consideration of a diversity of design vehicles that spoke towards a broader spectrum of users who are not normally considered in mainstream communication design.

The resulting design processes and attitudes formulated by the students provided a broad spectrum of engagement that could be applied to any mainstream client or communication. Projects used communication redundancies to address multiple types of users with multiple types of communication characteristics. For instance, creating a brand 'sound identity' to be used with an accompanying visual or by itself, began to address issues surrounding low and no vision communities at an undergraduate level of design education. The result was an engaging form of communication that allowed both users with vision, and those with no vision, to partake in traditional communications. Another approach resulted in logos that varied in scale in order to engage multiple reading dexterities. Adding variations in design characteristics when the logos were in different sizes increased readability whilst also creating visual interest for a fully sighted community. Having not just size changes but design variations in those sizes also increased visual interest. Another approach utilised tactile qualities within the visual identities that acted as both a design signature and a unique identity.

3.5 Conclusions

Ultimately, this work provided students with the tools to conduct investigations into the broader scope of social context, and interaction with potential user groups as a way of successfully achieving that. This was done in a way that did not exclude 'inclusive designs' as a boutique practice or special process. Instead, it was used as a vehicle for rethinking and reinvigorating the creative process, allowing students to experience the practice of inclusive design in any mainstream design discipline.

Though methods vary between these undergraduate and postgraduate courses there are a number of points that are common to the success of both. The picking of the right user research method is essential, as is the selection of the right type of user for each project. It is important to evaluate the resulting design artefact as well as the process that the student underwent. The key to measuring the successful integration of inclusive design practice into design education lies in delineating the amount of meaningful interaction the student had with user groups and in particular, with 'critical' user groups, such older people or visually impaired people who are generally ignored by mainstream design. A further measure of success lies in seeing how many students take these principles forward into their professional practice.

The willingness of users to engage with the design process is another point to note. Most people, especially those outside the consideration of mainstream design are eager to take part, but they do have to be briefed as to what is expected of them, and the process has to be tightly monitored as many will not have encountered a design-rich environment before. However, this can start to become counter-productive if the same users are approached repeatedly, as they start to move from commenting on their lifestyles, needs and aspirations, to a position as amateur design critic.

Users have to be carefully sourced. Many students rely on relatives or friends, but objectivity can be compromised. Teaching institutions and design courses therefore need to build up links with groups of 'critical' users such as older people and people with disabilities who are willing to work with their students. By choosing a level of engagement, users can either be take part in anonymous questionnaires, an afternoon focus group or become more deeply involved in the design project. Choosing the right method and then finding a suitable, willing participant can then become a much more viable process. Where access to users is limited or impossible, an introduction to inclusive design principles and theoretical experience of research methods would work towards establishing a framework that students could work with in practice.

Students have spent afternoons in wheelchairs trying to navigate the city and visited older people in their homes to see how they live. They have rapidly bonded with users, moving from a distant understanding of their needs to close engagement with their lifestyle and aspirations. This has helped to trigger design innovation and challenge design preconceptions, empowering the aspiring designer to engage these topics as part of their everyday practice.

3.6 References

Coleman R (1994) The Case for inclusive design - an overview. In: Triennial Congress, Toronto, 3: 250-252

Beyer H, Holtzblatt K (1998) Contextual design: Defining customer-centered systems. Morgan-Kaufmann

DTI Foresight (2000) Making the future work for you. Department of Trade and Industry, London, UK

Keates S, Clarkson J (2003) Countering design exclusion. Springer-Verlag, London, UK

Nicolle C, Rundle C, Graupp H (2003) Towards curricula in design for all for information and communication products, systems and services. In: Include 2003, London, pp 3-101

Nussbaum B (2001) Breaking boundaries: Include 2001: newsletter for the Include 2001 Conference. The Helen Hamlyn Research Centre, London, UK

Warbuton N (2003) Everyday inclusive design. In: Inclusive Design – Design for the Whole Population, Springer-Verlag London, pp 15-256

Chapter 4

Comparing Product Assessment Methods for Inclusive Design

C. Cardoso, S. Keates and P.J. Clarkson

4.1 Introduction

New emerging technologies and increasingly competitive design markets are strategically planned to satisfy 'mainstream' consumer needs. However, two population trends seem to have been ignored by this mainstream market perception: first, the economic power of the growing older adult consumer population in most developed countries; and, second, the increasing awareness and legislation about the rights of the disabled community (Coleman, 2001). Both groups are continually disadvantaged or even excluded from using many everyday design solutions, which impose functional capability demands beyond their acceptable limits (Keates *et al.*, 2000). As these 'non-mainstream' consumers become aware of their economic and legislative influence, there is clearly a need and opportunity to develop more inclusive design solutions (Yelding, 2003). The scarcity of commercially successful inclusive design solutions suggests that these users' wants and needs have not been properly included during the design process. Designers are either not familiar with these population trends or lack the methods to address this problem in real-life circumstances.

The aim of this research is to encourage designers to enhance the objectivity of their assessments, avoiding generating needless discomfort or exclusion for a wide range of potential consumers. A case study on the assessment of three different kettles is presented to illustrate the advantages and disadvantages of three different assessment methods: User Observation, Self-observation, and Simulation.

4.2 With or Without Users?

Assessment methods in general are divided in two broad groups: methods that involve the participation of users, such as: User Observation; Interviews; Questionnaires; Focus Groups; User Trials; or Ethnographic Studies (Wilson and

Corlett, 1995); and methods that do not comprise user participation – Self-observation; Brainstorming; Expert/Heuristic Evaluation; Tasks Analysis; Simulation (Jordan *et al.*, 1996; Nielsen, 1993).

Design consultancies have distinct preferences regarding the methods of assessment they adopt into their design process. While methods that involve users are likely to provide more realistic feedback about the usability and accessibility of everyday products, these methods are usually time-consuming and expensive to carry out (Dong *et al.*, 2002). Consequently, while for instance User Observation is indisputably one of the best methods for learning about users' experiences when interacting with products and their surroundings, some companies will not be able to carry out such studies. These companies will have to recur to in-house expertise to predict problems that users may encounter. This is not a problem if the target audience they are trying to reach is very similar in terms of background, knowledge and functional capability to the typically young male designers within the company. However, if the aim is to extend the range of the target consumer, it is likely that many people might be disadvantaged or even excluded. Whilst designers' intuition and creativity is essential to the development of innovative solutions, the proper identification of the usability and accessibility shortcomings needs more formal and thorough procedures.

4.2.1 Problem Categorisation

The problems identified during the three assessment methods presented in this study were categorised into three ways: *difficulty* in performing an action; use of *coping strategies* to perform an action; and *failure* to complete an action.

Difficulty in performing an action happens when the participant is able to carry out a particular part of the interaction the way that would be expected, but experiencing discomfort in doing so. Varying levels of difficulty may occur and it is important to capture these, especially the most difficult actions.

Coping strategies occur when the participant does not perform the action the way that would be expected (i.e. the way it was designed for), but resorts to alternative strategies to accomplish the required action. Such strategies may be the result of different circumstances, for instance the participant may adopt a coping strategy because the action was too difficult to carry out the expected way, thus the capability demands of the device exceed the participant's capability. Alternatively it was not very clear how the action should be performed or the participant just prefers to do things in a certain way, even if the action was not particularly difficult to accomplish in the way it was designed for.

Failure to carry out an action happens when the user cannot (or will not) perform a certain action, and it can arise from a number of different circumstances. For example, the participant may not understand what needs to be done – due to a mismatch between the participant's sensory or cognitive capabilities and the feedback provided by the device.

Such a mismatch may be caused by the device characteristics (the participant is not familiar with certain designs) or an external environmental influence, such as the level of luminosity or noise. Alternatively, the participant may not be physically able to carry out the action because of the demands placed on the user by the product, or due to an anthropometric incompatibility, or a combination of both. Lastly, the user may refuse to carry out an action – i.e. there is not motivation to do it – as a consequence of any of the above mentioned problems, or personal or cultural preferences.

The results derived from evaluations of the three assessment methods will be compared and discussed both in terms of total number of problems and the types of problems identified (e.g. *difficulty*, *coping strategy* or *failure*).

4.3 Case Study

The case study of the assessment of three different electrical kettles was divided into three different stages: 1) User Observation with a small group of users; 2) Self-observation with a group of five industrial designers; and 3) Simulation with the same group of industrial designers.

4.3.1 User Observation

User Observation (Drury, 1990) involves watching people interacting with the device being assessed in a real-life environment (e.g. the user's home) or in a controlled setting (e.g. usability laboratory). Observations carried out in real-life circumstances are likely to provide more realistic insight into the problems users may experience, since they are usually more comfortable in a familiar environment.

Despite the higher validity of this method, it is important to take into account that people's behaviour may be affected because they are aware of being observed (e.g. the so-called *Hawthorne Effect*). At the end of the observations, interviews can be employed to elucidate and give more insight into issues that were not clear to the assessor.

User Observation evaluation involved watching the participants interacting with the three different kettles to identify the types of problems each one experienced. It involved the participation of a group of six older adults (65-85). Two of the participants were wheelchair users exhibiting limited dexterity and reach and stretch capabilities – one due to a back injury that limited the strength in the arms, and the other due to severe arthritis in the hands. The other participants exhibited some level of capability loss, particularly a decreased strength in their hands and arms, either caused by arthritis or the natural ageing process.

The observations took place in a day-care centre in Cambridge. All the users were observed using the devices in the same environment – i.e. the kitchen of the day-centre. At the beginning of the observations the objectives of the study were clearly explained to all of the participants. There was only one researcher observing and videotaping the sessions. The assessor's presence may have had an influence on the participants' behaviour, although it has been observed that people get accustomed to observers over time (Stanton and Young, 1999). Making sure participants were fully aware of the objectives of the study, made them progressively more comfortable about verbalising any difficulties they encountered. At the end of each interaction the participants were asked a few questions, when clarification about the observed events was needed.

4.3.2 Self-Observation

Self-observation, or Self-modelling, is a commonly employed assessment method whereby designers consider themselves or a colleague as the user and act out the interaction process. Designers use their daily experience and intuition to try to predict how users will use the device and what type of difficulties they might encounter. One of the main advantages of this approach is that it is usually a low-cost and quick method, which does not involve the use of special resources. It can be easily implemented throughout the design process, being particularly suitable when the time and budget available for a project is limited.

However, an obvious limitation of this approach is the designers' assumption that they can be representative of a wider, heterogeneous population. In order to achieve realistic results, and assuming that the aim is to extend the market range, the designer would have to be familiar with a wide diversity of user capabilities and behaviours. A large number of users exhibit unique capability characteristics, which may result in unexpected behaviours or even prevent them from using certain products. Therefore, this usually informal approach may succeed in terms of enhancing user-product interaction for those who could already use a certain product, but it is likely to continue excluding large numbers of consumers who do not possess the 'required' capability profile.

Self-observation, which formed the second phase of this case study, involved asking a group of designers to assess the ease of use of the three kettles using their everyday experience with such devices. Five novice industrial designers participated – two female and three male, all of whom were able-bodied with ages between 24 and 30 years old. The sessions took place in the designers' studio at Central Saint Martins - The London Institute.

The designers were briefly presented with the objectives of the study and provided with a spreadsheet where they were asked to annotate their comments during the assessments. Designers were asked to perform the evaluations individually and not exchange or discuss any ideas among themselves. There was no limitation on the time available to perform the evaluations, but they were asked to keep a record of how long it took to assess each device. None of the designers were familiar with the concepts of Inclusive Design or similar philosophies. Each designer produced a list of comments about good and bad usability features and even some aesthetic considerations. Results from the Self-observation assessments are presented and discussed later on this chapter.

4.3.3 Simulation

Simulation (Steinfeld and Steinfeld, 2001) involves designers being outfitted with physical simulators to reproduce the symptoms of physical impairments. Designers are provided with, for instance, special gloves, goggles, weights for their upper or lower limbs and earplugs, to simulate a decrease of their motor or sensory capabilities. The main objective is to make designers feel what it would be like to have certain impairments, caused either by specific medical conditions or as a result of the ageing process. While it is practical to simulate physical impairments, cognitive impairments are more complex to simulate. Despite the interactive experience of feeling the limitation caused by certain impairments, the temporary use of simulators is unlikely to allow designers to fully understand the social consequences of being constantly impaired.

Simulation was the third phase of this study and it consisted of having designers use specific physical simulators to find out if they would experience the same types of problems users had encountered during the earlier User Observations.

The same group of designers who participated on the Self-observation phase took part on the Simulation assessment. The Simulation took place in Cambridge at the Engineering Department in a kitchen that resembled the one where the User Observations were carried out. Each designer performed the Simulation separately with the presence of a researcher who videotaped the sessions. At the beginning of the sessions the designers were briefed with the objectives of the assessment, and then provided with the physical simulators. The simulators were calibrated according the descriptions provided by the capability scales of the Office of National Statistics (ONS) (Martin *et al.*, 1988). The physical wearables focused on three particular physical constraints:

- glasses that simulated *"users who have difficulty seeing to read ordinary newspaper print"* – level S9/0.5 ;
- gloves that were aimed at simulating *"users who have difficulty picking up and pouring from a full kettle or serving food from a pan using a spoon or ladle"* – level D5/6.5;
- weights on the forearms that tried to simulate *"users who have difficulty putting either arm in front to shake hands with someone"* – level RS5/6.5.

The selection of these specific levels of capability was based on the nature and magnitude of the capabilities exhibited by the participants during the User Observations. The objective was to try reproducing the same type of impairment and find out if designers would experience the same number and types of problems that the users had come across. Designers were asked to use the three kettles. They were encouraged to verbalise what they were experiencing throughout the inter-action (the Think-Aloud Protocol), especially any difficulties encountered due to the use of the simulators. Occasionally the researcher would ask specific questions regarding the interaction where the observable behaviour was not clear. At the end of each interaction there was a debriefing session about the difficulties experienced during the kettle usage. At the end of the whole session the designers were asked further questions regarding their opinion about the use of the simulators.

4.4 Results

The results from the User Observations are shown in Figure 4.1, where the total number of problems encountered is shown. The number of problems shown for each kettle are unique problems – i.e. if one or more users experienced a problem with a particular kettle on a specific step of the interaction, it is counted as one problem.

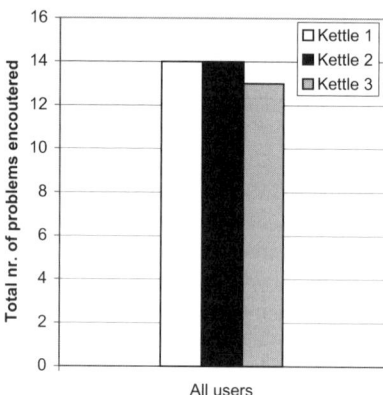

Figure 4.1. User Observation results – total no. of problems encountered for each kettle

For each kettle at least one user encountered problems in almost every step of interaction (e.g. a *difficulty*, a *coping strategy*, or a *failure*). This amounts for the apparent similarity in results between all three kettles. Of the 15 steps of interaction that were observed, only one step was entirely problem free for Kettles 1 and 2 and only two steps were entirely problem free for Kettle 3.

The results from the designers' Self-observation and Simulation assessments are shown on Figures 4.2 and 4.3, respectively. Both figures show the total number of problems encountered per designer for each kettle. Feedback from the designers' assessments is shown individually. Such presentation allows the identification of how many problems each designer found using the two different methods. It can be seen from these figures that Simulation allowed designers to find out more problems than Self-observation. In general, designers doubled or even tripled the number of problems encountered through the use of simulators. Designers 2 and 3 found seven times more problems for Kettles 3 and 2, respectively, compared with their previous results from Self-observation. Interestingly, during the Simulation assessment Designer 3 seemed to have found no extra problems with Kettles 1 and 3, when compared with the earlier Self-observation assessment.

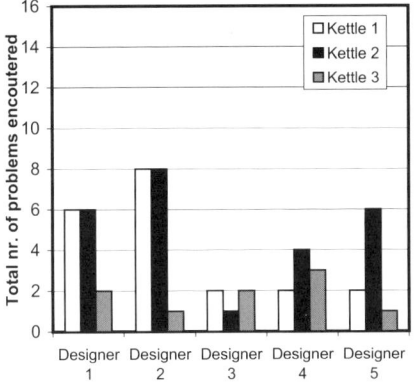

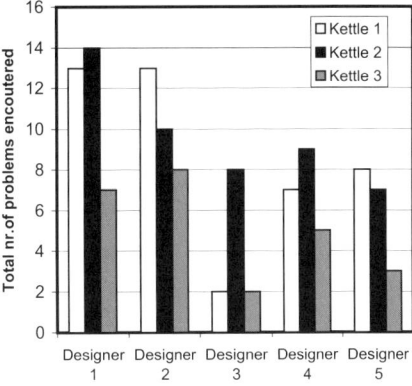

Figure 4.2. Self-observation - total no. of problems encountered for each kettle

Figure 4.3. Simulation - total no. of problems encountered for each kettle

This suggests that this designer, who was one of the males, was either not sensitive to the use of physical simulators or he was physically "too" strong to feel the constraints imposed by the simulators. This also raises the issue that simulators not only need to be adjusted to represent a particular level of impairment, they also need to be calibrated for the person wearing them – i.e. someone who is stronger may require more constraining simulators to feel the effects of the impairment being reproduced.

Figure 4.4 shows an example of the average number of problems encountered by each method categorised in terms of type of problem. These results are from the assessment of Kettle 2, but results from the other two kettles were very similar in terms of the ratio between the results of the three assessment methods. It was possible to learn from the list of problems that designers produced from the Self-observation, that all problems identified by this method were *difficulties* encountered and not the use of *coping strategies* or *failure* to complete an action as shown in the graph. The fact that fact designers were all young and fully able-bodied may have unable them to predict the occurrence of *coping strategies* or *failure* to complete an action.

Conversely, the use of simulators enabled designers to not only feel varying levels of difficulties, but also to experience the use of coping strategies and even some level of failure. These coping strategies and failures matched the type of problems that most of the users encountered. For instance, while wearing the special goggles designers could not clearly see how much water they were putting inside the kettles, either using the gauge or looking through the lid hole. On occasions, the designers had to position the kettles inside the sink or carry it with two hands, because it was *"getting too heavy to hold"* (in conjunction with the weights on their arms). The majority of the designers 'failed' when attempting to remove and replace the filters on the kettles due to the stiffness of the gloves. The users also experienced all these and other problems during the User Observation sessions.

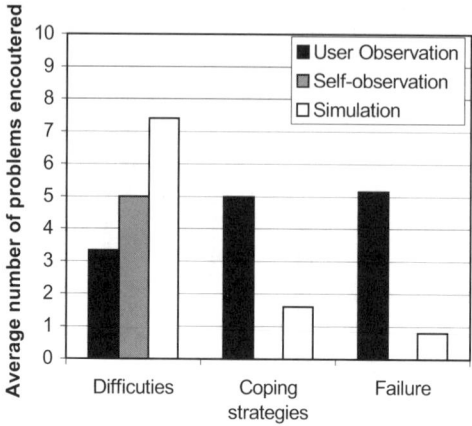

Figure 4.4. User Observation, Self-observation and Simulation results – average number of type of problems encountered

Although the designers experienced some *coping strategies* and *failures* to complete particular steps of the interaction, users resorted to, on average, three times more coping strategies and experienced five times more failures. This suggests that despite the use of physical simulators, designers managed to 'force' the physical constraints and carry out the interaction.

The result was a higher number of difficulties identified using simulators leading the designer to experience double the number difficulties encountered by the users for this particular kettle. It is possible to see from the Figure 4.5, which shows the average number of problems encountered for each assessment method, that User Observation allowed the identification of the highest number of problems.

It also shows that Simulation doubled the average number of problems encountered compared with the Self-observation approach. Yet, Simulation did not allow designers to identify all the problems users experienced during the observation sessions. This suggests that the calibration of the simulators may require some further adjustment. Increasing the level of constraint imposed by the simulators may enable the designers to experience the same usability problems as users.

Regarding the time spent for each method, 'user observation' was by far the most time-consuming with an average of two hours per kettle. 'Self-observation' took on average 10 minutes to perform and 'simulation' 50 minutes. In terms of problems found per unit of time per method:

- user observation: 1 problem/11 minutes;
- self-observation: 1 problem/3 minutes;
- simulation: 1 problem/6.3 minutes.

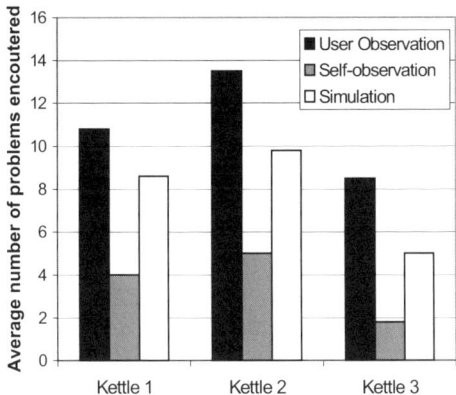

Figure 4.5. User Observation, Self-observation and Simulation results – average number of problems encountered

At first glance it seems that Self-observation is the fastest and best method since it allows designers to find a problem every 3 minutes. So, if there is only 30 minutes to carry out an assessment on the kettles, this method can potentially be the most effective of the three approaches. However, the ratio between the number of problems found and the time spent performing the assessment is likely to diminish over time. It is probable that there will be a point where designers will run out of ideas about all the possible different ways of interacting with a product. There will also be a limit on the number and variety of users that designers can imagine, and consequently on the prediction of the usability problems that users may encounter.

Alternatively, Simulation can almost always allow the designers to find more problems if the simulators are calibrated to higher levels of impairment, or to different combinations (e.g. vision – medium severity; dexterity – low severity; reach and stretch – high severity; etc.). Equally, User Observation can allow the designers to find out more about usability problems if more, or different, users are involved. Furthermore, a more thorough 'dissection' of the videos from the observations can also give insight into more subtle interactions, which may have been missed by earlier analysis.

From these results it seems that a balanced combination between User Observation and Simulation assessments could allow designers to gain more realistic feedback into the types of problems users may experience. Since User Observation appears to be the most fruitful yet the most time-consuming (and costly) method, it is suitable for implementation at milestones stages of the design process for more 'authentic' feedback. Simulation can be applied more flexibly and frequently during the design process.

In addition, simulators can every so often be re-calibrated with the capability profiles of the users involved in the User Observations. Such adjustment ensures that the simulators reflect the users' capabilities throughout the design process on the absence of the real user.

4.5 Conclusions

Methods that involve user participation, and particularly User Observation, can be robust and inspiring methods when it comes to designing more inclusively. However, in many real-life design project circumstances the use of such methods will not be feasible due to time and cost constraints.

Designers' common response to these constraints is to resort to usually informal Self-observation approaches when assessing the designs they create. However, a simple case study of the assessment of three different kettles shows the limitations of such approaches for predicting the types of problems real users may encounter. An alternative method to the costly and time consuming User Observation and the informal, insufficient Self-observation assessment is Simulation evaluation. Simulation is a fast and flexible method that could potentially be implemented throughout the design process when it is not possible to involve users directly. Feedback from the designers in this case about the use of simulators was positive. Designers said that even for situations where they managed to carry out an action, they could understand what the simulator was trying to reproduce. This gave designers insights into the sort of problems some users might experience for particular steps of the interaction.

The methods suggested here are not intended to be rules for showing designers how to design. Instead, the aim is to encourage the use of more objective approaches to the assessment of design usability and accessibility throughout the design process.

4.6 References

Coleman R (2001) Designing for our future selves. Universal Design Handbook, MacGraw-Hill, New York, pp 4.1-4.25

Dong H, Cardoso C, Cassim J, Keates S, Clarkson PJ (2002) Inclusive design: Reflections on design practice. University of Cambridge, CUED/C-EDC/TR 118

Drury CG (1990) Methods for direct observation of human of performance. In: Evaluation of Human Work. Taylor and Francis, London, UK

Jordan P *et al.* (2000) Usability evaluation in industry. Taylor and Francis, London, UK

Keates S, Clarkson PJ, Harrison LJ, Robinson P (2000) Towards a practical inclusive design approach. In: Proceedings of the 1st ACM Conference on Universal Usability, Arlington, VA, pp 45-52

Martin J, Meltzer H, Elliot D (1988) The prevalence of disability among adults. Office of Population Censuses and Surveys, Social Survey Division, HMSO

Nielsen J (1993) Usability engineering. Morgan Kaufman, San Francisco, CA

Stanton N, Young M (1999) A guide to methodology in ergonomics: Designing for human use. Taylor and Francis, London, UK

Steinfeld A, Steinfeld E (2001) Universal design in automobile design. In: Universal Design Handbook, MacGraw-Hill, New York, pp 50.1-50.13

Yelding D (2003) Power to the people. In: Inclusive Design: Designing for the whole population, Springer–Verlag, London, pp 104-117

Wilson J, Corlett N (1995) Evaluation of human work, 2nd edition. Taylor and Francis, London, UK

Chapter 5

Virtual Learning Environments: Improving Accessibility Using Profiling

S. Schofield, N. Hine, J. Arnott, S. Joel, A. Judson and R. Rentoul

5.1 Introduction

There is growing interest in and use of virtual learning environments in the delivery of course material, given their claimed advantages of temporal and spatial independence. The UK Special Educational Needs and Disability Act (UK Government, 2001) both strengthens the right for students with special educational needs to be educated in mainstream schools (integration) and ensures that these students are able to receive equivalent pedagogical experiences (inclusion). The impact on the teaching profession is a serious issue – the main concern expressed by English head-teachers regarding inclusion of special education needs students in primary schools was that of resource allocation (Archer et al., 2002).

This chapter looks at how the use of virtual learning environments can be both disadvantageous and advantageous to students with disabilities (Sloan et al., 2000), (Sloan et al., 2003). It outlines a profiling system to improve course-delivery, aid classroom management and reduce course-development costs.

5.2 The Adaptive Learning Environment

5.2.1 What is an ALE?

A virtual learning environment (VLE) is a computerised mode of delivery of teaching materials (Minshull, 2002). These materials are broken down into elements, and the movement of the student through the course monitored and recorded by means of an electronic bookmark. The results of each assessment are stored in a central database, giving instant and accurate feedback to both students and tutors. The VLE should also contain online tutor and peer group support, with general communication channels including email, group discussion and web access.

Course elements are made up of re-usable learning objects (RLOs) which are described by a set of metatags, such as those defined by ADL in the sharable content objects reference model (ADL, 2001). The aim of the standard is to ensure that RLOs are transferable from one VLE to another, enabling educational establishments to use educational brokers to purchase learning materials as well as cross-establishment transference of materials.

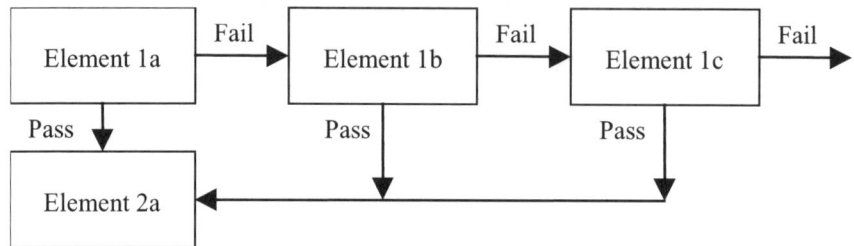

Figure 5.1. Simple navigation through an ALE-delivered course

In traditional teaching, the teacher is continually assessing the students, either formally or informally, and adapting the course material. An adaptive learning environment (ALE) is a VLE which adapts the elements delivered in response to virtual assessment results (Carchiolo *et al.*, 2002). Figure 5.1 shows a simplified progress through an ALE-delivered course. The student views element 1a and completes a computer-delivered test, itself an RLO. If the student passes the test, they are presented with element 2a. If the student fails, they are presented further information on element 1 (1b), at the end of which they take another test. The number of additions per element is dependent on the course-author, and there may be a point where the system alerts the teacher to the student's problems for teacher-intervention. This gives one-to-one student-driven learning.

5.2.2 Advantages

Web-based ALEs are spatially and temporally independent. This means that all the course material is available whenever and wherever the student has access to the web, and reviewable as many times as the student chooses, advantaging the cognitively impaired student. The teacher can be sure all material is as written, removing the problems of miscopied notes (particularly difficult for dyslexic children) and notes missing due to absenteeism. Indeed, the independent delivery means that absent children could continue with their work so long as they have access to the web. There is no statutory provision for children in hospital, but most hospitals employ teachers to provide tuition to school-aged in-patients. If a student is in hospital for more than a certain time (the length of time varies between educational authorities), the teacher liaises with the school. This inevitably leads to a break in continuity of education. With an ALE, the hospital teacher can see where the student is, and work can commence with minimal delay.

The information can be delivered in a multitude of ways. There has been much work done on a universal design, for example the IMS's 'Guidelines for

Developing Accessible Learning Applications' (Barstow *et al.*, 2002). Providing these guide-lines are followed, the content should be accessible to people who are blind, have low-vision, have colour-blindness, are hard-of-hearing or deaf, have physical disability or have language or cognitive disabilities. Following these guidelines has been found to also advantage people in general.

Student interaction can be fostered and supported by use of IT, enabling some who have been previously unable to interact to do so, for example a signing deaf student conversing with non-signing colleagues via text or a hospitalised student taking an interactive part in an on-line discussion via video-conferencing.

The student's progress can be monitored by the student and by anyone with administrative rights to that student's account, for example the student's parent / guardian or hospital teacher. These can be used statistically by the school or other interested parties without costly and error-prone score transference.

5.2.3 Disadvantages

The success of the system depends on the student being able to access the RLOs and the test assessing what is intended. Teachers will need to be trained to write for the system and courses restructured. Hardware and software may need to be upgraded, and users of the system trained in their use. For hospital and home use, sufficient bandwidth must be available. Unless a student has a dedicated machine, they will need to spend time resetting browser preferences each time they change machine. The school will need to ensure the necessary hardware and software are available, and the teacher will need to manage the resources.

5.3 Profiles

5.3.1 Why Profiles?

In his plenary talk on trends in software accessibility, Bill Haneman (2003) urged that:

> *'We should think less in terms of "one size fits all"; our message should be "we've got your size".'*

This leads to the question, how do we know we have the student's size? The course author could produce each RLO in everyone's size, but this would be expensive in time and resources, and incur redundancy. For example, pilots are tested for colour-blindness, so a set of duplicate RLOs rewritten to be accessible to students who are colour-blind would not be used by a class of pilots. Also, the onus of choosing the right RLO should not fall on the child. They may be unaware of which RLO would suit their accessibility needs, and may indeed be unaware of a particular disability or unwilling to draw attention to themselves by asking for an alternate RLO. The system therefore needs to assign the correct RLO to the student automatically. It is therefore recommended that a user profile recording the accessibility requirements for the individual be developed, with an equivalent profile for RLOs. Tools should be developed within the ALE to compare the profiles of the students registered for a particular course with the profiles of the RLOs making up that course. This should generate a report of any RLOs needing adaptation, and a duplicate made of that RLO, which could then be tailored to be suitable for the student. Alternatively, there should be the possibility for the course to skip that particular RLO if an alternative would not be suitable.

5.3.2 Multiple Profiles

There may be occasions when a student wishes to have more than one set of accessibility metatags stored. For example, a student may have very different needs when working alone to when working with their learning support assistant (LSA), or may have different needs when working on a personal digital assistant (PDA) to when working on a desk-top. The administrator could set up a different account for each case, but this is disadvantageous for several reasons:

- the user will be required to remember more than one login;
- the electronic bookmark will remain at the point reached last time that account was used; and
- marks from all accounts for that user will need to be collated when viewing a student's progress.

Instead, multiple profiles are proposed. On setting up an account, a default profile is set up. If the student does not require more profiles, on logging in the default profile is used. However, if the user has more than one profile, they will be offered a choice of profiles (Figure 5.2).

Figure 5.2. Logging in with more than one profile

A student account may require different access rights dependant on the profile selected, for example if they are working with their LSA. There may be occasions when an additional password is required for a profile.

5.3.3 Constructing the Profile

Each disability could be recorded, but more useful would be the implications to the individual student. For example, a student may be blind, but it would be better to record whether they need a Braille display and whether they require a screen-reader. In some cases, the requirement may be essential, but in other cases the requirement may be preferential. For example, a dyslexic student might prefer to use a tinted screen, yet be able to cope if one is not available. By storing this information, a tool could be incorporated within the ALE to help the teacher manage resources.

5.4 Some Disability Issues

Traditional teaching methods present a number of barriers for students with disabilities. Much material is delivered in written form, for example books, worksheets and wall-boards. These are problematic to students with visual impairments, and orally-delivered work is inaccessible to those with impaired hearing. Assistive means are sought to address barriers such as these. A review of literature on disability and assistive technologies (Schofield, 2003) gave an overview of student needs in this context.

Students with low vision may require screen-magnification, for example; this would need to be recorded in the student profile, and may require a higher-resolution RLO or an audio description. Colour, font type and size, as well as graphic elements can all cause serious problems for students with impaired vision. For audio material, the student using an ALE should be able to choose their own mode of delivery, for example earphones to reduce background noise and give control over sound volume, or audio clips can be described textually if required. The student's profile should contain information on delivery requirements, for example a need for a signing avatar and which sign language is required.

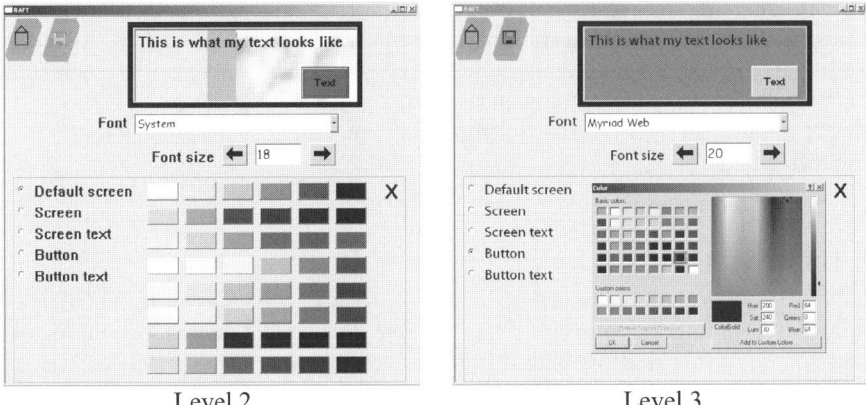

Level 2   Level 3

Figure 5.3. Screen-formatting form for levels 2 and 3

Physical disability can have implications; for example those with reduced fine motor skills may find drag-and-drop tasks problematic, so keyboard alternatives may be required, or a slower delivery / feedback time. Fatigue may require students to take lessons and tests in small sections.

The language of the user and language level should both be stored on the profile, allowing the interface to adapt to the cognitive level of the user. The cognitive level can also be used to decide on preferences for the interface. For example, a student of level one may be offered a choice of four colour-combinations, a student of level two a selection of colour-tiles, and a student of level three the full palette (see Figure 5.3).

5.5 Computer Aided Assessment

As indicated earlier, the ALE depends on the results of the assessment of each course element to deliver the next element. Because the assessments are RLOs, the same accessibility profiling can be used. RLOs highlighted as unsuitable for individual students can be adapted or replaced. For example, a test requiring identifying a musical instrument aurally may be replaced by a pictorial test, or may be deemed unsuitable for the profoundly deaf child.

Great care must be taken that the assessment is testing what the teacher intends. A child may fail a test due to the mode of interaction being employed rather than a lack of understanding of the test. In a pilot test, a group of children were observed using interactive reading software; one child was seen to be unable to move the mouse quickly enough to interact correctly with the program, and was therefore unable to progress to the next level. Aural testing found the child to be capable of recognising all of the letters, however; the child was disadvantaged because physical operation of the mouse was problematic (Schofield, 2003).

There will be some cases where certain characteristics of an RLO should not be changed. If a student is being tested for red-green colour blindness, it would not make sense to alter the Ishihara plate to be red-green insensitive. However, if the plate is being used in a genetics lesson to demonstrate how red-green can be tested, a modified RLO would be useful for the red-green colour-blind student. Also, the use of certain assistive technologies will not always be suitable for a test. For example, a screen-reader should not be used when testing reading. The RLO's profile should therefore contain information on any assistive technologies not applicable to the RLO.

5.6 Conclusions

Adaptive Learning Environments have a role to play in facilitating automated course delivery for students with different accessibility needs. Systems can be set up for comfort and usability under the control of a user profile, and management of additional hardware and software can be achieved more easily. Accessibility meta-tags inserted into re-usable learning objects will enhance the inclusion of students with disabilities, and, with the development of means to address potentially problematic learning objects, will assist in the efficient production of new ones.

5.7 Acknowledgements

This work is funded by the Commission of the European Communities under the IST 5th Framework.

5.8 References

ADL (2001) Sharable Content Object Reference Model v.1.2. Conformance Requirements. Advanced Distributed Learning (ADL) Initiative, USA, October 2001. Available at: http://www.adlnet.org

Archer T, Fletcher-Campbell F, Kendall L (2002) Annual survey of trends in education. National Foundation Educational Research, Digest No. 13, Autumn, Slough, UK

Carchiolo V, Longheu A, Marlgeri M (2002) Adaptive formative paths in a web-based learning environment. Educational Technology and Society 5(4): 64-75

Fletcher-Campbell F, Kendall L (2002) Annual survey of trends in education. National Foundation for Educational Research, Digest No. 13, Autumn, Slough, UK

Barstow C, Rothberg, M (2002) IMS guidelines for developing accessible learning applications. Version 1.0 IMS Global Learning Consortium. Available at: http://www.imsglobal.org/accessibility/accessiblevers/sec2.html

Hanemann B (2003) Trends in software accessibility. Assistive Technology – Shaping the Future, IOS Press, pp 66-70

Minshull (2002) Virtual Learning Environment (VLE) Functional Specification. Joint Information Systems Committee, Briefing Paper No. 3, London, UK

Schofield (2003) An accessible interface for WINDS, MSc Thesis, Applied Computing, University of Dundee, UK

Sloan D, Rowan M, Booth P, Gregor P (2000) Ensuring the provision of accessible digital resources. Journal of Educational Media 25(3): 203-216

Sloan D, Gibson L, Milne S, Gregor P (2003) Ensuring optimal accessibility of online learning resources. In: Usability evaluation of online learning programs, Information Science Publishing, London, UK

UK Government (2001) Special Educational Needs and Disability Act 2001. Her Majesty's Stationery Office, London, UK

Chapter 6

Assessment, Insight and Awareness in Design for Users with Special Needs

R. Adams and P.M. Langdon

6.1 Introduction

User-Centred Design (UCD) has to take into account insight and awareness shown by potential users as a key part of the process. Other important factors (listed below) also depend upon insight and awareness.

This chapter distinguishes first between insight and awareness, and second between individuals with head injuries and others with muscular skeletal injuries. Awareness is defined as an individual's short-term ability to monitor and correct current performance, whilst insight indicates the long-term ability to learn from past performance and to develop specific knowledge about strengths and weaknesses. Nine case studies are reported examining in-depth assessments of users with acquired disabilities and the degree of insight and awareness they display. We examine the tacit hypothesis that overall insight and performance awareness share the same underlying mechanism in both musculo-skeletal and brain injuries.

6.2 Background and Objectives

Effective modelling of user requirements (Stary, 2001) is a vital aspect of UCD, and is necessary if advanced, assistive technology is to be designed well enough to support a move towards universal access and the effective personalisation of IT systems. User modelling depends critically upon a number of vital factors including:

- general guidelines and standards (Stephanidis *et al.*, 1987);
- the development of automatic user interface adaptation methods (Stephanidis and Savidis, 2001);
- user capability and psychology models (Jokela, 2000);

- a robust theoretical framework (Langdon *et al.*, 2002);
- task analyses with some psychological validity (Card *et al.*, 1981; Adams *et al.*, 2002);
- broad applications to task contexts e.g. work, home, in public. (Capobianco and Carbonell, 2002);
- the specific needs of users with disabilities and other groups in the population (Jacko and Vitense, 2001);
- vocational contexts and objectives (Adams *et al.*, 2002);
- learning and help requirements (Capobianco and Carbonell, 2002);
- research and assessment methods (Kujala and Mantyla, 2000);
- the levels of insight and awareness of the individual user (Sherwin and O'Shanick, 1998).

This chapter focuses on the last factors of insight and awareness, since almost all the other factors listed above depend critically upon them to some extent. There is growing evidence that many individuals with brain injuries will show lack of insight into their deficits resulting from their injuries (Sherwin and O'Shanick, 1998).

Three issues or assumptions are important here. First, we explore the implicit assumption that insight problems are confined to those with head injuries and avoid those with other types of disability.

We suspect that individuals who present with musculo-skeletal disabilities may have comparable problems, though for different reasons, including failure of coping mechanisms (Cohen and Lazarus, 1980) and stress. Second, it is typically assumed that insight (long term) and awareness (short term) are the same phenomena. The data in this chapter challenges that assumption. Third, it is by no means certain that all insight problems will involve underestimation rather than overestimation of abilities.

Clearly, there are important benefits if system users can achieve significant insights into their performance potential and good awareness of their current performance. They would be able to say what they are good at and what design options would suit them.

This would aid significantly in the evaluation of new systems and their prototypes, as well as providing valuable feedback for self adaptive systems which could track the needs of users. Conversely, many system design methodologies implicitly assume that users possess high level insight into their strength and weaknesses, as well as effective awareness of their current and potential performance.

Indeed, the system expert may significantly underestimate the difficulties faced by the user since the expert possesses an unrepresentative level of familiarity with the system. When these assumptions are not realised, the results of such studies and their consequent design recommendations may be unreliable.

On this basis, nine case studies are reported, involving individuals with a range of disabilities, including but not limited to brain injuries. The following case studies are drawn from on-going programmes of vocational assessment of individuals with a range of acquired, career threatening disabilities, including muscular skeletal and brain injuries.

6.3 Case Studies

6.3.1. Case Study A(1.1)

This individual was involved in a road traffic accident leading to a below the knee amputation. No head injuries were reported. He reports some phantom pain and back pain. He is concerned that he will not be able to meet the demands of physical work and will need to develop new vocational objectives. He feels that he lacks confidence and has always had a very poor memory. He is using significant pain-killers. He considers that his memory limitations will reduce his job prospects.

Assessment. His overall cognitive aptitude was evaluated with a task which measures abstract reasoning, in which he performed well, producing an estimated IQ of 112, a high average score. His numeracy and literacy were tested. His personality profile indicated an introvert personality with average anxiety levels. Overall, his performance was average to weak average, despite his stated concerns. He reported that he found all of these tasks to be very demanding. At his request, subsequent work was conducted with this individual on his memory and allowed him to obtain and sustain good memory performance.

Conclusions. This individual's overall profile indicates significant potential despite his stated lack of confidence, work skills and self-esteem. There were some slight indications of average to weak memory performance on a range of tasks, but this may be due, in part to a lack of training and awareness as to how best to use memory. There are significant differences between his comments and his actual task performance. An interview, questionnaire or a discussion would not have been sufficient to identify his strengths or weaknesses without performance measures. There was some indication too of performance awareness problems, such that he reported some memory tasks to be difficult even when he produced good scores.

6.3.2. Case Study A(1.2)

He has had five strokes since 1997, resulting in mild left side hemiplegia and mobility problems. He is keen to improve his mental abilities and skills. His confidence and self - esteem are low.

Assessment. His overall aptitude was evaluated by means of a standard IQ test, in which he performed reasonably well, producing an estimated IQ of 103, an average score. He reported that he found these tasks difficult, however his performance scores indicate a weak/average memory, they do not support the conclusion of a poor memory. Again, self-report and performance are discrepant.

Conclusions. This individual shows average to low average performance on a range of cognitive tasks. Further work should look at his ability to concentrate over longer time scales (most tasks used here lasted less than an hour) , since there was some indication that the effort to concentrate was sometimes problematic. Again, there are significant differences between his comments and his task performance. Again an interview or a discussion would not have provided an accurate picture of his strengths or weaknesses, overestimating the extent of his performance problems.

6.3.3. Case Study A(1.3).

He sustained a head injury as a result of a road traffic accident twelve months ago. The resulting closed head injury involved the left frontal lobe and left parietal lobe, producing right hemiparesis and mild left hemiparesis. He initially had no insight into his deficits, with impaired memory and concentration. After two months, he showed slightly improved insight, better memory but with significant cognitive problems.

Assessment. A structured interview was conducted to explore the key issues with him. He felt that he sometimes had problems "with his mind" and added that he sometimes did not think well enough for what he wanted to do, but that this was not a bad problem. Given his background profile of problems, these responses are all consistent with a lack of full insight into his cognitive problems, significantly underestimating them. His overall aptitude was evaluated by two IQ tests producing an IQ estimate of 69 and 75. The NART test was used to estimate his pre-morbid IQ (using the pronunciation of irregular words) which turned out to be 105.

Clearly his pre-morbid IQ was significantly higher than his currently estimated IQ. In view of his history of memory problems after the accident, his current memory performance was examined, using a simple free recall task for short digit sequences (four digits per sequence, 25 sequences per task). To assess his cognitive skills, his performance on a version of the Stroop task was considered (Hartley and Adams, 1974). This task involves the use of colour names printed in different coloured inks.

The participant is required to examine one item and to select one item from four options which matched it according to a predefined rule. The nature of the rule is varied to produce different versions of the task. His performance was very slow, completing approximately 25% of the number of items typically completed in the time allowed. He learned to do each task, but his performance actually declined from the practice session to the main session in every case In two cases out of four, this decline was big enough to be statistically significant on a t-test for proportions (p< 0.001) with the non-significant comparisons going in the same direction.

This result is consistent with a difficulty with his ability to organise the demands of the tasks, even though he had been given ample opportunity to learn them i.e. a problem with executive functioning, a predominantly frontal lobe function. His performance declined significantly across the different versions, suggesting that his ability to organise each task declined with exposure to different variations of the task.

Conclusions. This individual has very significant problems with executive functioning. In contrast, performance of passive tasks like memory for brief digit spans was unimpaired. His current IQ appears to be significantly depressed when compared to an estimate of his pre-morbid IQ. He is unable to pace himself in an externally un-paced task (e.g. 16PF). Again, there are major differences between his comments and his task performance. An interview or a discussion would not have provided an accurate picture of his strengths or weaknesses. He showed both lack of insight into his problems and lack of awareness of his current performance.

Double Dissociation. This individual performed very well in the memory task but very badly on tasks which measure cognitive skills. In contrast, cases A11 and A12 showed exactly the opposite profile performing relatively well on cognitive tasks but less well on the memory tasks.

This is an important observation, since it means that differences between the two types of task cannot be explained simply in terms of their relative difficulty. This contrasting pattern of results indicates a double dissociation. A double dissociation is said to occur when two dissociations occur between two task but in opposite directions.

6.3.4. Case Study A(1.4).

This individual, a student, was involved in a road traffic accident, with resulting frontal lobe damage and surgical removal of portions from both frontal lobes. He is reported to exhibit inappropriate social behaviour.

Assessment. His overall IQ was estimated to be 109. He also completed a task to assess his pre-morbid IQ (NART) which produced a significantly higher estimated IQ of 118. This reduction is highly likely to be related to his accident rather than being a chance result. His perceptual speed and accuracy were also measured by means of a DAT subtest.

He performed well on this task, completing 43 items out of 43 without error. In the Stroop task it was observed that he required significantly more time to learn each version of the task, but when he had learned each task he performed them relatively well. This suggests that he faces problems with his executive processes, whilst his basic information processing skills seem to be intact. He reports concerns with his memory and so this function was assessed using two versions of a simple word recall task. He performed well in both versions of the task, ruling out any significant memory problems. His metamemory was tested by means of a simple procedure in which his memory for prior events was tested. Whilst his basic memory seems to be functioning well, his metamemory, has been dramatically impaired. This is a striking contrast between working memory and metamemory.

His basic, low level cognitive skills like simple memory, concentration and attention seem to function well, whilst his higher functions like IQ, executive functions, structuring new tasks and metamemory are significantly impaired.

His perceived personality was also assessed (MBTI and 16PF) and there were indications that his underlying personality tendencies and his post injury behaviour were different. His frontal lobe injuries seem to be implied in his passive approach to tasks, his executive function problems, his competent memory and basic attentional processes, lack of drive and social inhibition.

Conclusions. This individual has significant executive function problems as shown by reduced IQ, an inability to organise new tasks, lack of drive, socially inappropriate behaviour, poor metamemory yet functional low level memory and attentional processes. He reported a poor memory, performed well on a simple memory function task, yet displayed poor metamemory. He expected to perform poorly on the Stroop task, but did well. His perceptions of his own personality contradicted his own behaviour as observed and reported by reliable others.

6.3.5 Case Study A(1.5)

This individual problems with language skills and possible dyslexia.

Assessment. A number of dyslexia related tasks were employed to explore his linguistic skills. i.e. Adult Check List. This twenty-item questionnaire explores possible areas of everyday errors. When an individual selects most of the items on this questionnaire, they are advised to seek further help. He selected only five questions, indicating a more limited set of problems. The Bangor Dyslexia Test covers ten areas of potential linguistic problems, it is based on indicative performance in each area. Again, there is some indication of linguistic problems but not a broad spectrum dyslexia.

His IQ was assessed to be 98, which does not explain the above linguistic difficulties. He completed a computer battery of tasks. He did well in; communication, numeracy, spatial ability, verbal memory. He did less well in; visual memory, logical reasoning. This profile indicates of inconsistent performance, but not a purely linguistic problem.

Conclusions. These scores are complex and do show some problems and inconsistencies in his cognitive skills, but there is no clear indication of dyslexia related problems. In fact, there were some tasks which he did well which a diagnosis of dyslexia would preclude. He was concerned that he might be about dyslexic but these fears were not confirmed. Specific linguistic and cognitive problems were found, but they were found to be limited to certain tasks and may indicate inconsistent performance rather than profound deficits.

6.3.6. Case Study A(1.6)

He experienced a subarachnoid haemorrhage eight years ago. He reports intermittent problems with concentration and with left side hemiplegia.

Assessment. His overall aptitude was estimated at IQ 100 (an average score). His perceptual speed was weak (18th percentile), his perceptual organisation was relatively strong (99th percentile) as was his working memory (73rd percentile).

Conclusions. As a result of his brain injuries, this individual has experienced significant cognitive deficits which, fortunately, are limited in range. He has retained an average IQ, his working memory and his perceptual organisation are relatively unscathed. Perceptual speed, however, appears to be significantly impaired and so his general speed of cognitive working will be impaired. He showed a general insight into his concentration problems, though was not able to specify the exact nature of those problems as indicated by his performance, i.e. lack of perceptual processing speed.

6.3.7. Case Study A(1.7)

She was presented as having mild learning difficulties from birth, but it turned out that she had problems communicating, indicating a more serious level of difficulty.

Assessment. It soon became obvious that she was not able to respond validly to the questions, responding only with the last option heard. This profile was consistent with a short-term memory problem in general and an auditory recency effect in particular. It was as if earlier information was being lost from auditory memory. To test the above explanation of her difficulties, a simple free recall for brief digit sequences (four digits per sequence) was used. The digits were presented auditorily, visually or in combination.

As predicted, she showed a marked recency effect in auditory short-term memory. The pattern for visual presentation was very different. A more typical serial position curve was proposed with the first and last items being well recalled. It seems that her learning problems may be due, in part, to a limitation in her short-term auditory memory.

Conclusions. This individual has significant learning difficulties, though it was shown that she can acquire work like tasks. Initial indications of a deficit in auditory short term memory were confirmed strongly by a simple free recall task. This individual could not articulate her memory problems. However, she did show a significant learning curve in a simple manual task.

6.3.8. Case Study A(1.8)

This individual has cerebral palsy, which effects his left side and his speech. He also reports some learning difficulties.

Assessment. In an initial interview, he showed good insights into his strengths and weaknesses, and career objectives. He completed a digit symbol substitution task, in which digits are replaced by symbols according to a set plan, measuring perceptual speed and accuracy. He completed all 100 items correctly, indicating an unimpaired perceptual speed. He also attempted a series of IQ tasks, averaging around 80. His language skills are relatively stronger than his basic number operations.

Conclusions. This individual is developing his specific aptitudes starting with a weak basic IQ. He is developing basic work skills and IT presents a potentially valuable career area for him. In this case, the individual shows a good level of insight into his strengths and weaknesses. This implies that insight is not closely related to intelligence. Other cases present significant over or under estimates of their deficits. For recently acquired disabilities, lack of awareness of the extent of disability appears more frequent.

6.3.9. Case Study A(1.9)

This individual is schizophrenic, with his condition controlled by medication. He is concerned about his concentration and his abilities to carry out work activities efficiently.

Assessment. He is a pleasant and quiet individual who appears keen to work well and to be employed. He appears to be aware of expressed concerns about the quality of work, but he does not seem so aware directly of his problems. He was first given a measure of his overall aptitude (RSPM) which produced a score of 30th percentile of the general population. The Cognitive Failings Questionnaire (CFQ) explores the frequency of everyday mistakes. It requires the individual to report on the perceived frequency of their errors. He produced a low score of 34 (as compared with a middle range score of 100). This indicates that he is either unaware of his mistakes or that his mistakes fall into a narrow band, or both.

The above findings suggest serious problems with cognitive skills, a hypothesis which is tested by use of the Stroop test, a task requiring the matching of colour words in different inks according to preordained rules. This task requires the individual to organise and acquire new tasks and to attend and implement them well. This individual seemed to experience no problems in learning how to learn the tasks.

However, he appeared to experience significant negative transfer from one task to another. This is an important result since he apparently cannot deal with conflicting demands of two simple tasks. This hypothesis was tested by means of a free recall task for words. In one version, errors were not permitted. In the second version, errors were allowed. The results were very clear. Under error making conditions, he performed significantly worse than under error free conditions.

Conclusions. This individual needs to learn under error-free conditions or he will retain errors after training. He cannot cope well with similar tasks with competing demands. He shows problems both of lack of long term insight into his difficulties and lack of short-term awareness of his current performance problems.

6.4. Summary of Results

It was surprising that the majority of these cases showed significant associated difficulties of insight (Table 6.1). Of the nine case studies, seven showed significant difficulties of insight, with an additional one showing minor insight problems. In addition, we found that not all insight problems were of the same kind. Some individuals seemed to be totally unaware of their difficulties, except for some nominal acknowledgement acquired from a third party, to those who knew that they had problems but were unsure of their exact nature. In some cases, individuals underestimated their skills rather than overestimated them.

6.4.1. Awareness

We also looked at the individual's awareness of their own performance (Table 6.1). It turned out that performance awareness and insight into deficits were not completely coincident. Of the nine case studies, four seemed to have problems associated with a lack of awareness of their own performance. In one extreme case, the individual appeared to be unaware of his performance problems. He was unable to cope with the conflicting demands of different tasks but was not able to articulate any of his problems. Left to work alone, his work output would begin to slow and become more error prone. A second individual with learning difficulties also showed no awareness of her performance problems.

Table 6.1. Insight and Awareness

Case study	Insight (* indicates problem)	awareness of performance (* indicates a problem)
A1.1	* underestimates abilities	* slightly underestimates
A1.2	* underestimates abilities	* slightly underestimates
A1.3	* no insight into problems	OK
A1.4	* insight problems, miss-estimation	OK
A1.5	* only minor insight problems	OK
A1.6	* only minor insight problems	OK
A1.7	* no insight into problems	* low awareness
A1.8	OK	OK
A1.9	* no insight into problems	* low awareness

The other two individuals, who both presented with insight problems, such that they underestimated their abilities, also reported tasks to be very hard even when they were performing very well. Their perceptions of their performance therefore appeared to be inaccurate.

A lack of performance awareness might have been expected to be an integral part of lack of insight, but this did not turn out to be the case. Even where an individual showed a significant insight deficit, they could often carry out set tasks and be aware if their performance was good or bad. If so, it may be a reasonable question to ask someone "How are you doing / did you do on that task?" If this analysis is correct, however, many of our clients will find questions of the kind "Are you good a this type of task?" to be very difficult to get right. Lack of insight may render their answers uncertain. If so, we need to look carefully at the methods used to elicit user views of new systems and prototypes. Questionnaires, focus groups, protocol analysis and interviews all rely on user's insights and the present study suggests they should be used in conjunction with experimental and metric performance measures wherever possible.

6.4.2. Performance and Insight: Conclusions

The relationship between performance awareness and overall insight seems to be more complex than originally anticipated. Clearly, insight and awareness do not share the same underlying mechanisms; the tacit hypothesis tested in this chapter. Many clients with acquired disabilities gradually develop a degree of insight into their difficulties, but it is clear that that this development can be slow and painful.

If an individual can possess some awareness of his current performance, he can use that awareness to build up his insight of his strengths and weaknesses. It is surprising, therefore, that four of the five in-depth case studies considered here showed poor insight accompanied by good awareness. Clearly, the link between awareness and insight is not simple. Perhaps in these cases, much more time will be required to build insight upon awareness.

A second and less positive view would state that these individuals might have suffered damage that not only impacted on insight but also on the link between awareness and insight itself. On either view, considerable effort would be require to build an adequate level of insight. We suggest that these results make a good case for the construction of metric insight and awareness assessment test that can be administered as part of a user-centred design methodology. Such a test would be based on normalised measures of performance awareness and overall insight treated as interacting cognitive dimensions.

6.5 References

Adams R, Langdon P, Clarkson PJ (2002) A Systematic Basis for Developing Cognitive Assessment Methods for Assistive Technology. In: CUWAAT'02, Springer-Verlag, London, UK

Card SK, Moran TP, Newell A (1981) The keystroke level model for user performance time with interactive computer systems. Communications of the ACM 23: 396-410

Cohen F, Lazarus RL (1980) Coping with the stresses of illness. In: Health Psychology - A Handbook. San Francisco : Jossey Bass

Hartley LR, Adams RG (1974) Effect of noise on the stroop test. Journal of Experimental Psychology 102: 62-66

Jacko JA, Vitens HS (2001) A review and reappraisal of information technologies within a conceptual framework for individuals with disabilities. Universal Access in the Information Society 1: 56-76

Jokela T (2000) User capability models - review and analysis. In: People and Computers XIV - Usability or Else, HCI 2000, Springer-Verlag, London, UK

Kujala S, Mantyla M (2000) How effective are user studies? In: People and Computers XIV - Usability or Else. In: Proceedings of HCI 2000. Springer-Verlag, London, UK

Langdon P, Adams R, Clarkson PJ (2002) Universal access to assistive technology through client-centred cognitive assessment. In: ERCIM'02, Lecture Notes in Computer Science, Springer-Verlag, London, UK

Sherwin ED, O'Shanick GJ (1998) From denial to poster child: Growing past the injury. In: Traumatic Brain Injury Rehabilitation, Butterworth Heinemann

Stary C (2001) User diversity and design representations: Towards increased effectiveness in Design for All. Universal Access in the Information Society 1: 16-30

Stephanidis C, Akoumiankis D, Ziegler J, Faehnrich K-P (1997) User interface accessibility: A retrospective of current standardisation efforts. In: ECAI 94, Amsterdam, The Netherlands

Stephanidis C, Savidis A (2001) Universal access in the information society: Methods, tools and interaction technologies. Universal Access in the Information Society 1: 40-55

Chapter 7

New Cognitive Capability Scales For Inclusive Product Design

P.M. Langdon, S. Keates and P.J. Clarkson

7.1 Introduction

Existing capability scales, such as that of the UK Office of National Statistics (ONS) are based on a practitioner defined concept of intellectual function that is not compatible with current psychology. This chapter addresses the design requirements of a set of putative cognitive capability scales from a psychological perspective. In order to assess capability for product design, a scale should address all aspects of cognition that may be involved in product use.

As a starting point, we aimed to develop new scales to assess the cognitive capability of individuals starting with items from the existing UK ONS scale, re-analysed in terms of cognitive requirements. The new scales were constructed by classifying test items with reference to a simple cognitive user model representing an overview of cognition constructed from well-established findings in mainstream cognitive science (Langdon *et al.*, 2002). Using the data from 7,500 interviews in the original survey, new scorings were re-calculated from the resulting scales. These new scales are then quantitatively and qualitatively compared with the existing scales.

7.2 Background and Objectives

The rights of older and disabled people are growing in prominence. Increasing awareness of this challenge is reflected in legislation, such as the 1996 Disability Discrimination Act. By 2020, almost half the adult population in the UK will be over 50, with the over 80's being the most rapidly growing sector.

Recent research into inclusive design (Keates and Clarkson, 2002) has investigated the relationship between capabilities of the population at large and guidelines for the design of features of products. This research suggests that a good representation of the capability range of individuals can be made on a three-axis scale derived from the basic psychological dimensions of sensory, motor and cognitive capability.

Existing scales for the assessment of intellectual capability ranges, such as those compiled by the UK Office of National Statistics (Grundy *et al.*, 1999), focus on intellectual function as a combination of a number of items and sub-scales devised by health practitioners and validated using panels of judges. To our knowledge, no other methods for assessment of everyday cognitive capability exist although the cognitive considerations behind information displays and cockpit designs has been investigated in the human-factors area in the context of workload (e.g. Endsley *et al.*, 2003). While effective in other areas, these scales may not reflect cognitive capability of individuals as they were derived from practical needs in healthcare without any unifying system or theory. We addressed the need to derive scales giving accurate capability estimates for product design by re-analysing the existing survey data in the light of modern cognitive psychological theory.

7.2.1. The Cambridge Inclusive Design Model

The development of a systematic basis for cognitive assessment for the purposes of matching individuals to products should make reference to an overall approach to accessibility and disability in the population at large. The simplistic model, to be outlined, is intended to tackle in more detail a number of specific issues more generally addressed by the Cambridge Inclusive Design Cube (Keates and Clarkson, 2002). Based on early psychological theories of keystroke interaction with basic character-based computer terminals, the Design Cube is a representation used for analysis of human interaction with computers, such as may take place while using computer–based assistive technology products. The three axes of a 3D cube are used as imaginary scales of degree of capability with the fully able user being represented as the origin corner. Clearly, in this representation, the cognitive scale is a summation of the effects on the individual's capability of a range of fundamental cognitive competencies. The simplistic model, to be outlined below, allows the nature and relative importance of those competencies to be examined at a general level. Furthermore, the model allows interactions between sensory, motor and core cognitive functions to be specified in order to address specific tasks and skills. It also follows that the cognitive simplistic model can also be used to unpack the detailed considerations that correspond to user perception, cognition, and motor function.

7.2.2 The Sources of Data

In order to assess the ranges of capability in the UK population pertinent to features of product designs, a source of data is required. Data is readily available for the range of sensory and motor scale dimensions but the cognitive dimension is often poorly addressed, in this case, by only one scale, that of intellectual function.

We address the underlying considerations for construction of a scale of cognitive capability both for the purpose of individual and product assessment and as a basis for the creation of guidelines for inclusive product design.

There are many sources of capability data such as: Older Adult (Smith *et al.*, 1998), which focus on anthropometric-based capabilities; the RNID for data on deafness (RNID, 2000); and the RNIB for data on visual impairments. We used one of the most complete representative data sets; the disability follow-up to Great Britain Family Resources Survey (FRS) (Semmence, 1998) designed to establish the prevalence of disability in the UK. In the following section we examine the methodology used to derive the scales used, focussing in particular, on the "intellectual function" scale.

7.2.3 The Scales of the Disability Follow-up Survey

The Great Britain Disability Follow-up Survey (DFS) was based on a measure of severity of disability established through the consensus of judges assessing the capability limitations of a variety of disabilities and their combinations. To give an overall severity score a one-dimensional interval scale was constructed from these judgements and used as an estimator.

7.2.3.1 The Methodology of the DFS

Survey items based on the ICIDH (International Classification of Impairments Disabilities and Handicaps) definitions of disability (WHO, 1980) were used in the field collection of data from 7500 interviews using a stratified probability clustering sample, prior to any scale development. The original items were designed to cover all the disability areas at all levels. The DFS methodology utilised panels of judges for 10 areas of disability identified from the original items. This was done on the basis of criteria such as: inclusion in the survey; avoidance of inter-correlation; simplicity; and, elimination of over inclusive items. The 100 judges were selected from professionals such as doctors, physiotherapists, occupational therapists, clinical psychologists, independent researchers and disabled representatives of voluntary organisations. Judges were required to place cards denoting limiting activities on a scale from 1 (least limiting) to 11 (most limiting) without regard to handicap, prognosis or age but with regard to activities of daily living. Items with low reliability were removed at this stage and statistical measures of between-judge agreement were used to assess consensus. Judges out of line with the majority were excluded. The resulting scales were highly correlated with each other (greater that 0.81) apart from that of intellectual function (0.19). This was due to poor agreement between more than half of the judges. As a result of this a new scale was constructed by asking judges to rate the severity of impairment arising from 11, 8 and 4 items expressing an intellectual limitation. It was assumed that there was a linear relationship between severity and number of problems without regard for the nature of the "intellectual" impairment.

It seems likely that this assessment scale, dependent as it is on diverse original test items that confounded a range of cognitive functions, does not reflect cognitive capabilities in a systematic way. For this reason, we aimed to carry out a reassessment and reclassification of the original selected test items in terms of their categorisation in terms of well-accepted elements of mainstream cognitive theory.

The DFS survey finally recognised thirteen capability scales of which seven are most relevant to product evaluation: locomotion, dexterity, reach and stretch, vision, hearing, communication, and intellectual functioning. Each of these scales, ranging from 0 (fully able) through 0.5 (minimal impairment) to 12.5 (most severe impairment), were aligned by 57 judges to ensure that equal scores broadly related to equivalent levels of disability (Martin and Elliot, 1992).

The DFS explored all thirteen of the capabilities, giving the interviewee a score for each. These scores were moderated to provide a common scale across all capabilities, i.e. a score of 5.5 on locomotion was judged to represent the same loss of capability as a score of 5.5 on vision. As a result, the severity scores are not evenly spaced, indeed neither are the definitions consistent in their language of description. In this case locomotion includes consideration of walking, bending and straightening, falling and balance, and climbing steps and stairs. This is typical of all the scales and reflects the validity considerations inherent in using the data for anything other than population estimates. In addition, the DFS assessed the prevalence of multiple capability losses by obtaining judges' ratings of severity resulting from a selection of representative profiles of 2 to 4 multiple disabilities occurring together, and relating the resulting scales using a linear-regression model of influence on overall severity. The resulting alignment of the severity scales allows for the combination of scores to give an overall severity category. This is derived as a weighted sum where:

$$\text{disability score} = \text{worst} + 0.4 \times (\text{2nd worst}) + 0.3 \times (\text{3rd worst}) \qquad (7.1)$$

This weighted sum was then re-scaled into a final overall severity category using the mapping shown in Table 7.1.

Table 7.1. Correspondence between disability scores and severity category

	Least severe										*Most severe*
Disability score	0	0.5-2.95	3-4.95	5-6.95	7-8.95	9-10.95	11-12.95	13-14.95	15-16.95	17-18.95	19-21.4
Severity category	0	1	2	3	4	5	6	7	8	9	10

7.2.4. The Simple Cognitive Model

Cognitive psychology can provide a rich variety of architectures for working models. For example, simplistic architectures like Broadbent's Maltese Cross (Broadbent, 1984) capture an overview of cognition but do not attempt to be complete, whereas more complex models like the Interacting Cognitive

Subsystems approach (Barnard *et al.*, 2000) consists of an information processing, parallel approach that attempts to be complete and to address the complexity of realistic cognition. Whilst any of these could be used to model the assessment of cognitive skills, we adopt a parsimonious approach based on Broadbent's (1984) simplistic model because of the advantages of simplicity as a framework for research and practical assessment. A more detailed rationale for choice of this model is given in Langdon, Adams and Clarkson (2002).

The overall structure adopted in shown in Figure 7.1. It consists of a set of four memory stores that are linked by a central processing system. One of the roles of this central system is to transfer or copy memory traces from one store to another. The processing system also acts as a selection filter. This initial formulation (Broadbent, 1984) leaves out any indication of input and outputs, implying some form of selection or filtering before the sensory memory store. More recent adaptations of this model (Revelle and Loftus, 1990) incorporate a selective filter before sensory memory. However, the present model also allows for more advanced forms of selection when information is transferred between memory stores and allows for memories to be present in one or more stores, either partially or fully.

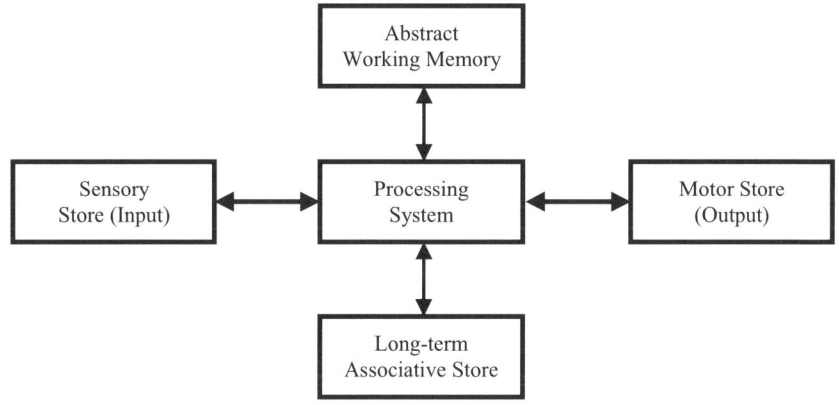

Figure 7.1. The overall structure of the simplistic model

Sensory Store: This is a limited capacity memory store that accepts transfers from the other stores as a translation or change of code. This store mainly receives a relatively raw input from the senses. It is divided up in terms of the physical dimensions that describe sensory inputs.

Output Store: This store holds sequences of motor output programmes, including sub-vocal speech sequences and is normally the last stage before responding. However, these programmes need not issue into overt actions but can feed back into another store.

Abstract Working Memory: Interference between memories may not depend on similarity of later input, but rather on the sheer numbers of items. It is a temporary, limited capacity memory. Memories could be crowded out by a very large volume of information if a large amount of central processing is performed.

Long term Associative Store: This is not concerned with events themselves but with the running totals of the co-occurrence of stimuli. The model assumes that with practice the individual builds up stronger associations between the relevant items in the task being learned.

Processing System: The processing system or central executive has the principal role of transferring information from one memory store to another. Thus this system need to have its own long term memory, since these rules are not stored in the long term associative store. The Processing System must also have some form of shorter term memory to keep track of current and recent actions.

7.2.5. Implications for Cognitive Scales

It is clear that the simple cognitive model divides a number of cognitive distinctions that reflect findings in experimental psychology but are not preserved within the DFS question items or the intellectual function scale. Rather, the items of the original scales confound and confuse cognitive capabilities in the same way that they combine physical capabilities such as reach and stretch, dexterity and locomotion. The principal gain from using the model in this context is that it supplies a coherent theory based on established findings that can be used to contextualise the construction of specific scales. In principal, the model subsumes at least the following areas of capability: (1) *Executive Function:* input, output and central attentional processes; visual cognition; visual search; attention and executive function; reasoning and abstraction; meta-cognition: (2) *Memory:* input, output and working memory; task learning; visuo-spatial memory; memory structures: categorisation and output processes; meta-memory.

7.3 Experimental Validation

The individual survey questions from the ONS scale were categorised according to the area of cognition they addressed using the simplistic framework for guidance (Adams, Langdon and Clarkson, 2002). This categorisation was then used to construct a number of new scales corresponding to cognitive categories using the original SPSS data from the survey. The new cognitive scales were embedded within the Cambridge capability-scaling tool (Keates and Clarkson, 2002) and the calculated scores compared with those generated by the original intellectual functioning scale for a range of age groups.

7.3.1. Capability Analysis

The Cambridge Inclusive Design capability tool uses derived data from the scaled scores of the original DFS data to calculate comparative charts of prevalence of varying capabilities, as represented in the individual scales, for differing age groups, sex, and capability bands.

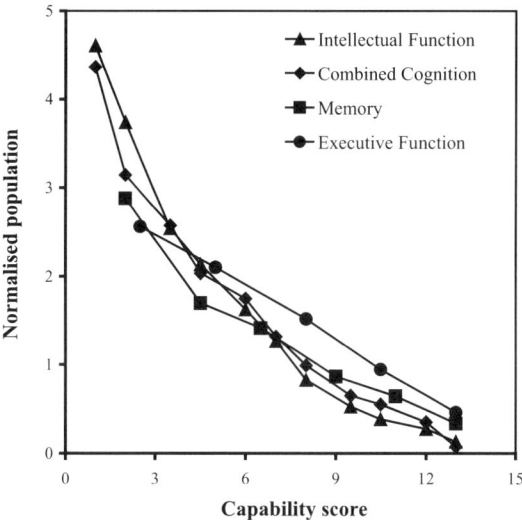

Figure 7.2. Visualisation charts of prevalence of impairment

Figure 7.2 shows the relationship between the new and existing scales, highlighting the differences between three new scales and the original intellectual function scale in terms of the numbers of the population scoring at differing degrees of impairment, as indicated by the scale. Three new scales were tested: (1) Combined cognitive scale combining the memory and executive function scales, (2) the new memory scale and (3), the new executive function scale. For all three scales, the impairment score was arrived at by adding the number of capability problems that were reported as discussed above. It is clear from the graph that while the scales are broadly correlated (as are all the scales in the DFS), the combined cognition and the intellectual function scale are very similar as would be expected since they both account for most of the capabilities involved in mental life. However, interestingly, the memory scale shows a trend towards less problems than either at mild impairment levels and the executive function a trend towards more problems at the higher impairment levels.

This implies that the sample reported either a few memory impairments with some attention and organisation problems or reported serious executive function problems combined with accompanying memory difficulties. The distribution of these impairments with age band and their relation to other impairments are examined below.

It would be expected that the latter would be more frequent in old age and the former associated with neurophysiological injury. The relationship of any one capability scale to another can be visualised using a graph such as that shown in Figure 7.3. This clearly shows that, statistically, good motion capability is present in individuals with normal to slightly impaired sensory capability but that it is greatly impaired at a sensory threshold of scale level 2. This implies that full motion is not easy once the senses are impaired beyond a certain level.

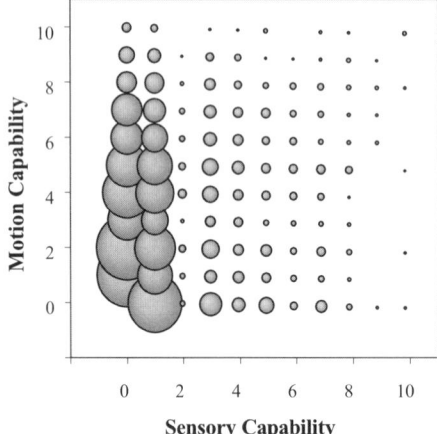

Figure 7.3. Prevalence of co-occurrence of motion and sensory impairment

This type of analysis can give us information about the nature of cognitive impairment with different capability scales. For example, Figure 7.4a and 7.4b show the relationship of cognition to motion and sensory scale scores. To some extent, the relationship reflects the prevalence of multiple impairments. For example, the co-occurrence of sensory and motion disorders with cognitive disorders may occur in neurological injury and stroke.

Figure 7.4a suggests that large degrees of deterioration of cognitive capability is not accompanied by sensory impairment at high levels but in the main is more frequently associated with mild to moderate sensory impairment. In contrast, 4b shows that high degrees of motion impairment are associated with only mild cognitive impairment. The former could represent the situation with stroke and ageing whereas the latter suggests a strong influence of the range of medium to strong motion impairments that do not affect the brain.

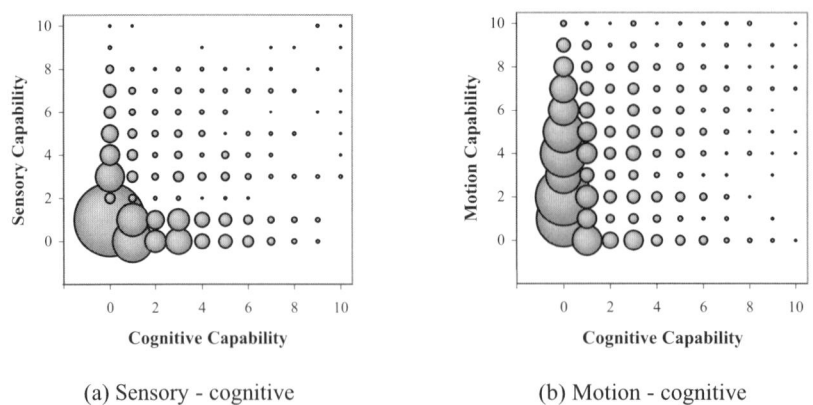

(a) Sensory - cognitive   (b) Motion - cognitive

Figure 7.4. Sensory (a) and motor (b) impairment prevalence compared with cognitive capability impairment.

These comparisons with the existing cognition scale and the associations they suggest could be further explored using the newly calculated memory and executive function scales in order to probe the micro-structure of cognitive impairment. In particular, age related cognitive impairments and commonly co-occurring multiple impairments may coincide with specific medical populations or disorders. These populations, once identified may be used for quantitative and qualitative product design assessments (Keates and Clarkson, 2003).

7.3.2 Discussion

In the light of the comparison with the cognitive theory derived scales, the original ONS intellectual function scale confounded many aspects of cognition in individual question items. This is not surprising as the question items were devised by health practitioners in order to reflect common disabilities in the ICIDH classification. In addition, the scale operates by simply counting the number of intellectual impairments reported and scales this as a measure of overall impairment, ignoring the interrelations between impairments. The comparisons suggest that this scale would be poor predictor of the cognitive usability of product designs. The new cognitive scales, however, appear better able to differentiate between product features but only in as much as they were able to do so using the existing question items.

A general conclusion, therefore, is that the new derived scales are more accurate cognitively but cannot go beyond the original items. Formation of more accurate capability assessments will require the development of new question items. This process will require careful development of questions by cognitive psychologists aiming to avoid confounding different cognitive functions and will be informed by the considerable body of experimental cognitive psychology findings that already address these distinctions. Ideally, further scales to be used in future surveys would be normalised with reference to known impairment sample groups and re-scaled for equivalence to the other scales used.

Two new scales could be superimposed on the ONS survey items: *executive function* and *memory*. One important conclusion resulting from the use of the simple cognitive model is that there are a number of desirable and important aspects of cognition identified by the model that were not addressed at all by the ONS scales. These include visual cognition and reasoning; categorical memory, meta-cognition and further executive functions such as information filtering and multiple-tasking. The effectiveness of new scales enhanced using these new cognitive aspects for forming capability and product assessment, as well as identifying multiple impairment groups or medical populations, are currently being evaluated.

7.4 References

Adams R, Langdon PM, Clarkson PJ (2002) A systematic basis for developing cognitive assessment methods for assistive technology. In: Universal Access and Assistive Technology, Springer-Verlag, London, UK

Baddeley AD (1996) Your memory: a user' guide. Prion, London, UK

Barnard PJ, May J, Duke D, Duce D (2000) Systems interactions and macrotheory. Transactions on Computer Human Interface 7: 222-262

Broadbent DE (1984) The Maltese cross: a new simplistic model or memory. Behavioral and Brain Sciences 7: 55-94

Endsley MR, Bolte B, Jones DG (2003) Designing for situation awareness. An approach to user-centred design, Taylor & Francis

Grundy E, Ahlburg D, Ali M, Breeze E, Sloggett A (1999) Disability in Great Britain. Department of Social Security, UK

Keates LS, Clarkson PJ (2002) Defining design exclusion. In: Universal Access and Assistive Technology, Springer-Verlag, London, UK

Langdon P, Adams R, Clarkson PJ (2002) Universal access to assistive technology through client-centred cognitive assessment. Proceedings of the 7th ERCIM Workshop. In: Lecture Notes in Computer Science, "State-of the-Art Surveys". Springer-Verlag, London, UK, pp 555-567

Lee FJ, Anderson JR (2001) Does learning a complex task have to be complex? A study in learning decomposition. Cognitive Psychology 42: 267-316

Martin J, Elliot D (1992) Creating an overall measure of severity of disability for the office of population censuses and surveys disability survey. Journal of the Royal Statistical Society 155(1): 121-140

Revelle W, Loftus DA (1990) Individual differences and arousal; implications for the study of mood and memory. Cognition and Emotion 4: 161-190

RNID (2000) Statistics on deafness. Available at: http://www.rnid.org.uk

Smith S *et al.* (2000) Older adult: The handbook of measurements and capabilities of the older adult - data for design safety. Department of Trade and Industry, London, UK

Semmence J, Gault S, Hussain M, Hall P, Stanborough J, Pickering E (1998) Family resources survey, Great Britain 1996-97. Department of Social Security, Corporate Document Services, London, UK

WHO (1980) International Classification of Impairments Disabilities and Handicaps. World Health Organisation, Geneva, Switzerland

Part II

Enabling Computer Access and New Technologies

Chapter 8

An AAC-Enabled Internet: From User Requirements to Guidelines

C. Nicolle, K. Black, A. Lysley, D. Poulson and
D. Hekstra

8.1 Introduction

Ensuring that WWW pages are accessible and usable for people with complex communication needs provides a particular challenge for WWW page designers. Despite advances in commercially available assistive technologies, people using augmentative and alternative communication (AAC) comment on continuing difficulty and frustration in physical access to technology and subsequent reliance on non-disabled partners (Clarke *et al.*, 2001; 2002).

The EU WWAAC (World Wide Augmentative and Alternative Communication) project, which began in January 2001, has been engaged in a number of research and development activities in order to overcome some of these problems, including the:

- development of Internet applications, including an adapted Web browser, tailored to the needs of people who use AAC;
- contribution to the development of Web accessibility guidelines;
- development of a communication infrastructure and protocol to support symbol-based communication on the Web, based upon open-sourced concept coding;
- development of a Dreamweaver extension to enable Web developers to symbol embellish their Web pages via the on-line concept coding database.

This chapter will concentrate on the first 2 activities to demonstrate how the design, development and evaluation of an adapted Web browser with people who use AAC will lead to more accessible and usable software.

This work is also contributing to the development of WWW accessibility guidelines, which will feed into the work of the World Wide Web Consortium–Web Accessibility Initiative (W3C–WAI). It is important, however, to consider these activities in light of the concept coding stream of the work, which is briefly described below.

Concept coding will facilitate the sharing of symbol-based content between different symbol users using different symbol language systems. It will also enable symbols to be converted into text and vice versa. This might mean, for example, that a person who uses AAC could open an Internet bank account by completing an on-line form using their own symbol system.

The vision of concept coding is that instead of images and symbols having to be transferred from one computer to another, it is possible to share a unique code designating the meaning of the symbol needing to be transferred. In addition to efficiency in handling images used for communication purposes, this concept would also allow personalised or idiosyncratic symbols specific to one person to be used by them in Internet-based communication. An open source concept coding, in combination with more accessible and usable software, is the driving force behind the WWAAC project.

8.2 Survey of User Requirements

The primary target population of end users defined by the project are people between the ages of 12 and 25 years who use graphic symbol-based AAC in face-to-face interaction, and who are professionally supported in their use of AAC and the Internet within school/college or receiving non-professional support at home. However, the developments may well be applicable to people of all ages who use graphic symbol-based AAC, and to those who use text-based AAC. They may also be applicable to a broader range of groups such as people with learning disabilities who use symbols as aids to literacy, people with aphasia, and the elderly. This is something that will be explored during a later stage in the project.

During the survey of user requirements, interviews were held with 51 service providers (e.g., Speech and Language Therapists and Teachers) and 10 software manufacturers/distributors. In addition, individual interviews were held with a sample of 28 people, with relatively high receptive abilities, who use AAC from England, Sweden, Finland and Spain. Details of this investigation are reported in Clarke *et al.* (2001; 2002). The interviews were designed to gain a better understanding of the use of Web browsing and email by people who use AAC, their particular problems, and what their needs and preferences might be, both with regard to the technology itself and future services.

The survey testified that access to the Internet is problematic for people who use AAC, and an analysis of the user requirements provides some insights into the likely needs not only for the users but also for the designers and developers of Web pages. These needs include:

8.2.1 Integrated Speech Output

The most common need identified was for good text to speech systems that would read email and WWW pages to those with complex communication needs, and for the speech output to be integrated into such applications.

8.2.2 Simplified Content

Recommendations were needed to ensure that short and simple text was used on WWW sites and that keywords were clearly identified. The issue of layout and use of graphics was seen as being important to address, particularly in relation to the size of images and the use of animation.

8.2.3 Improved Accessibility for Switch Users

Advice on making the Internet accessible to switch users was also seen as being needed. In addition to the issues of physical and sensory access, cognitive issues also need to be considered, e.g., simplifying materials and providing cues to users to assist them in navigating a site.

8.2.4 Improved Access for People who Use Symbols

A significant number of comments related to the development of WWW services for people who use symbols, as well as the need to both improve access to general web-sites for these end users and to develop a greater number of symbol-based sites.

8.3 The Simulator Studies

A simulated off-line Web browser was developed to test out design ideas, first with experts internally within the project and then with professional experts outside the project (see Figure 8.1). Preliminary impressions of the software by experts were very favourable and it was perceived to be much better than other Web browsers for the primary target population due to its flexibility. Specific concerns were addressed, and the robustness of the software was improved before the trials with people who use AAC could begin.

The simulator was then evaluated with users of AAC during 3 main phases: Preliminary evaluations with 9 people in the United Kingdom, the Netherlands and Sweden; a workshop with 8 people, held at the ISAAC 2002 Conference in Odense, Denmark; and a workshop with 4 people, held at the Communication Matters Conference in Lancaster, UK. All the workshops started with a demonstration of the software to the users and their facilitators, either individually or in small groups. A default interface was used, as well as showing other configurations of the icons and layout which would meet individual needs and preferences. Once the appropriate switches/scanning interfaces/other hardware were set up by the project's technical suppprt, the users then had 'hands-on' experience with the simulated browser for at least one-half hour, during which time the project team were there to answer questions and observe the users' behaviour and interaction with the system.

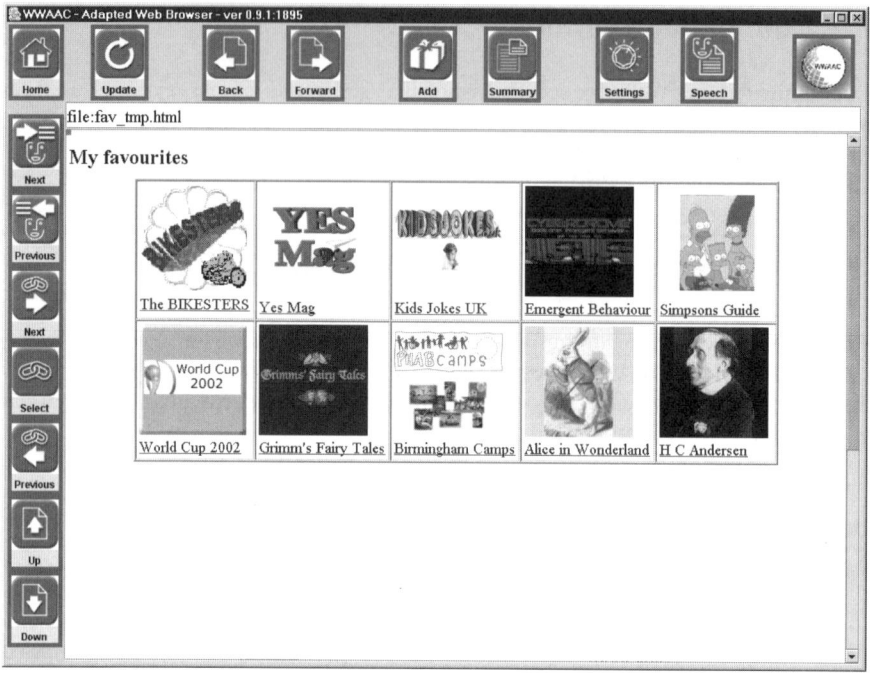

Figure 8.1. The simulated Web browser

Although the main focus of the evaluation was the simulated Web browser, it was also possible to obtain valuable information on the use of symbols to support Internet access (Nicolle *et al.*, 2002). These preliminary evaluations with users suggested that the software was a significant step towards independent use of the Internet by people who use AAC. More specific comments made by the users, their facilitators and family confirmed the importance and the benefits of particular features of the WWAAC browser, including:

- a graphical based, easy to use favourites page;
- speech output, synchronised with the visual focus on the screen;
- a summary page enhanced with symbol support;
- compatibility with the person's own switch(es) and/or AAC system; and,
- flexibility to configure the interface to meet the needs of individuals.

8.4 Development and Evaluation of the Alpha Browser

The user requirements and evaluation activities described above led to the development of the Alpha version of the prototype software, which incorporated the functionality of the simulator.

In addition, the Alpha version had the following key features:

- integrated speech output to support text presentation of site content suitable for AAC users;
- full accessibility from the keyboard;
- built in simple scanning interface to allow single or two switch/button entry;
- some configurability of displayed controls and layout;
- simple icon-based access to page favourites;
- filtering of Web page content to provide simple text summaries and lists of available links;
- go anywhere capability.

Some of these Web browsing features are available from other commercial products. In addition, other systems under research and development, such as the AVANTI Web browser (Stephanidis *et al.*, 2001) and BrookesTalk (Zajicek and Morrissey, 2001), are exploring ways of providing more adaptable and usable interaction for people with disabilities. However, it is in the area of symbol support that the WWAAC project will be providing a unique contribution. Additional aspects of the development work are to provide symbol support both for the conversion of symbol to text (for emails and on-line form filling) and for assistance in reading Web content (using symbols to support text and speech output).

The Alpha evaluation of the WWAAC browser involved 4 end users in the UK (two direct-access users, and two switch users), 2 end users in Sweden (both using direct access), and 1 direct-access user in the Netherlands, along with additional comments from teachers and facilitators.

Following introduction to the project and the demonstration of the browser's functionality to the end-user and his or her facilitator, the evaluation of the software was conducted on a one-to-one basis with 2 evaluators, one with the task of working with the user and the other observing and recording. Following the user's familiarisation with the browser, a range of tasks were performed, including for example, selecting a Web site from the favourites page, reading some text, and then selecting a link. A template was provided for the evaluator to record problems observed and specific comments for each task. Each participant was then interviewed following a short pro-forma established for the project. Talking Mats™, also used during the user requirements phase, often proved helpful in eliciting the views of end-users on abstract issues which they do not often address in their everyday conversations (Murphy, 1998; Clarke *et al.*, 2001). The workshop lasted for about 5 hours in total, over two sessions, as well as about an additional hour for detailed discussions with local facilitators and experts.

Some of the key points which emerged from the user testing and further expert interviews have been summarised under the headings that follow.

8.4.1 Speech Mode

The speech synthesiser (very different in many respects to conventional screen readers for visually impaired users) was considered by many end users and experts to be one of the key features of the browser. It was felt that end users need to be able to choose the most appropriate mode (word by word, line by line, sentence by sentence, or continuous reading). Some suggested that the speech support would help with the development of literacy skills.

8.4.2 Summary Page

Even in its present simplistic form, end users found the summary helpful to identify the main content of the site and to view and make use of the list of available links on the page. There is a need for symbol embellishment of the text summaries.

8.4.3 Favourites

End users liked the large icons on the favourites page, commenting that they would like an easy way to add a clear image to identify a new favourite site. Control over the size of the image and text on the favourites page was felt to be important.

8.4.4 Icons

In some cases understanding the icons that signified particular functions was a problem. It was suggested that while a good default set of icons was needed, the facility to import your own would be useful. Potentially, these icons could be selected from the person's own symbol set.

8.4.5 Button Layout/Appearance

It was noted that it would be useful to be able to hide some of the buttons for certain end users, to create one's own layout, and to be able to use different colours on the buttons to indicate different groups of functions. A layout editor is needed to configure the display to meet individual needs.

8.4.6 Alternative Scanning Interface

The browser must be compatible with other commercial keyboard/mouse emulators such as SAW and The Grid. If someone is using their own scanning interface, the browser's own buttons should be able to be hidden.

8.4.7 Entering URLs

End users need help to enter new web-sites.

8.4.8 Navigating Through and Selecting Links when Scanning

It is necessary to improve navigation on pages for non-mouse users where there are a large number of links. The current method of scrolling through links one-by-one was seen to be tiring and frustrating. Some form of 'fast forward'/'rewind' buttons was suggested.

8.4.9 Output/Display

An easy facility is needed for people who use AAC to change the size and colour of the text on the Web page.

8.4.10 Scrolling

Even though some end users were able to use the scroll bar, for others the browser's scroll up/down buttons proved very helpful.

8.4.11 Training

With such a diverse end user group, there was much variety in use: after a morning familiarisation, one person was able to make use of a number of the browser's features independently that afternoon.

However, another person required support throughout the day to remember what button to use when.

8.4.12 Comparison with Alternatives

End users and their facilitators were aware only of the standard Internet Explorer browser. They expressed a preference for the WWAAC browser over the standard browser.

8.5 Formulating New Web Accessibility Guidelines

The user requirements activities and the evaluation of the WWAAC project's adapted Web browser has provided valuable and unique insight into the guidance that is needed by developers to make the Internet simpler to access by people with complex communication and physical needs.

Table 8.1. Draft guidelines under discussion in the WWAAC project

Draft Guidelines	Rationale
Provide a clear representational image on the site's home page	Identification of the most representative image would enable people with complex communication needs (and others) to more readily guess what the site is about. Tagging the most representative image in the content could be used in automatic creation of a thumbnail image for the favourites page
Provide a page-graphic tag which can be used to retrieve a thumbnail image of the page itself (min. 64 × 64 pixels)	For people who use AAC and the envisaged usage of the WWAAC browser, a small graphic on the favourites page may not be enough. A graphic of the entire page, in a larger size (min. 64 x 64 pixels) may facilitate recognition of the Web site on the favourites page by end users
Provide Alt tags which give prime information for the user and distinguish between salient (most prominent) and non-salient content	End users with complex communication needs should be spared extraneous information. Some non-text content relates only to decorative images, and for some users, this just provides unnecessary clutter. The WWAAC project would recommend that graphics without content (such as a line, spacers, background) are marked as such. In addition, images that are not essential for the content of the site are also identified as, for example, background, decorative, advertising, etc.
Provide simple page descriptions as meta data (i.e., Alt-Content)	Some users will benefit from a simple summary of Web content, displayed according to their preferences in simple text and/or symbols. Alt-Content would potentially be a useful way of providing a simple summary and would also support symbol translation. This could be produced for the page, or parts of a page, by the Web author, and stored within the page itself. This would be done with 'in-page annotation,' using existing or emerging document formats, to support access to the content.

Whilst it is not realistic to expect Web developers to create symbol-based Web pages as standard, access to Web pages by symbol users can be facilitated by careful design. The WWAAC project is, therefore, contributing to the W3C Web Content Accessibility Guidelines, by suggesting guidelines for developing symbol-enabled Web pages for people with complex communication needs (Poulson and Nicolle, 2002; Poulson and Nicolle, in print) - see Table 8.1. A selection of draft guidelines under discussion in the project is given below, with rationale based on the user requirements and evaluation work. Many of these ideas will support best practice when designing Web pages for people who use AAC, as part of Guideline 3.3 in draft WCAG 2.0, which recommends that 'Content is no more complex than is necessary and/or is supplemented with simpler forms of the content' (W3C–WAI, WCAG 2.0 Working Draft).

8.6 Conclusions

The WWAAC project team is planning to assess some of these draft design guidelines with experts and end-users in the remaining months of the project, in particular the provision of Alt-Content and ways of providing summary information, for example, by means of a concept encoded Dreamweaver extension for symbol embellishment. In addition, the results of the Alpha evaluations described above have now been fed into the development of the Beta version of the software to improve its accessibility and usability.

Evaluation of the Beta browser and email software will run from October to end-December, 2003. These will be conducted in a similar fashion to the Alpha evaluation activities. However, following our experiences it is possible to make certain refinements to procedures, for example, advising evaluators to ensure that non-verbal communication from the end-user is captured, and the interview templates now provide a reminder to record this.

These Beta evaluations of the adapted browser will be followed by longitudinal case studies with 3 to 4 end users in each of three countries early in 2004 and by a series of informal end user and expert consultations. This final evaluation phase will demonstrate integration with the concept coding aspects of the project and hopes to prove a big step forward in making the Internet more accessible and usable for people who use AAC. The current adapted browser will be made freely available via various web-sites, but it is hoped that a sustainable commercial version will follow in late 2004.

8.7 Acknowledgements

The authors are grateful to the European Commission for the funding received within the Information Society Technologies (IST) Programme and also wish to thank the entire WWAAC Consortium for their comments and contributions to the study, including Handicom (The Netherlands); The ACE Centre Advisory Trust (United Kingdom); Loughborough University (United Kindgom); Dundee University (United Kingdom); DART Regional Children's Habilitation, Sahlgrenska University Hospital (Sweden); Department of Speech, Music and Hearing, Kungl Tekniska Hogskölan (Sweden); Modemo (Finland); MITC (Denmark); and Femtio Procent Data (Sweden).

8.8 References

Clarke M, Lysley A, Nicolle C, Poulson D (2002) World Wide AAC: Developing internet services for people using AAC. In: Proceedings of ISAAC 2002, Odense, Denmark

Clarke M, Nicolle C, Poulson D (2001) User requirements document. EU IST WWAAC project (Deliverable No. 2). Available at: www.wwaac.org

Murphy J (1998) Helping people with severe communication difficulties to express their views: A low-tech tool. Communication Matters 12: 9

Nicolle C, Poulson D, Clarke M (2002) Simulator study report and additional evaluation activities. EU IST WWAAC project (Deliverable No. 7)

Poulson D, Nicolle C (2002) Guidelines for developing an AAC-enabled world wide web. In: Proceedings of ISAAC 2002, Odense, Denmark

Poulson D, Nicolle C (in print) Making the internet accessible by people with cognitive and communication impairments. In: Springer International Journal Universal Access in the Information Society (UAIS): Special Issue on Guidelines, Standards, Methods and Processes for Software Accessibility

Stephanidis C, Paramythis A, Sfyrakis M, Savidis A (2001) A case study in unified user interface development: the AVANTI web browser. In: User Interfaces for All – concepts, methods and tools. Lawrence Erlbaum, Mahwah, New Jersey, pp 525-568

World Wide Web Consortium – Web Accessibility Initiative Web-site. Available at: http://www.w3c.org, WCAG 2.0, Working Draft 24 June 2003 at http://www.w3.org/TR/2003/WD-WCAG20-20030624/, and Working Draft 27 October 2003 at http://www.w3.org/WAI/GL/WCAG20/WD-WCAG20-20031027.html

WWAAC (World Wide Augmentative and Augmentative Communication) project Web site. Available at: http://www.wwaac.org

Zajicek M and Morrissey W (2001) Speech output for older visually impaired adults. In: Proceedings of IHM-HCI Conference, Lille, France

Chapter 9

Gathering Requirements for Mobile Devices Using Focus Groups with Older People

J. Goodman, A. Dickinson and A. Syme

9.1 Introduction

Dedicated mobile devices have considerable potential for supporting older people in their day-to-day lives; devices such as memory aids, security alarms and navigation aids gain much of their utility from the security they provide by being with the user all the time. The imperative for developing such devices stems not only from their potential for supporting older people in maintaining their independence and quality of life, but also from the economic realities of the ageing population and the large new market it provides.

However, there are significant obstacles to the development of genuinely useful and usable mobile devices for older people, particularly to eliciting high quality requirements. Examining the use of mobile devices in the context in which they will be used can be time-consuming and complicated, particularly with older participants, who often tire more easily. It is therefore important to consider methods that can be used within stationary settings.

Such methods include interviews, surveys and focus groups. Although all of these methods can be useful, focus groups have several advantages: they allow interaction between potential users, producing more information and more ideas (see Section 9.3.2), allow greater numbers of people to be consulted in less time than interviews take, but with more in-depth information and discussion than is possible in a survey. This chapter therefore considers the use of focus groups, although some of the techniques can also be used with other methods.

Focus groups are widely used to elicit requirements for technological devices, but the implications of using a stationary setting to encourage people to envisage and discuss mobile experiences is rarely recognised. Focus groups on mobile devices are seldom reported in the academic literature and their methods are rarely discussed (Kjeldskov and Graham, 2003).

There are some exceptions and there are lessons that can be learnt from other fields such as Psychology, but the need remains to draw together a methodology for such work. In this chapter some of the methodological issues are discussed, and a range of techniques is suggested for focus groups on mobile devices.

While these issues and techniques are relevant to most groups, we believe that they are particularly useful in requirements gathering with older people. Stationary methods are especially useful for this user group because older people often tire physically more easily. The techniques we describe are of particular value because failing memory necessitates more effort to help participants to remember and imagine situations, and less technological knowledge means that greater effort is required to communicate concepts and ideas.

This chapter draws on observations from our work as part of the UTOPIA project (Eisma *et al.*, 2003b), in which we have worked with a wide range of older people to develop more effective methodological approaches to requirements gathering with such groups. In particular, the techniques suggested in this chapter were evaluated during a focus group on mobile navigation devices. This session was a variation on a classical discussion focus group, and included a number of activities taken from other areas of usability and psychological research designed to aid the process of requirements gathering in such groups.

9.2 A Focus Group on Navigation

The techniques described in this chapter were used during a focus group on navigation and the experiences in this group are used as examples of the successful, and unsuccessful, application of these methods throughout this chapter.

The potential advantages of appropriate navigation devices for older people are considerable, helping them to maintain independence and quality of life. Older people are likely to experience more difficulty navigating sucessfully than younger people do, due to declining sensory and cognitive abilities, and a mobile navigation aid could help them to overcome these difficulties. Such an aid can provide information appropriate to the location, present only the information that is necessary at the time and alter its display parameters to suit particular users' needs.

The focus group was part of the requirements gathering process for the design of such a device, with the specific aims of understanding more about how older people navigate and how navigation information should be presented to them. It involved seven participants over the age of 60 and used a range of methods, as described below:

- discussion sessions, some prompted by photographs of navigation situations, as described in Section 9.4.1;
- photographs were taken at regular short intervals along two routes. These were shown using a data projector, stepping through the photographs as if travelling along the routes on foot. Questions were asked and discussion took place at certain points along these routes (see Section 9.4.2);
- smaller groups of two or three, each with a facilitator, in which participants gave travel directions to each other and described routes and places that they used to be familiar with in the past. More details can be found in Sections 9.4.3 and 9.4.4.

These methods were successful to varying degrees in eliciting information from participants, as described in further detail below.

9.3 Some Observations on Focus Groups

There are some issues that need to be considered when running any focus group and these apply in particular ways to focus groups on mobile devices with older people. This section discusses some of these issues and the factors involved.

9.3.1 Choice of Participants

When running a focus group or workshop, the choice of participants is extremely important as it will affect the dynamics of the group and the usefulness of the results. Unlike some other methods, focus groups are not used to generalize results to a population, meaning that randomised sampling is not necessary and other factors should be considered in the choice of participants (Morgan, 1997).

One such factor is the homogeneity within the group. Most researchers suggest that this is desirable "in order to capitalize on people's shared experiences" (Kitzinger, 1995). Morgan (1997, p35) suggests that "meeting with others whom they think of as possessing similar characteristics or levels of understanding about a given topic, will be more appealing than meeting with those who are perceived to be different." This is particularly important for focus groups about navigation and mobile devices, as they are likely to contain discussions of topics about which participants may feel embarrassed or not confident, such as descriptions of times when they got lost and discussions about unfamiliar technology.

One way to obtain such homogeneity is to use "naturally occurring groups". Kitzinger (1995) suggests that these have the added advantage that participants can "relate to each other's comments to incidents in their shared lives, and can also challenge each other on contradictions ..." Examples of such groups within the older population are social and educational clubs targeted at retired people.

In addition, navigation around an unfamiliar environment is often performed in small groups, particularly couples, as well as by individuals. We feel that the inclusion of such navigation-specific "naturally occurring groups", such as older couples, can provide important insights into the navigation experience, which would otherwise be missed. In addition, it is likely that some future mobile devices will be shared between couples, and it is therefore important to consider the opinions of both halves of the "couples" and not just those of one half.

Patton (1990) suggests that purposive or theoretical sampling is an appropriate sampling strategy for focus groups, and that it is important to set predetermined key characteristics of group members to suit the purpose of the study. Suitable characteristics for a study of mobile devices include social and financial status, as the target market for a mobile device would have to be able to afford such a device. It is also important to select participants with a reasonable level of mobility as mobile devices are of more use to those who travel and are physically active.

There are also characteristics that are useful to include as heterogeneous variables in order to gain a sufficiently wide insight into the differing experiences of the target population. For example, gender may be such a characteristic as gender differences have been shown to occur in navigation (e.g. Lawton, 1994).

For the focus group described in this chapter, we therefore chose participants who already knew each other as they came from the same social group. We included a mix of both genders, two pairs of married couples and chose participants with sufficiently high social and financial status and mobility levels to be interested in a mobile application.

The composition of a focus group or workshop is very important to its success or failure and, whilst the final composition of the group may be ruled by other factors such as difficulties in recruiting and cancellations, the importance of getting the right group composition should not be underestimated.

9.3.2 Different Sizes of Groups

One advantage of focus groups over one-to-one interviews is the wide range of responses elicited from the interactions of the group members where responses are not directed exclusively to the facilitator (Catterall and Maclaren, 1997). Whilst this method is effective, it may require adaptation for particular groups and particular topics. For example, Morgan (1997) suggests a group size of between six and ten participants, but there is some recent evidence that the optimal number for involving older adults in focus groups may be lower (Lines and Hone, 2002).

In addition, eliciting information on some particular topics may not be well suited to a traditional focus group. There are some kinds of information that are difficult to elicit from groups of six or more. For example, personal, in-depth information, especially in narrative, is better suited to individuals relating their experiences to a facilitator than to discussions involving several people. In the context of navigation, examples of this kind of information include descriptions of navigation incidents, e.g., where the participant got lost or confused, and examples of how participants give directions and navigate round environments.

Obtaining such information in a focus group setting may require participants to be more passive, with less opportunity to contribute, leading to loss of interest and consequently an elicitation of data which is of poor quality or at least not as insightful as it could be.

It is therefore useful to adapt the traditional focus group method by dividing the group into smaller groups, each with a facilitator, for parts of the session. This allows a smaller group interview approach to be used for specific exercises, such as the navigation exercises described in Section 9.4.3.

Schensul et al. (1999) suggest that the success of a focus group depends on "balancing depth and breadth of participation". We therefore suggest that different sizes of groups be used within a single session. The main group can be divided into smaller groups for certain activities and brought back together for others, which benefit from the interaction of the group as a whole. This mixture of group sizes means that a variety of activities can be used within a single session and that different kinds of information can be obtained.

9.4 Focus Group Methods for Exploring Mobile Settings

There are many possible methods that can be used within focus groups, including standard discussions, participatory design (Forlizzi and McCormack, 2000) and hands-on sessions (Eisma *et al.*, 2003b). This section describes some methods that we believe to be particularly useful in the requirements gathering stage of the design of a mobile device.

They are not all separate methods and can be used in combinations within a group. We discuss how they can be best used to bridge the gap between the stationary focus group setting and the mobile situations under discussion, particularly for older people. These methods were used in the focus group described in Section 9.2 and we give examples of their successful and unsuccessful application from that group and other areas of our research.

When considering which methods to use in practice, the choice is affected by the topic under discussion, the researchers' aims, the stage of exploration, the participants involved and practical and time constraints. For example, unstructured discussions can be used more effectively when the topic is "intensely shared" by the group members, while more structured discussions are more generally suited to cases where there is a "strong, pre-existing agenda" (Morgan, 1997). The discussions of methods in this section include descriptions of some situations where they can be used effectively.

9.4.1 Visual Probes

It is important for participants in a focus group to be able to remember and imagine situations and experiences in order to relate them to the rest of the group. This is particularly difficult when investigating mobile situations because participants have to imagine themselves in a completely different context. The challenge for those running such groups is to aid this remembrance and to make the situations and issues salient to the group members.

This can be dealt with to some degree in discussion, with verbal and textual prompting. However, additional cognitive prompts or probes, such as images, can encourage participants to remember experiences and situations relevant to the topic under investigation (Seale *et al.*, 2002). Visual probes are particularly important when investigating mobile settings, because experiences are often closely tied to the location in which they occurred.

One form that such probes can take is that of photographs and other images of locations and mobile situations, as shown in the example in Figure 9.1. These can be displayed on cards, perhaps with captions, in handouts and using PowerPoint presentations, as well as through other means.

In our focus group, we used photographs of locations where people might get lost, such as hospitals and shopping centres, in order to prompt participants' memories of incidences when they did get lost. These were attached to cards with captions.

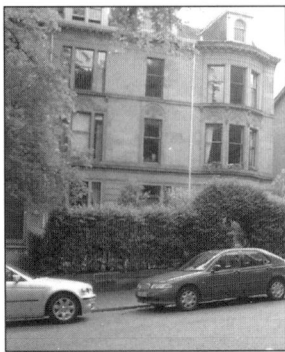

Figure 9.1. An example of a visual probe

Such card probes have proven successful in the past, both in other people's research (e.g. Seale *et al.*, 2002) and, to a limited extent, in our own. However, in this study, they proved ineffective in encouraging discussion. There are several possible reasons for this, including a poor match between the choices of situations and photographs and the situations in which the participants had actually had difficulty. Another possible reason is the lack of a structured exercise or task involving the cards. For example, Seale *et al.* (2002) used a structured sorting task, which may have been an important factor in their success. Both of these are important factors to take into consideration if using card probes in a focus group.

It is also helpful to consider other presentation methods, such as a PowerPoint or other similar presentation. Elsewhere in our project, we found that such a presentation was more successful than displaying the same images on cards. This could be related to the more focused aspect of formal presentations, which helps all of the group to focus on the probes together, and in which the facilitator takes the lead in the activity, leaving the participants able to focus more fully on the topic.

9.4.2 Scenarios

Another technique for eliciting requirements for mobile devices from stationary settings is the use of scenarios. Carroll describes scenarios as "informal narrative descriptions... stories about human activity" and notes that they are used "to conduct analysis and design in a vocabulary that permits end-user participation" (Carroll, 2000a, p 41). Scenarios are often specifically defined situations including a particular setting, a central character or "agent" and a plot, consisting of a sequence of actions and events (Carroll, 2000b, pp 44-45).

Scenarios are extremely flexible tools and can be used in a variety of ways within usability engineering. In particular, they can be used within requirements gathering, where they permit people to discuss situations without reference to specific technologies. This is particularly valuable when working with older people as their frequent lack of knowledge about technical language and different technologies can be often prove a barrier in requirements gathering (Eisma *et al.*, 2003a). Scenarios are also particularly valuable when investigating mobile settings because, like visual probes in Section 9.4.1, they help the participants to imagine a setting that is very different from the stationary focus group.

Using real locations in the scenarios helps to tie them more closely to reality and thus generate descriptions of how the participants would actually behave. This likelihood is further increased if known locations can be used, and also enables the participants to better imagine the context surrounding the depicted locations and scenarios - context which is particularly important in the use of mobile devices. Known locations may also help to elicit descriptions of actual past behaviour rather than how participants believe that they might behave.

Scenarios can be described in different ways, including text, speech, photographs and video clips. For the investigation of mobile settings, visual means are particularly important as discussed in Section 9.4.1. A visual description of a location is much more powerful and evocative than a written or verbal one.

These visual descriptions can be presented using a video or data projector to step through photographs taken at short intervals along a route, as shown in the example in Figure 9.2. This method has been used in psychology to investigate navigation, e.g., (Lipman, 1991), but can also be used in requirements gathering for technological systems. Although a video may provide a more stream-lined overall picture of the route, stepping through photographs has some important advantages. It is easier to move around in the presentation and the presentation can also be paused more easily with a higher quality of image remaining on the screen, facilitating discussion of that point in the route or that part of the location. Such discussions can help to elicit information on particular features in an environment, how participants know which way to turn, or other location-specific issues.

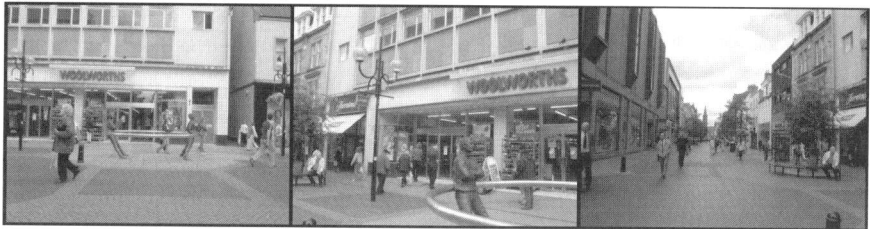

Figure 9.2. Three consecutive images used to depict a route in a scenario

A variety of scenarios are appropriate for requirements gathering for mobile devices. In our investigation of navigation, we found one scenario in particular to be valuable, although others are also likely to be useful. In this scenario, the central character (the agent) navigates along a route. We varied this theme to create two sub-scenarios, using first a familiar and then an unfamiliar route.

In the first sub-scenario, the actor found his (or her) way along a familiar route in a familiar location. We paused at various decision points on the route (when the actor must decide which way to go) and asked participants how they would know the way to go. A route familiar to most of the participants was used to help them to imagine the scenario most accurately and to relate their own experiences.

The second scenario involved the actor navigating along an unfamiliar route. At the decision points this time, we gave participants examples of methods that could be used to indicate the way (see Figure 9.3). These examples tied into the specific scenario under discussion. This strategy was successful, allowing participants to comment on what sort of directions they would find useful in a specific situation.

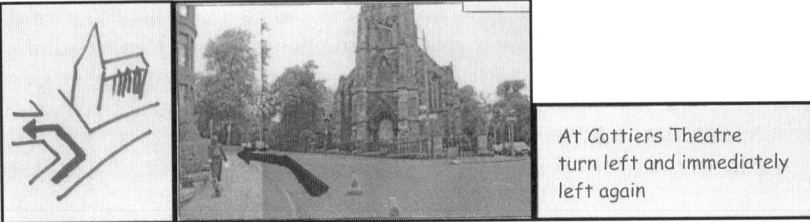

Figure 9.3. Examples of methods of giving directions used in the focus group

9.4.3 Exercises

Another useful focus group method is setting the participants exercises or tasks to do. This is not a completely separate method from those previously discussed and can be used effectively in combination with both card probes and scenarios. Its use within scenarios is discussed further in Section 9.4.4.

There are a wide range of such exercises that can be suitable, including some of those used within cultural probes (Gaver *et al.*, 1999) and in interviews. However, in focus groups, some exercises, such as taking photographs of meaningful objects, are no longer applicable, others, such as indicating places on a map, can be used without modification, and some can be used with some alteration. Other exercises can also be used, taking advantage of the interaction opportunities provided by the presence of several people as well as the ability to use speech and movement as well as visual techniques such as writing and drawing.

For example, Bradley and Dunlop carried out an exercise with participants in an interview setting where they asked them to give directions to certain set locations, both verbally and in writing (Bradley and Dunlop, 2002). In our focus group, we adapted this exercise to take advantage of the group setting. Participants were divided into groups of two or three, in which they firstly gave each other directions and later described locations to each other.

The group setting allowed questions and prompts from the other participants. In the first exercise, it was hoped that this would mimic better the actual setting of giving directions in which the enquirer can ask for clarification. However, this did not always work in practice, perhaps due to lack of adequate explanation in advance and the fact that other group members were often also familiar with the route being described. In the second exercise, the group discussion generated more information about the locations as participants asked each other questions.

These exercises introduced more variety into the focus group, helping to engage interest, and allowed varying group sizes with their corresponding advantages as indicated in Section 9.3.2. They also helped to elicit more personal and more detailed information by encouraging participants to consider situations in more detail and from different angles.

9.4.4 Using Scenarios in Exercises

It can be very profitable to use scenarios to help set the scene for exercises and tasks in a focus group. For example, as described in Section 9.4.2, participants were given the scenario of finding their way along a specific unfamiliar route. They were then given the task of choosing their preferred method of being given directions at decision points along that route out of a selection shown to them.

However, scenarios can also be used in a different way in an exercise, by using the outline of a scenario rather than a full description. For example, participants can be asked to describe or imagine a particular scenario that fits a more general description, or to fill in the details in an outline of a scenario.

In the navigation focus group, we used this method to generate scenarios with more personal relevance for each participant. For example, participants were asked to imagine themselves in a familiar place and to give directions to the rest of the group about how to get to a place nearby. By letting the participants themselves choose and then give the details of the scenario, places that they were familiar with could be used, making it more likely that they would visualise an actual route rather than talking about the ways in which they *believed* they navigated and gave directions. In addition, an easily-remembered and familiar location avoided many of the potential disadvantages of discussing mobility and navigation in a stationary setting; participants needed little prompting because there was less mental effort involved in visualising and describing a place that the individual was familiar with.

9.5 Conclusions

Focus groups can be a valuable method for obtaining requirements for mobile devices from older people, despite difficulties caused by the gap between the static focus group setting and the mobile context under investigation. There are a variety of techniques that can be used to bridge this gap and so improve their use and the quality of information obtained from them.

This chapter has described and discussed some of these techniques, as well as some other important aspects of such focus groups. We believe that these methods constitute an effective range of techniques for the successful investigation of mobile situations in focus groups, and that our experience of using them in the focus group described in this chapter provides an initial framework for identifying which techniques can be used immediately and which need to be adjusted for use with this particular user group in this situation.

However, further work on techniques is needed. We plan to continue to evaluate and develop the techniques described in this chapter as well as other methods as part of our on-going work on navigation aids for older people.

9.6 Acknowledgements

This work was funded by SHEFC through the UTOPIA project (grant number: HR01002). We would also like to thank all the participants in the focus group and the Perth branch of the University of the Third Age (U3A).

9.7 References

Bradley NA, Dunlop MD (2002) Understanding contextual interactions to design navigational context-aware applications. In: Proceedings of Mobile HCI 2002, Springer-Verlag, London, UK

Carroll JM (2000a) Introduction to the special issue on "Scenario-Based Systems Development". Interacting with Computers 13(1): 41-42

Carroll JM (2000b) Five reasons for scenario-based design. Interacting with Computers 13(1): 43-60

Catterall M, Maclaran P (1997) Focus group data and qualitative analysis programmes: Coding the moving picture as well as the snapshots. Sociological Research Online 2(1)

Eisma R, Dickinson A, Goodman J, Mival O, Syme A, Tiwari L (2003a) Mutual inspiration in the development of new technology for older people. In: Proceedings of Include 2003, Helen Hamlyn Research Centre, Royal College of Art, London, UK

Eisma R, Dickinson A, Goodman J, Syme A, Tiwari L, Newell AF (2003b) Early user involvement in the development of Information Technology-related products for older people. To be published in Universal Access in the Information Society, Dec 2003

Forlizzi J, McCormack M (2000) Case study: User research to inform the design and development of integrated wearable computers and web-based services. In: Proceedings of DIS 2000, ACM Press

Gaver B, Dunne T, Pacenti E (1999) Cultural probes. Interactions 6(1): 21-29

Kitzinger J (1995) Qualitative research: Introducing focus groups. British Medical Journal 311: 299-302

Kjeldskov J, Graham C (2003) A Review of Mobile HCI Research Methods. In: Proceedings of Mobile HCI 2003, Springer-Verlag, London, UK

Lawton CA (1994) Gender differences in way-finding strategies: Relationship to spatial ability and spatial anxiety. Sex Roles 30: 765-779

Lines L, Hone KS (2002) Research methods for older adults. In: A New Research Agenda for Older Adults, Workshop at HCI 2002, London, UK

Lipman PD (1991) Age and exposure differences in acquisition of route information. Psychology and Aging 6(1): 128-133

Morgan DL (1997) Focus groups as qualitative research, 2nd edition. Sage Publications, London, UK

Patton MQ (1990) Qualitative evaluation and research methods, 2nd edition. Sage Publications, Paerk, CA

Schensul JJ, LeCompte MD, Nastasi BK, Borgatti SP (1999) Enhanced Ethnographic Methods. Audiovisual Techniques, Focused Group Interviews and Elicitation Techniques. Altamara Press, London, UK

Seale J, McCreadie C, Turner-Smith A, Tinker A (2002) Older people as partners in Assistive Technology research: The use of focus groups in the design process. Technology and Disability 14(1): 21-29

Chapter 10

Devices and Desires: Identifying the Acceptability of AT to Older People

C. McCreadie

10.1 Introduction

There is now a vigorous body of opinion that has recognised both the major demographic transitions that have taken, and continue to take, place in most countries in the world, and the ways in which the design of both products and the built environment can either aggravate or ameliorate the impact of some of the disabling conditions that come with ageing (Clarkson *et al.*, 2003). Furthermore, there is recognition of the fundamental importance of research with older users, and of understanding the interaction between individual and environment or "technology" in its broadest sense. This chapter reports on a component of a multi-disciplinary research project that was concerned with the introduction and use of a wide range of AT* in existing (older) housing occupied by older people. The main aims of the research were, in conjunction with ten housing partners, to investigate the feasibility and cost of introducing AT in relation, on the one hand, to user needs and, on the other, to the age, type and standard of property. However, the extent to which AT can narrow the gap between the home environment and individual capacity, depends upon the willingness of older people to use AT. If AT is to be introduced on any significant scale to support care in the community of older people, it must be easy and effective to use, and be positively welcomed by older people themselves. A key element in the research was therefore to explore with older people their use and experience of a range of AT.

10.2 Methodology

The ten housing partners were drawn from both local authorities and registered social landlords and included both specialist and generalist housing associations. They were widely spread geographically. Seventy-two tenants were interviewed in nine out of the ten areas between May and November 2001. In three areas, the provider selected or partially selected the respondents, largely with a view to gaining user views on some of the latest electronic technology. In the remaining six, a screening questionnaire was used to recruit respondents. It was sent, either directly by the provider, or by the researcher in close association with the provider, to forty tenants all of whom had had some AT installed in the previous two years. The overall response rate was 54%. Respondents, who indicated that they were prepared to help further with the research, were selected to give a good range of both AT ownership and of age, gender and living arrangements.

The interview schedule comprised both closed and open questions. The closed questions focused very largely on what Assistive Technology the respondent had. Open-ended questions were used to investigate the user's experience of AT. The AT was divided into five sections: entry and movement; baths and W.C.; communication, safety and alarms; electrical; and other. Questions on functional capacity drew on the EasyCare assessment system. (Sheffield, 1997).

Questions used from the assessment schedule covered both activities of daily living (using stairs, bathing and getting dressed) and instrumental activities of daily living (housework, meal preparation, going shopping) as well as using the telephone –i.e. functional criteria bearing on people's physical capacity to manage everyday life in ordinary housing. Shopping and meal preparation have been identified as particularly important for older people in maintaining a sense of independence (Godfrey and Callaghan, 2000).

Two questions about sight and hearing were also taken from the EasyCare schedule. Use of this system enabled us, using the respondents' self-reports, to give an approximate score of disability to respondents. In total, 67 respondents over the age of 70 were interviewed.

10.3 Findings

10.3.1 Respondents

Respondents were largely in their seventies or eighties (range 70 to 97), and were predominantly female. Nearly 60% lived in flats/maisonettes and just over half were in sheltered housing. Most lived alone but were in touch with their family, who generally offered considerable support. Three-quarters were estimated to suffer from moderate or severe disability. By far the most common disabling condition was arthritis. Only a few were receiving formal care.

10.3.2 AT Provision

The provision of AT, although not the subject of the research, appeared to be variable and dependent on local systems and individual occupational therapists. The general impression gained was that AT was prescribed to meet a specific need, rather than addressing a wider range of options to promote independence. The AT provided is shown in Table 10.1.

Table 10.1. Assistive Technology in interview respondents' homes. n=67

Item of Assistive Technology	n	%
Telephone	64	95
Remote control for TV	64	95
Smoke detector	57	85
Grab rails in	54	81
Community alarm	48	72
Grab rails/ramps out	40	60
Walking stick	36	54
Electric plugs/sockets changed	30	45
Door entry phones	29	43
with video	8	12
W.C. raised seat/frame	27	42
Level access shower	21	31
Over bath shower	21	31
Wheelchair	19	28
Walking frame	16	24
Low access shower	14	21
Stair lift	8	12
Mobile hoist	2	
Overhead track hoist	1	
Additional lighting	4	
Environmental alarms	6	
Remote controls (except TV)	0	

The most commonly found AT, included as AT because of its immense importance for communication, social life and social participation, was the telephone, and running very close to it, remote control for TV. Smoke detectors and indoor grab rails were found in more than 80% of cases, community alarms in more than 70%. Half our respondents used walking sticks and a quarter each used walking frames or wheelchairs. 80% of respondents had a shower of some kind; getting on for a half had door entry phones, largely reflecting living in blocks of flats. About 1 in 8 had stair-lifts, although this rose to 50% in houses. Some AT was rarely found in the respondents' houses – hoists, and despite a deliberate attempt to include them, environmental alarms, using sensors. Despite the considerable number of people with visual impairment, additional lighting was rarely found, and there was no example of colour contrast decoration. Remote controls, while used nearly universally for TV, were used for any other activity such as door opening (except door entry phones) window opening or curtains.

10.3.3 Explaining the Acceptability of AT to Older People

Respondents were overwhelmingly concerned to manage as much of every day life for themselves as possible, but there were examples in the research of individuals who were managing effectively in difficult circumstances but did not see themselves as needing help. After extensive analysis of the qualitative interview data, we developed a model of the factors that go toward making AT acceptable to older people.

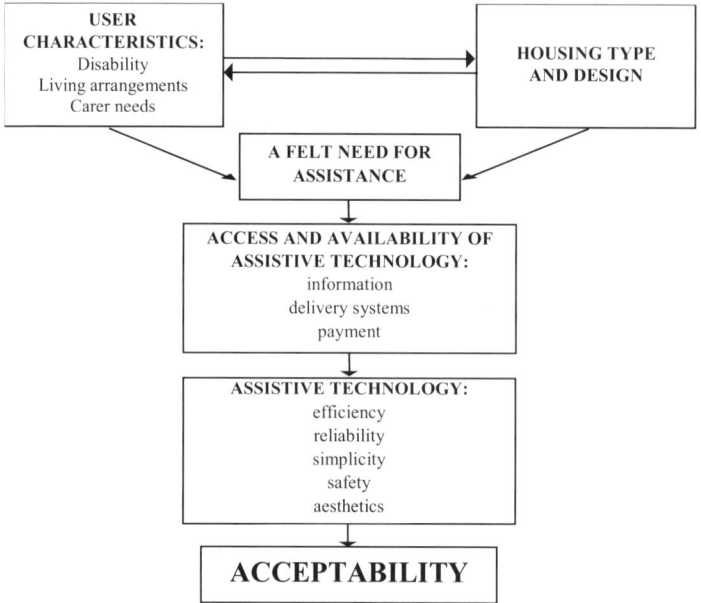

Figure 10.1 A model for acceptability of Assistive Technology

The model suggests that the acceptability of AT to older people depends on three main factors: firstly. their "felt need for assistance", which depends in turn on a various user characteristics and the way these interact with the older person's housing, secondly. a range of factors associated with the AT itself and thirdly on the systems for making AT accessible and available. The key "user factors" are the older person's disability and health, their living arrangements and family support, the needs of carers in their own right and personal motivations and preferences.

These interact with the type of housing in which the person is living, its design, location and internal layout. This however is only one side of the equation. The other side relates to the AT itself. The factors that were found to be important were: "operational efficiency", reliability, simplicity, safety and aesthetics. The next part of the chapter details some of our findings in respect of these factors.

10.3.4 "Operational Efficiency" of AT

Since people were dependent to a greater or lesser degree on the AT, it was fundamental that it worked properly. Various examples were given of AT that did not work properly, due to either design or installation failings. Mrs Joyce was 86, very mobile and suffering from a severe hearing and visual impairment, but this did not seem to have been allowed for in her community alarm:

"There is a problem with the alarm. When they speak to Mrs Joyce it's not loud enough, and she can't hear them. They had a panic the other day 'cos they couldn't communicate with her, and thought obviously something was wrong. It was just that she couldn't hear it."

(Mrs Joyce's carer)

In another case, a vertical lift had been installed, but although it went up and down satisfactorily, it did not sit flush with the floor. The carer, whose wife was severely incapacitated by a stroke and dependent on a wheelchair, had considerable difficulty getting the wheelchair on and off the lift:

" (The lift) is a good thing, I'll give that you, but you want it in working condition don't you? … Social services should come and check it to make sure that it is a perfect finish. Especially for one of them to go on (the lift) ".

(spouse carer of Mrs Black, 81)

In another example, Mr Castle, in his mid 80s, had requested a handrail to help him get around his flat. One had been installed without battens on a plasterboard partition wall and had come away in his hand, causing him to fall. He was so irritated by this workmanship that he had simply put the rail away and a neighbour had filled in the holes in the wall and repainted it.

10.3.5 Reliability of AT

Reliability, that is, a consistent standard of performance was a particular problem with stair lifts, smoke alarms and with the newer type of electronic alarms. Most people with stair-lifts had experienced a problem, despite regular maintenance. Generally, service engineers attended promptly and rectified the problem, but there were examples where the lift was out of action for some time, or broke down again. Because people were dependent on the stair-lift, they had considerable difficulties when the stair lift broke down. Mrs Morrison, at the time of the interview had been waiting six weeks for her stair-lift to be working again, although various engineers had tried to repair it. Meanwhile, she was having great difficulty getting up and down, sometimes having to go on her hands and knees and had hurt her shoulder trying to get up and down stairs without it:

"It's been terrible. A nightmare ... I didn't walk up those stairs from the day it was put in until the day it broke down ... you know, you sort of forget something and go up for it. ... [There's]) been a lot of to-ing and fro-ing, people coming and looking at it, scratching their heads and going, 'Oh,' again, getting it going and it's kept conking out. Anyway the last time it went finally at the top of the stairs. ... So anyway, a man came last week, he was here for five and a half hours ... and then all the fuses blew. ... And when he looked at the wiring, he found it was only telephone wire, instead of proper."

It also made them understandably nervous about a recurrence:

"It's been a help up to now. But it broke down recently ... we've had huge pantomimes with it. We've had a broken spring about a year or so ago, in the March, I had to spend the night on the settee because I couldn't get upstairs."

(Mrs King, 78)

Reliability was important in relation to various kinds of environmental alarm, but the problem took the form of "over-sensitivity" – that is, the alarm would go off when people did not want it to. Smoke alarms attracted many comments similar to the following:

"If I'm doing toast, it goes off."

(Mrs Rivers, 72)

Respondents were not happy about setting off their alarm accidentally even though the call centre personnel in various localities were always very reassuring if this happened:

"Once or twice I've had a bit of an accident with [the pendant], you know. You know if I've been leaning over some things you know, and I've accidentally caught it [laughing], I've had to apologise. [laughing so much she cannot talk here] Well to be honest with you I told a little white lie. Oh I said God will forgive me for a little white [laughing]. I said it was my little grand-daughter, she pulled the cord, she thought it was the light I was so ashamed to have to tell them that everything was all right."

(Mrs Wheeler, 82)

The result was that people could be reluctant to wear the alarm:

"It's a wrist thing, I haven't got it on. The kids are always telling me off 'cos I haven't got it on ... I know it's silly, I shouldn't ... actually the reason I don't, because it's so cumbersome on my wrist, I'm liable to knock it and set the alarm off. And there is a pendant thing, and I didn't fancy that. But I may say to them I might get that, if it's not too cumbersome. "

(Mrs Nicholls, 80)

"[I wear it] if I don't feel well. Otherwise you just walk round and you just touch something, like your glasses, and it's off, you know."

(Miss Penney, 82, living alone)

Mr Murphy, aged 91 and living on his own, had not worn his fall detector which was integrated to a belt, because he had set it off too easily:

"I never put it on until this morning, because it was that sensitive when I was touching it, I was always alerting these people and I didn't think it was right. ... I don't mind wearing it, but as I say, I take it off so often, because 5 times it alerted, and yet it wasn't an emergency at all."

10.3.6 Simplicity of AT

The simplicity of technology was appreciated. Mr Murphy (91) for example very much liked his Tunstall telephone with the pre-coded numbers:

"So I can just touch these buttons, if I press this button, the neighbour will come in, and if I press that, my daughter will come, but I've never done that because she's working, press this and my son would come. ... They've done everything they can for me, they've been very, very helpful."

Part of the research was with a small group of respondents from a housing association, which had installed a new door entry system and internal communications system in a sheltered housing block. Respondents were generally very positive about this system, which involved the use of a key fob to enter themselves and use of their TV screens to show them who was standing at the front door. The technology was simple to operate and served a felt need for safety.

10.3.7 Safety of AT

Safety was very important to people. Although level access showers were very popular, a number of respondents commented on feeling nervous about the shower chairs whether these were fixed to the wall, or free-standing.

"And I had a stool, but I can't use the stool because I slip off. ... Well it's got two little arms, but you know when I'm sort of washing myself I'm slipping off."

(Mrs Todd, 70+)

10.3.8 Aesthetics of AT

Although the aesthetic aspects of AT were not often raised by respondents, there were comments that related to the need to design in harmony with people's surroundings. Grab rails were one of the most common items of AT, but were invariably white plastic, and it was notable that people commented on the quality of good rails:

"I got a wood one there, it was there when I came here. That's all right. I ain't worried by that. It's a nice one, polished one he is. We've never painted it, we always kept it polished. They look nicer like that."

(Mrs Perry, 79)

A good number of respondents with steps at their front and back doors needed rails to help them up and down. Here, addressing fears of safety and security, by unobtrusive design may be important, since older people sometimes fear attracting the attention of unscrupulous callers by any advertisement of disability. Another item is the chair raising device that can be placed under an ordinary armchair to raise it. Both well designed attractive and singularly non 'inclusive versions of this were observed. Raised toilet seats and frames were among the least attractive products and, while found invaluable by some people, were also rejected by others if they were at all able to dispense with them. The following comments were typical:

> *"I sent that back, because they're so awful those things. They do help when you can't lower yourself down, to start with. But I don't need that now."*

(Mr Castle, mid 80s)

> *"It's on a frame. I don't like it, so I don't use it."*

(Mrs Hollick, 74)

Many people did not wear their pendant alarm because they did not really feel they needed to, and it is questionable whether design can address these respondents' needs. However their reluctance to do so raised the question of design:

> *"I've got a press button. I can't get used to wearing [it]. At the moment I just don't feel as if I want to wear one of them."*

(Mrs Steller, 71)

10.4 Discussion

Four areas have been chosen as particularly relevant to the theme of "Designing a more inclusive world": reducing the "medicalisation" of AT; problems relating to "smart" solutions, enabling people to access "solutions"; and the relationship between ageing and disability.

10.4.1 Reducing the "Medicalisation" of Assistive Technology.

Alan Newell (2003) has pointed out that "assistive technology often has an institutional air about it." This was noticeable in the research in respect of a number of products, notably, grab rails, wheel chairs, chair raisers, W.C. seats and frames and pendant alarms. The ubiquity of white and beige plastic conveys, as Newell says, the feeling that the product has been designed for a hospital ward, rather than for a person's home. The evident pride of the vast majority of respondents in their home, and the attention that was paid to making them comfortable and aesthetically pleasing was quite striking. It seems likely that people would welcome products that were less visibly "medical" in design.

10.4.2 Problems of "Smart" Solutions if Reliability Problems are not Fully Solved

Reliability of AT was of the greatest importance to respondents. Much is heard these days about "smart" technology, although "smart homes" are still at an experimental stage and none were seen in the research. Those few respondents who had more than the basic social alarm were enthusiastic to the extent that the technology worked reliably. All alarm systems depend on human back-up, and it was clear that, in most cases, respondents preferred not to use an alarm rather than generate false alarms. Whether alarms are portable or fixed, they present designers with a significant challenge: to design an alarm that is acceptable to people in terms of wear and ease of use but does not go off by mistake.

10.4.3 Enabling People to Access "Solutions"

During the course of the interviews, a number of issues arose that related to accessing AT. In general, respondents did not appear well informed about the kinds of technical help that might benefit them. Many appeared short of items that might have helped them. This supports findings of national surveys (Grundy *et al.*, 1999) and suggests that the resources available to help people are limited. In a surprisingly large number of cases, respondents, or their family, had bought AT privately. Examples included expensive items like electric wheel chairs, adjustable beds, and riser chairs. Age Concern England (2002) has recently drawn attention to the dangers of commercial marketing of these kinds of product. One conclusion that might be drawn from our research is that there is considerable scope for improved ways of enabling people to find out about how they might address their particular "felt needs". People need more and better information and this is partly a question of design, so that catalogues, and displays of AT in retail outlets, or specialist disability centres, are visibly addressing people's social, as opposed to medical, needs.

10.4.4 Age or Disability?

As all the respondents were recipients of a housing adaptation, they were all disabled to a greater or lesser degree. It was evident that there is a tension in addressing older people's needs in terms of disability, when their perception is that they are "older" rather than "disabled". This is a sensitive and difficult issue because it might be seen as implying a pejorative view of disability. Yet it is disabled people who have identified clearly the importance of the environment in creating disability, and whose campaigning efforts are benefiting older people. "Mainstreaming" AT and promoting inclusive design may go some way towards addressing this tension.

10.5 Conclusions

The powerful desire of older people to continue to "manage" and "do things for themselves" so as to maintain independence confirms the likely benefits of technical solutions to some daily living problems. Respondents in this research did not display aversion to the AT that they had in their homes. They welcomed technical solutions that addressed their needs, as they experienced them and felt them, in an efficient way. There was little evidence that chronological age was relevant to people's responses. These were more complex and nuanced, depending on an interaction between user characteristics, housing and subjective understanding on the one hand, and on access to efficient, reliable and straightforward AT on the other.

10.6 Acknowledgements

The research reported in this chapter was part of a larger study funded by the Engineering and Physical Sciences Research Council (Project GRN 33218). The author is grateful to colleagues in the research team, including: Professor Anthea Tinker and Rachel Stuchbury, Institute of Gerontology, King's College London; Professor Keith Bright, Professor Peter Lansley, Sue Flanagan and Kate Goodacre, Research Group for Inclusive Environments, University of Reading; Dr Alan Turner-Smith, Dr Donna Cowan and Alex Bialokoz, Centre of Rehabilitation Engineering, King's College London.

10.7 References

Age Concern (2002) Sharp selling practices in the sale of assistive products to older people. Age Concern, London, UK

Clarkson J, Coleman R, Keates S, Lebbon C (eds.) (2003) Inclusive design: design for the whole population. Springer-Verlag, London, UK

Godfrey M, Callaghan G, (2000) Exploring unmet need. Joseph Rowntree Foundation, York, UK

Grundy E, Ahlburg D, Ali M, Breeze E, Sloggett A (1999) Disability in Great Britain: Results from the 1996/7 disability follow-up to the family resources survey. Corporate Document Services, London, UK

Newell A (2003) Inclusive design or assistive technology. In: Inclusive Design: design for the whole population. Springer-Verlag, London, UK

Sheffield Institute for Studies on Ageing (1997-9) EASYcare Elderly Assessment System. UK version (1999-2002), Sheffield Institute for Studies on Ageing, Sheffield, UK

Chapter 11

Beyond Functionality – Product Semantics in Assistive Device Design

J.L. Allen

11.1 Introduction

This chapter discusses work carried out on a Ph.D. study addressing the design and development of a wearable communication aid for people who are illiterate and cannot speak. People with such disabilities often depend on electronic Augmentative and Alternative Communication (AAC) devices for interpersonal communication. However such products, and products intended for people with disabilities more generally, have characteristics that inadequately attend to users' needs – in particular many devices pay insufficient regard to the psychological and sociological impact the devices have upon their users. The chapter briefly discusses an empirical case study to design and develop the Portland Communication Aid (PCA). The process of establishing user requirements, and in particular the notion of designer-facilitated participatory design, is discussed. The resulting prototype of the PCA is briefly explained along with a discussion of the importance of product semantics in the design of assistive technology.

Products catering for people with disabilities have a crucial role in determining the quality of life for their users. These products must perform both functional and communicative goals if they are to satisfy users' needs, wants, aspirations, abilities and capabilities (Jonas, 1993). That is to say, the design of disability products must address not only technical functions but, as Buchanan describes, the "more thorough and diverse interpretation of the physical, psychological, social, and cultural relationships between products and human beings" (Buchanan, 1992).

Regarding disability products in general, Paul Hogan, then Chairman of the European Institute of Design and Disability (EIDD), states:

Most of the products on display are engineered and not designed. No thought appears to have been given to the psychological impact of the design on those who have to use them. The majority of products ... are ugly, shiny and say in the most emphatic way to the purchaser, "You are a cripple".

(Hogan, 1994)

This is a damning statement and highlights a profound problem. Technology is capable of granting people with disabilities greatly increased independence and quality of life, affording opportunities to perform tasks that would otherwise be impossible. A product's success is, however, often marred by a lack of consideration of how its technology is packaged. In many cases, the very devices intended to assist people with disabilities in fact do damage: they compound people's disabilities by drawing attention to impairments.

So how can this be addressed? The author sought to answer this question in part, through the design and development of the Portland Communication Aid (PCA), a prototype product designed to empower its user by more sensitive and perceptive design. The design work, commenced in 1995, was carried out as part of a Ph.D. study (Allen, 2002) in the Department of Design and Technology, Loughborough University, in conjunction with Portland College, an independent college for people with disabilities in Mansfield, Nottinghamshire. Portland College had identified the need for an improved communication aid for non-vocal, illiterate and ambulant young adults. Although considered to be state-of-the-art, the electronic communication aids used by their students presented a number of shortcomings. The process of establishing user requirements and the resultant design work are discussed here.

11.2 Establishing User Requirements

There is a limited, but growing body of literature on designing for people with disabilities, but at the time of the study there was little - particularly on its application in practical situations. Whilst some authors present guides to the selection of particular methods (e.g. Stanton and Baber, 1996; Poulson *et al.*, 1996), and some note the problems and issues specific to selecting methods of assessment for people with disabilities (Galer, 1983; Nicolle *et al.*, 1995), little is discussed with regard to communication disabilities. The designer is therefore faced with a problem: how to uncover and thoroughly understand the perspectives of people with disabilities, along with their needs, wants and aspirations for disability devices.

For the study it was imperative to involve AAC users in the process of designing. There were particular difficulties of doing this however. Traditional techniques for assessing user needs and wants typically rely on the user providing some form of feedback. AAC users cannot talk but instead typically rely on a communication aid to convey their thoughts. The very fact that an AAC aid is used in the communication process in assessing user needs can also detract from the quality and efficacy of the results. Further, many AAC users lack co-ordinated motor control, and so the representation and exploration of their ideas through non-verbal media such as sketches and models (techniques typically used by industrial designers), was limited.

A number of techniques were used in the designing to establish user requirements, including, literature reviews, observation, participant interviews (formal, informal, video recorded), expert interviews, questionnaires, 'days-in-the-life-of' participants, photographic studies, sketching, modelling and prototyping. This chapter focuses upon interviews and the role of design work (sketching, modelling and prototyping) in those interviews to establish user requirements.

Informal but semi-structured, one-to-one interviews were carried out with AAC users at Portland College. The interviews were conducted under the guise of chats so as not to intimidate the interviewees, and to allow the interview to be participant-led. An interview protocol was followed when conducting the interviews. Open-ended questions were first offered in order to encourage the AAC users to respond as freely as possible. As the AAC users' communicative abilities varied, the same basis of the questions was usually posed in a closed format to prompt and encourage responses. Often the ordering of questions would change to ensure the interview sounded more conversational than set. Where possible the questions were adapted to focus upon issues raised by the interviewees. A set of questions was posed to determine:

- users' needs of a communication device;
- users' wants and desires for a communication device;
- users' perceptions of their machines, the relationship between themselves and their machines, and their perceptions of how others saw them and their machines based on their own experiences.

Over fifty interviews and discussions were conducted at the College over the period of the study, providing the opportunity to review findings in relation to the participants' circumstances and experiences at the time. Seasonal changes revealed different physical requirements of both the user and the AAC device (for example, in summer fingers may slip on keyboards due to sweating, whilst in winter hands operating a keyboard get cold and numb). Such findings may not have been apparent if only one 'snap shot' interview had been conducted. Interviewing the same participants periodically provided a more comprehensive account of their needs at different times.

A strong rapport developed between the author and the participants, permitting more open communication. This allowed, when necessary, sensitive and difficult questions to be asked with comfort, compassion and consideration, as mutual trust and respect had already been established. Thus, issues raised by the participants could be penetrated at depth (something more difficult and time consuming to establish with a greater number of participants). The interviews also provided the participants the opportunity to spend time talking with someone who was keenly interested in their ideas and concerns, and hence they felt valued. The interviews also provided the participants with a form of symposium by which issues central to their everyday lives could be expressed and explained.

Building a rapport with these students throughout the duration of the study provided the opportunity to experience in an intimate way their frustration, hopes and everyday interactions. Being accepted into their social activities gave the author an opportunity to see, at close hand, different sides to these students when compared to their behaviour in a classroom setting. In addition, over the year key events took place in their lives: birthdays, parties, achievements, relationships, illnesses and injuries, and so on. These events provided a more complete picture of what the users required.

11.2.1 Designer-Facilitated Participatory Design

The design activities of ideation, sketching and modelling had a significant role in establishing user requirements. In this instance, the author engaged in designer-facilitated participatory design whereby the author stimulated, interpreted and synthesised participants' ideas in the form of sketches and models in order to more accurately articulate their needs.

Sketches of concepts were shown in the interviews to solicit interviewees' thoughts and preferences. The author's ideas were deliberately left until last to ensure that the interviewees' perspectives and ideas were not shaped or manipulated by poor interview technique. In addition, it was important to reassure the interviewees that they were involved in the design of the device, and that their comments were valued. Sketching the students and placing design ideas upon the same drawing helped to put the concepts in context. (Figure 11.1 shows an example of one such sketch.) The sketches were then used, in part, to help focus the participants upon particular points being discussed in the interviews, and to solicit interviewees' thoughts and preferences. Moreover, the sketch work was used to help the participants think about alternative possibilities to their own preconceived ideas (there were often differences between participants' initial statements of what they wanted and those posed by the participants after exploring other options and design proposals).

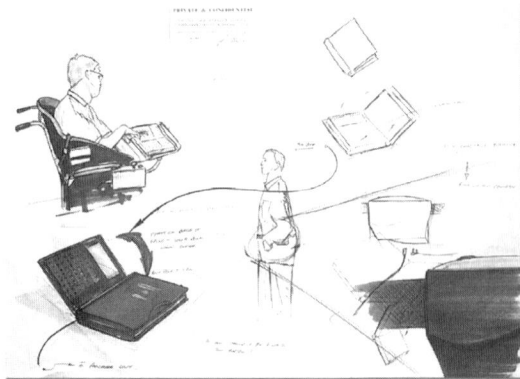

Figure 11.1. Sketching design ideas in relation to the actual participants of the study

Often the AAC users' statements of their needs and wants changed when presented with alternative ideas. It could be argued that these changes were the result of an imposition by the author. Rather than supplant the AAC users' ideas with those of the author, however, the author's ideas, typically presented though discussion or in the form of sketch work, provided an opportunity to further explore ideas coming directly from AAC users. Whilst there can be dangers of this approach, most notably that the designer is at risk of usurping the role of the participants, in this case there were distinct advantages. The ideas of the participants were often bound by their knowledge of what they believed to be possible or, counter to this, participants would propose possibilities outside the practical constraints of the project.

After each interview further sketching and ideation were conducted, with many of the ideas that participants suggested being incorporated into product proposals. The drawings would then be shown to the participants on later occasions for further evaluation. In turn, drawings would help in the articulation of user requirements by transforming users' own mental models into recognisable and feasible sketched design ideas.

However, physical (3D) models allowed the AAC users to more fluently comprehend design ideas, and proved to be much more powerful tools for evaluating and discerning user requirements than verbal presentations and sketches alone. The hard Medium Density Fibreboard (MDF) models accurately approximated the weight and feel of the intended designs, and although they were more time consuming to produce than softer foam models, the ruggedness they provided was necessary in this instance, as foam models were not durable enough to last the duration of the interview session. There is a great difference in how someone with cerebral palsy interacts with a hard or a soft material - typically the harder material can be used to help support the hand when performing a task. Hence, the MDF models were more useful in establishing whether certain tasks (such as reaching for a button) could be performed by AAC users.

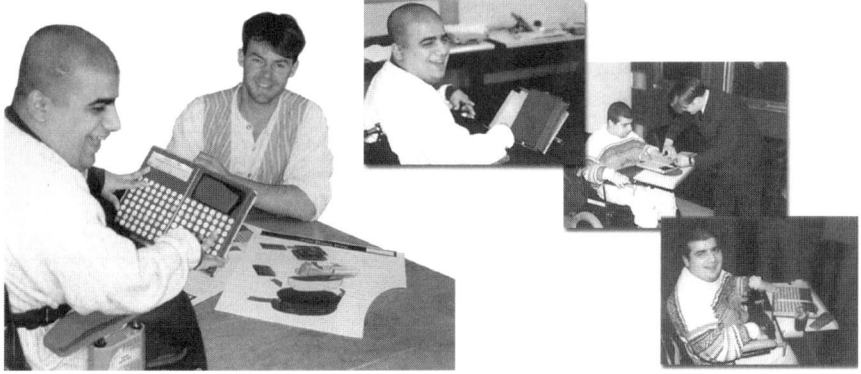

Figure 11.2. The use of physical models in a series of interview sessions with one participant

Developing ideas through working prototypes added an important sense of realness to design concepts. Owing to their interactive properties, the prototypes proved important tools for eliciting user feedback: an action on the user's part resulted in a reaction from the product. Visual models rely on interpretation and imagination to comprehend the final item, whilst working prototypes are easier to perceive and relate to as final production items. Presenting prototyped parts of the PCA to AAC users at the College, and allowing them to try them out and comment upon provided more detailed and empirical feedback on design details than either drawings or solid models could provide.

Presenting and re-interpreting users' ideas in the form of sketches and models whilst designing had many benefits. Working with AAC users in this way permitted them to learn about design, and so in time the participants developed a greater awareness of, and ability to articulate their needs and conceptualise their ideas (albeit through the hand of the author). Often the AAC users' statements of their needs and wants became more comprehensive after consultation with the author. Intervention and co-operation led to a comprehensive Product Design Specification - without it, the specification would have been patchy. The designer has the ability to articulate and "specify", in functional terms, what is required. In this sense, the designer, knowledgeable in many areas, has a vital part in articulating user needs. Further, the designer can facilitate participants in the design process by helping to:

- generate and develop more creative ideas (by prompting questioning, by visualising the participant's ideas);
- broaden options (an idea can be extrapolated to cover other, unthought of, areas, and the designer's knowledge of contemporary and emerging technology can expand options and possibilities);
- rationalise ideas (the designer's technical acumen (manufacturability, availability of technology, predicted costs, and so on) can help focus a participant's ideas into practicable concepts);
- articulate and define user needs.

11.3 Findings

A number of problematic issues facing AAC users were revealed through the study and were broadly categorised under 6 main headings:

- physical issues of devices (e.g. batteries running out of charge, or the aid being prone to knocks;
- perception of the devices;
- interface issues (e.g. fingers slipping on keys);
- system issues (ability to be programmed by users);
- situational issues (problems of use outdoors, in the dark);
- voice issues (in particular the intelligibility of the voice synthesiser, lack of intonation and expression).

The range of methods used in the solicitation of user needs also revealed much about users wants and aspirations for a new communication device. Moving beyond the problems of devices, to the possibilities for devices was an exciting and liberating step in the design of the PCA, and one in which the students at the college keenly participated. Indeed, whilst the functional limitations and problems of the students' AAC devices were an extremely important concern, many of these issues could be relatively easily addressed in the product design. In order to develop a truly useable and successful design of an assistive technology device, it was important to consider the wider psychological and sociological effects of the use of such disability devices upon their users.

11.3.1 The Importance of Product Semantics

Krippendorff and Butter define Product Semantics as "the study of the symbolic qualities of man-made forms in the context of their use and the application of this knowledge to industrial design. It takes into account not only the physical and physiological functions, but also the psychological, social and cultural context" (see Krippendorff and Butter, 1984). Erving Goffman (1973), in Stigma - Notes on the Management of Spoiled Identity, notes that, "first appearances are likely to enable us to anticipate ... 'social identity'" (Goffman, 1973), and hence, clothing, artefacts and personal possessions, in addition to physical appearance and manner, constitute the constructs of a stranger's social identity. Clothing is an obvious example where the individual is placed into social and cultural groups based upon the observer's value judgements. Attire can be used to establish or impart social standing, or to express an individual's tastes, interests, aspirations and attitudes. Dressing up or dressing down is also a very obvious way in which an individual can attempt to change his or her perceived social identity.

Material possessions, therefore, have an important role in establishing social identity as well as in the construction of selfhood (Goffman, 1973; Csikszentmihalyi and Rochberg-Halton, 1981; Dewey, 1938). It is, therefore, important to consider the effects of the use of disability devices by people with disabilities, and their relationship with those devices. The study revealed that AAC devices, and disability devices more generally, are seen as extensions of their users, and therefore the aesthetics and product semantics of these devices reflects upon their users and has a significant impact upon users' self-image. Self-image is very important, and often the very devices designed to help people in fact compound their problems by drawing unwanted attention to their impairments. "The main disadvantage mentioned by users of high-tech [AAC devices] was that their devices drew attention to them that they did not want" (Murphy, 1993); indeed, one user said, "people focus their attention on the machine, not me" (Murphy, 1993). This gives rise to a situation where many people are reluctant to use aids as the devices may contribute to their problems compounding a psychological stigma of inferiority. Other authors have cited that many products within the disability sector are rejected by their users (e.g. Ring, 1980; Jonkers, 1980; Murphy et al., 1995) due to their unreliability (Murphy and Collins, 1994), their appearance (Hogan, 1994/5; Collingsworth, 1993) and the handicapping aspects of the product (Ring, 1980; Hogan, 1994/5; Murphy and Collins, 1994). One could argue there is a paradox: disability products often disable their users, not necessarily in a physical sense, but on a psychological and sociological level.

11.4 The Portland Communication Aid

In pursuit of this design goal, the design approach was to modularise the Portland Communication Aid (PCA) and to design each part as a socially acceptable, even desirable item. The PCA is in three physical parts: the Book; the Bum-bag; and the Mobile speaker unit.

The principle idea for the Book was to camouflage the technology and to attach to the product an association of intelligence, whereby those using it would be perceived to be literate and, hopefully, intelligent. A book carries more than just the association of intelligence, however. The information or stories contained within books, rather than the physicality of them, stimulates emotive or reactionary responses. In this way, the intention of the Book was to draw the public's attention away from the 'machine' and to focus upon the content of what was generated upon it and spoken by the PCA (in other words, what the user was saying). The association of books with story telling was also apt for the PCA, in that a story-teller can captivate an audience by reading from a book. The correlation between learning and books was also intended to be explicit, as the PCA was intended to be used as an aid for learning.

The Book's resemblance to a personal organiser or a diary was by no means coincidental. Both objects are used to store personal information, and have significant value to their owners. Likewise, the Book sought to foster such an association. The design of the Book had additional virtues as discovered through concurrent evaluations with AAC users at the College:

- avoidance of unwanted attention drawn to the user (to all intents and purposes the user is reading);
- a means of keeping private material private (the Book can be closed);
- the act of closing the Book allows a very demonstrative statement to be made: "I don't want to talk to you".

Breaking the system up into discreet components is a distinct departure from the status-quo. It is tempting to suggest that advances in circuit packaging density, battery technology and power management will ultimately allow all the electronics to be housed within the PCA's Book. The separation of the various parts of the system, however, is an integral part of the design concept. The Bum-bag is seen as assisting the semi-ambulant user in maintaining a better posture and provides a secure repository for the more expensive parts of the system. The Mobile speaker concept allows the user's voice to emanate from the correct part of his or her body or to facilitate a private conversation. The advances mentioned will, though, allow the unit to be thinner and lighter and will certainly offer extended endurance.

More generally, the PCA has inherent design features and has incorporated key principles that are equally applicable to other projects in the disability sector:

- modularity of components;
- separation of interface, processor and output devices;
- camouflaging technology;
- affording meaning through semantics and metaphor;
- using remote links to other components;
- using noble materials (metal and leather) for their longevity and patina;
- making use of standard parts (such as batteries) to minimise costs and provide greater availability of replacements;
- utilising standard hardware (upgrading is simple);
- push towards software over hardware solutions.

The evaluation of the PCA was limited, given time and financial constraints. However, concurrent evaluations, heuristic evaluations, a questionnaire with new students at the College and an evaluation interview with one of the primary participants revealed encouraging and positive responses towards the device. More extensive evaluations and user trials are desirable.

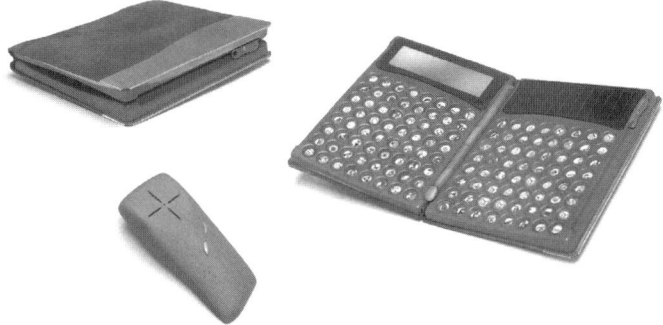

Figure 11.3. Two of the PCA components – the *Book* in open and closed states, and the *Mobile*

11.5 Conclusions

Through reading, observation, social intercourse, discussion and interviews, a comprehensive understanding of the needs, wants, abilities, capabilities and experiences of AAC users was established. Over time, a rapport was developed with the students of Portland College. The nature of this informal and unobtrusive approach to requirements capture provided a much-needed sympathetic comprehension of the nature of the problems faced by AAC users. The observational studies helped to foster an understanding and appreciation of the lives of the participant AAC users, and of how to conduct interviews with people with severe communication disabilities. The processes of designing and the 2-D and 3-D models thereby produced were important in the exploration and articulation of user requirements. Through consolidation of these user requirements, a prototype of the PCA was created that both embodied AAC users' ideas, and addressed their needs, wants and even desires for an AAC device. In this study both the process of designing and the subsequent outcomes of Industrial Design, had a valuable role in the empowerment and rehabilitation of AAC users.

It is the author's contention that many disability products have addressed, at best, only functional goals in solving problems associated with disability. Designers have shown insufficient regard for communicative goals that deal with how products are perceived. Such communicative goals include raising status, prestige, desirability, self-esteem, and pleasure for their users. It is proposed that disability products can be greatly improved by paying greater attention to such communicative goals. This is not just a case of re-styling, but an exercise in meshing needs, wants, aspirations, purposes, abilities and capabilities of potential users of disability products with technological and functional requirements.

11.6 References

Allen JL (2002) Some problems of designing for augmentative and alternative communication users: an enquiry through practical design activity. Ph.D. Thesis. Loughborough University, Loughborough, UK

Buchanan R (1992) Wicked problems in design thinking. Design Issues 8(2): 5-21

Collingsworth J (1993) Design for Disability: A Handbook for Students and Teachers. London Guildhall University, London, UK

Csikszentmihalyi M, Rochberg-Halton E (1981) The meaning of things - Domestic symbols and the self. Cambridge University Press, Cambridge, UK

Dewey J (1938) Experience and education. The MacMillan Company, New York

Galer M (1983) Methodology for the evaluation of aids for the disabled. Institute for Consumer Ergonomics, Loughborough, UK

Goffman E (1973) Stigma - notes on the management of spoiled identity. Penguin Books Ltd, London, UK

Hogan P (1994/5) Introducing the European Institute for Design and Disability. Usertalk 4(Winter): 2-3

Jonas W (1993) Design as problem-solving? or: Here is the solution - What was the problem? Design Studies 14(2): 157-170

Jonkers HL (1980) Aids for the physically disabled: Consumer conclusions drawn from a cost-benefit analysis. In: The Use of Technology in the Care of the Elderly and the Disabled. Francis Pinter, London, UK

Krippendorff K, Butter R (1984) Product semantics: Exploring the symbolic qualities of form. Innovation, the Journal of the Industrial Designers Society of America, Spring, pp 4-9

Murphy J (1993) The advantages and disadvantages of high tech AAC devices with voice output. In: Fifth Annual European Minspeak Conference. Mansfield, UK

Murphy J, Collins S (1994) Advantages and disadvantages of AAC systems. Communication Matters 8(3): 5-7

Murphy J, Marková I, Moodie E, Scott J, Boa S (1995) Augmentative and alternative communication systems used by people with cerebral palsy in Scotland: Demographic survey. Augmentative and Alternative Communication 11(1): 26-36

Nicolle C, Poulson DF, Richardson SJ (1995) A methodology for defining user requirements for rehabilitation and assistive technology. In: The European Context for Assistive Technology. Proceedings of the 2nd TIDE Congress. IOS Press, Paris, France

Poulson DF, Ashby MC, Richardson SJ (eds.) (1996) USERfit: A practical handbook on user-centred design for assistive technology. ECSC-EC-EAEC, Brussels

Ring ND (1980) Communication aids for the speech impaired. In: The Use of Technology in the Care of the Elderly and the Disabled. Francis Pinter, London, UK

Stanton N, Baber C (1996) Factors affecting the selection of methods and techniques prior to conducting a usability evaluation. In: Usability Evaluation in Industry. Taylor & Francis, London, UK

Chapter 12

Consensus-based Adaptive User Interface Implementation in Product Promotion

J. Sobecki and M. Weihberg

12.1 Introduction

In the recent years web-based systems are very often used in product promotion mostly for delivering up-to-date information about them. For most systems of this kind well designed user interfaces are of a great importance. These systems are, however, used by a highly differentiated population of users accessing these systems by means of various platforms. So, it is almost impossible to design a single interface that would be sufficiently usable for all of the users.

There could be various solutions to this problem. The traditional approach has been worked out by the area of the Human Computer Interaction (HCI) and suggests designing an interface according to the future user profile as well as the system platform characteristic (Newman and Lamming, 1996). Unfortunately these solutions could not be fully applied in the today's web systems, so various types of recommender systems are used instead.

Recommender systems that concern user interfaces are usually called adaptive (Langley, 1999) or personalised user interfaces (Montaner *et al.*, 2003). The personalisation could be made in many different ways (Mobasher *et al.*, 1999). Generally, the personalisation settings concern three basic elements of the system interface: the system information content, the way the information is presented to users and how the information is structured (Kobsa *et al.*, 2001). The recommendations are usually based on the user model that is usually represented as a user profile, containing both the user data and the usage data. The interface settings, on the other hand, are stored in the user profile.

In this chapter the implementation and verification of consensus-based adaptive user interface of web-based system from the field of product promotion is presented. The general idea of the consensus-based socially adaptive user interface is presented in work (Nguyen and Sobecki, 2003). It is based on the ideas of one of the type of recommender systems that are called collaborative filtering.

In the next section the system architecture is presented. In the following section the system implementation of an information system presenting the selected car model is described. The last section presents the test results that were conducted with over 75 users that to some extent could represent the real users of that system together with some final remarks.

12.2 Consensus-based Interface Adaptation

The system architecture is based on the general ideas of collaborative recommender systems. Generally, in these types of systems item ratings of other users are utilised to find the best fitting one for the particular user.

Collaborative filtering is able to offer novel items, even such that user has never seen before. We must remember however that the ratings delivered by the community are rather subjective. These properties of collaborative filtering are found to be advantageous over content-based recommender systems (Montaner *et al.*, 2003).

Collaborative recommended agents have also some disadvantages: the predictions are poor when the number of other similar users is small; the quality of service for users of peculiar testes is also bad; lack of transparency in the process of prediction and finally the user's personal dislike may be overcome by the number of other similar users' opinions.

The disadvantages of content based and collaborative recommendation could be overcome by applying the hybrid solution. It seems however that in the case of web-based systems user interface adaptation the collaborative recommendation may be sufficient because the disadvantages mentioned above do not influence it much. First, we can assume that web-based systems always have quite many similar users. Second, when the prediction does not fit the user, he is able to personalise the interface manually.

The system adaptation (see Figure 12.1) starts with registering each new user. The registration data are stored in the user profile. Then according to the user profile the user is assigned to the appropriate group. With each group of users there is associated a corresponding interface profile.

The user registration is not obligatory but in this case the default interface profile is delivered. According to the interface profile the actual user interface content, layout and structure is generated. The user may start to work with the system and if he or she wishes also modify the interface settings. Finally, these settings together with usability evaluation given by user are stored in the interface profile.

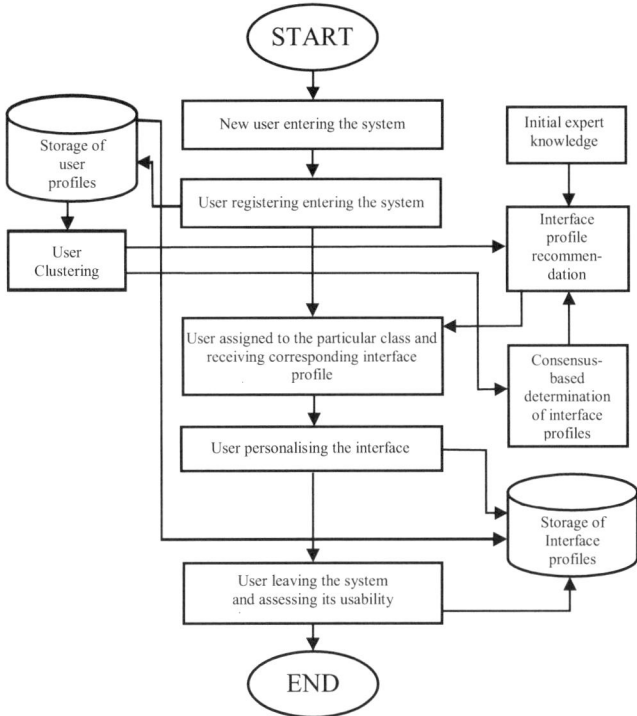

Figure 12.1. Architecture of the consensus-based user interface adaptation

When the system registers the required number of users, users are first clustered and then according to these clusters using consensus methods new interface profiles for recommendation are distinguished. These procedures may be repeated for the following occasions: many new users registering to the system or interface recommendations become poor usability ratings.

12.2.1 User Profile

User profile contains all necessary data to model the user in the adaptive system. Usually the user profile contains two types of data: user data and usage data (Kobsa, Koenemann and Pohl, 2001). The user data may contain different user characteristics:

- demographic data (name, sex, address, occupation, education, customer and psychographic data);
- user knowledge;
- user skills; and,
- user interests.

The user profile could also contain the usage data that may be observed directly from the user's interaction with web-based system. It should also contain the identification data such as user login and password, which is necessary for authentication purposes.

In the recommender systems the user profile could be represented by many different forms: binary vectors, feature vectors, trees, decision trees, semantic networks. In this chapter we propose to describe the user profile as a tuple defined in the following way: the finite set A^u of attributes describes each user and the set V^u contains attribute values, where: $V^u = \bigcup_{a \in A^u} V_a^u$ (V_a^u is the domain of attribute a). The tuple that is a function $p : A^u \rightarrow V^u$ where $(\forall a \in A^u)(p(a) \in V_a^u)$.

12.2.2 User Clustering Based on the User Profiles

Clustering problem could be defined as partition of the given set of user profiles into subsets such that a specific criterion is optimised.

We can use k-means clustering to minimise the average squared Euclidean distance between a profile and the corresponding cluster centre by partitioning the set of the profiles into k non-overlapping clusters that are identified by their centres.

This problem is known to be NP-hard, but still it is attractive because of its simplicity and flexibility (Kanungo et al., 2002). In our implementation we are using Dattola algorithm (Dattola, 1968), known from the field of Information Retrieval that is not NP-hard but produces the sub-optimal solution.

In order to cluster the set of users into k separate groups the initial centroids must be selected, in our case they are selected by experts. Then for each user profile the distance function (see below) between the profile and each centroid is determined.

The profile is joined to the group with the closest the centroid and also lower that assumed threshold, those above are assigned to the class of so-called isolated elements. Then for each group the centroids are recalculated and the process is repeated until no one profile changes its class assignment. Finally all profiles from the class of isolated elements are assigned to the group with the lowest distance function values or left as a separate group.

12.2.3 Interface Profile

The interface profile models the actual user interface together with its evaluation. Like in the interface personalisation (Kobsa et al., 2001) in the interface profile we can find the following information: the interface layout, the information content and its structure. In order to know whether the settings are appropriate for the particular user the interface profile also contain the usability value associated with this profile (Newman and Lamming, 1996).

The interface profile formal description reflects its complexity. For quite many cases, also for the car model information system, a tuple is sufficient for the interface representation. However for more complex systems also other structures, for example trees, may be considered (Sobecki, 2003).

In the interface profile represented as a tuple, A^i denote the finite set of attributes describing the interface instance for the particular user and a set V^i of attribute elementary values, where $V^i = \bigcup_{a \in A^i} V_a^i$ (V_a^i is the domain of attribute a). The interface profile is represented by a tuple that is a function $r : A^i \rightarrow V^i$ where $(\forall a \in A^i)(r(a) \in V_a^i)$

12.2.4 Distance Function Definition

The distance function between values of each attribute of the interface profiles is defined as a function $\delta^{at} : V_a \times V_a \rightarrow [0,1]$ where V_a denotes V_a^u or V_a^i for all $a \in B^u \subseteq A^u$ or $a \in B^i \subseteq A^i$. This function should be given by the system designer and fulfil all the distance function conditions but not especially all the metrics conditions. The distance function values could be enumerated or given in any procedural form.

The distance between profiles (user and interface) could be defined in many different ways. First, the distance between tuples i and j could be defined as a simple sum of distances between values of each attribute (t denotes p or r, and A denotes the subsets of A^u or A^i):

$$\delta(t_i, t_j) = \sum_{a \in A} \delta^{at}(t_i(a), t_j(a)) \tag{12.1}$$

or the root of the sum of squares of these distances. We also can indicate the importance of each attribute a by multiplying the distance by appropriate factor defined as a function $c : A \rightarrow [0,1]$:

$$\delta(r_i, r_j) = \sum_{a \in A} [c(a) * \delta^{at}(r_i(a), r_j(a))] \tag{12.2}$$

12.2.5 Representation of the Set of Interfaces

To solve the problem of finding the representation in the set of interfaces we must have the values of usability measure $u(j)$ assigned to each of the interface j. Let assume that the usability measure falls in the [0,1] interval and the value 0 denotes completely useless interfaces and 1 denotes ideally useful interface. Then to find the consensus (recommended interface for particular group of users G) we must find the interface i that's sum of the distances to all other interfaces j that were used and evaluated by users belonging to the same group of users G multiplied with their usability measure $u(j)$ is minimal (Sobecki, 2003):

$$\min(\sum_{j \in G} u(j) * \delta(\mathbf{r}_i, r_j)) \tag{12.3}$$

This problem could be computationally difficult, but according to (Ngu, 2001) we can reduce the computation by finding the minimal value for all attributes a of a tuple separately:

$$\min(\sum_{j \in G} u(j) * \delta(r(a)_i, r(a)_j)) \tag{12.4}$$

12.3 Adaptive System Implementation

In order to verify the consensus-based adaptive user interface architecture an experimental system of a selected car model presentation was implemented. We have chosen Renault Megane II (c) the model of the car that was awarded with Car of The Year 2003. That choice was made in order to attract as many users as possible and also because of the ease of acquiring all the necessary materials to build the system.

In this chapter we present the implemented user profile and interface profile with distance functions assigned to selected attributes, the initial user profiles centroids that represent the user groups with initial corresponding interface profiles assigned to them and finally description of the short description of the software implementation of the system.

12.3.1 User Profile Implementation

The car model presentation system is quite simple and so is the user profile. The data stored in the user profile are entered by the users during the registration process. The user data is reduced to only a few attributes of demographic information and one that characterises the user's interests.

The set of attributes A^u = {*login, password, name, surname, age, sex, education, number_of_inhabitants, type_of_information*}.

These attributes have the following set of values:

- V_{login}, $V_{password}$ are strings with maximal length of 10 characters;

- V_{name}, $V_{surname}$ are strings with maximal length of 15 characters;

- V_{age} ={less_than_18, from_18_to_25, from_25_to_50, over_50};

- V_{sex} ={male, female}, $V_{education}$ ={primary, secondary, higher};

- $V_{number\_of\_inhabitants}$ ={less_than_100.000, from_100.000_to_500.000, from_500.000_to_1.000.000, over_1.000.000};

- $V_{type\_of\_information}$ ={general, technical_details}.

The attribute names and their values are self explaining maybe except the last one, which describes the user preference concerning types of information about the car model, general or with more technical details. In Figure 12.2 the registration window is presented.

12.3.2 Interface Profile Implementation

The interface profile attributes in the case of already mentioned car information system are the following:

A^i ={login, main_menu, option_information, option_colours, option_gallery, option_version, option_files, toolbar, background, music_track, music_loudness, sound_effects, effects_loudness, language, type_of_information, usability}

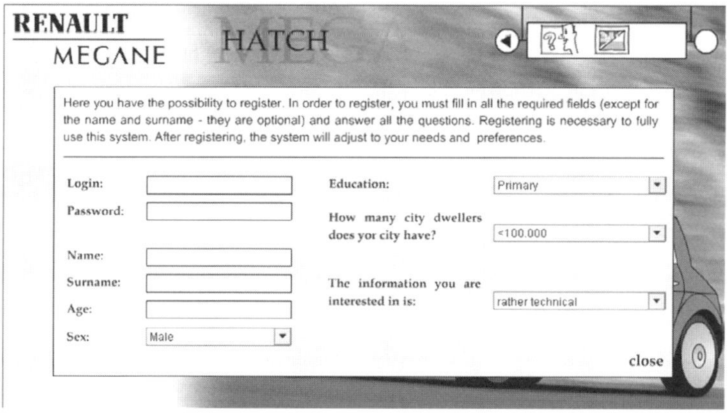

Figure 12.2. Registration window

The interface profile contains information concerning interface layout, information content and structure. The first attribute *login* as in the user profile presents the user login, which must be unique in the whole system.

Each of the following attributes: *main_menu, option_information, option_colours, option_gallery, option_version* and *option_files* represent elements (scenes) of the car information system, the main menu and five options that could be selected in the main menu: information, colors, gallery, version and files. All these attributes have five values denoted as 1, 2, 3, 4 and 5 and representing five different layouts of each option.

These values represent graphical layouts ordered from modern to traditional. They are implemented as separate movies in Macromedia Flash and loaded from the server according to the interface profile settings. The next two attributes *toolbar* (four different values) and *background* (five different values) are implemented in the same way. We have also five values for attributes *music_track* and *sound_effects*.

The values for loudness: *music_loudness* and *effects_loudness* are integer values from 0 to 100. The following two attributes: *information_type* and *language* concerns system content. The former has two values: *general* and *technical_detail* and the later: *Polish* and *English*. The *usability* value is an integer from 0 to 4, where 0 denotes the worst and 4 the best interface usability rate given by the users.

One of the windows with personalisation settings of the interface profile is shown in Figure 12.3.

In this window every interface setting has its thumbnail and every music track or sound set has a few seconds long preview. It helps the user to make sure that the new, selected layout is the expected one before applying the changes.

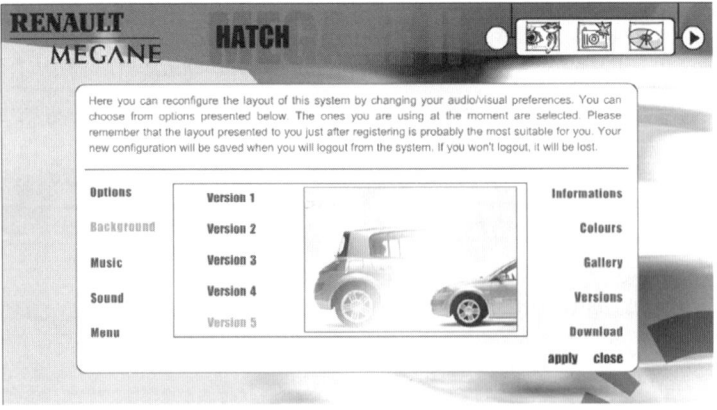

Figure 12.3. Window with the interface profile personalisation

12.3.3 Distance Functions in User Profile and Interface Profile

In order to calculate the distance value between either two interface profiles or two user profiles the distances between all atom values of every attribute had to be specified. In our system all values of each attribute are sorted, what means that if for example an attribute has five possible values, the distance between the first value and the second one is 0.25, between the second value and the third one is 0.5 etc. To calculate the distance between two profiles all distances between values of each attribute are summed up and the result is divided by the number of attributes.

12.3.4 Initial User Profile Centroids and Corresponding Interface Profiles

The attributes values of the initial centroids were selected by the experts so that none of them had all the extreme (maximal or minimal) values and the distance between consecutive centroids was similar. Below are presented the attributes values of the four initial centroids:

- male, less than 25 years old, primary education, from 500.000 to 1.000.000 inhabitants, technical information;
- male, over 50 years old, primary education, from 500.000 to 1.000.000 inhabitants, technical information;
- female, from 25 to 50 years old, secondary education, from 100.000 to 500.000 inhabitants, general information;
- female, over 50 years old, higher education, over 1.000.000 inhabitants, general information.

Each of these centroids had the corresponding interface profile that ware assigned also by the experts. The interface of the first centroid was rather modern, of the second one was designed for men (both presented detailed technical information), of the third one was designed for women and finally the last interface of the fourth centroid was rather traditional (both presented general information).

12.3.5 Software Implementation

The system was created in the 3-tier architecture, which allows separating the three main elements of a dynamic web application: presentation layer, business layer and data layer. In this architecture the system scalability is very high. Every layer is created separately in different technology. These technologies can be replaced at any time without any loss (for example as a database there can be used MS SQL Server instead of MySQL etc.). Also the business logic is centred in one layer so any changes to it are made in one place. The scalability was increased by using the XML mark-up language, which allows transferring data between the three layers in an ordered and well structured way.

In our system the presentation layer, which is displayed in a client's browser, was created with Macromedia's Flash. Its latest version, MX, offers a very advanced programming environment combined with a huge multimedia support. Flash allows combining information content with music, sound, movies and graphics in an interesting and efficient way, so the user will be attracted to the system and will spent more time with it.

PHP was used for implementation of business logic and data processing. It is a perfect solution for managing the data exchange between a presentation layer and a database via dynamically generated XML documents. It can process the information send by Flash and store it in a database and also extract the data from database by using queries and pass the results further.

12.4 Test Results and Final Remarks

The effectiveness of implemented consensus-based user interface adaptation was tested in controlled conditions by about 75 users, students of masters' degree and postgraduate studies at the Faculty of Computer Science at Wrocław University of Technology. The users were of different age, education, musical and graphical taste, preferences concerning the system layout and information content. The tests were conducted in three steps described below.

In the first step a group of the users registered themselves and they were joined to the appropriate group according to the smallest distance to the centroids. When the distance to all the centroids was greater than 0.4 the user was assigned to the default group. According to the group assignment corresponding interface profile was delivered to the users. In this step users were not allowed to personalise their interfaces and at the end the users were asked to fill-in the questionnaire concerning seven usability aspects, i.e. information content, visual content, interaction etc. Each aspect was divided into several questions, where the user could mark a particular element of the system (the scale was from 1 to 10) and write a comment. The answers were stored in a database.

In the second step a new group of users was asked to register themselves and personalise their user interface according to their preferences. Then they were asked to assess the general usability with four grades scale.

Before the final experiment step was made the users registered in the previous step were clustered and corresponding interface profiles were determined using consensus methods. With the new clusters the new centroids were also determined. Then the last group of users, as in the first step, was assigned to the appropriate groups according to their distance to the centroids. According to these assignments corresponding interface profiles ware delivered to the users. Again after working with the system and obtaining all desired information on the car model users were asked to fill-in the usability questionnaire.

Comparison of the all user interface usability aspects made in the first step and the third step shows that the interface adaptation results in receiving higher marks. The raise of marks was rather small (0.3 in average in the 10 point scale) but was encountered in all aspects, so user interface recommendations delivered by adaptive procedures were better than those delivered by experts, but both were rated very high - 8.42 before and 8.72 after the adaptation. The results obtained are not statistically significant but exhibit some interesting properties of the adaptive user interface recommendation.

12.5 References

Dattola RT (1968) A fast algorithm for automatic classification. In: Report ISR-14 to the National Science Foundation, Section V, Cornell University, Department of Computer Science, NY

Kanungo T, Mount DM, Netanyahu, NS, Piatko C, Silverman R, Wu AY (2002) An efficient k-means clustering algorithm: analysis and implementation. IEEE Transactions On Pattern Analysis and Machine Intelligence 24(7): 881-892

Kobsa A, Koenemann J, Pohl W (2001) Personalized hypermedia presentation techniques for improving online customer relationships. Knowledge Engineering Review 16(2): 111-155

Langley P (1999) User modelling in adaptive interfaces. In: Proceedings of the Seventh International Conference on User Modelling, Banff, Canada

Mobasher B, Cooley R, Srivastave J (1999) Automatic personalisation based on Web usage mining. Technical Report TR99010, Department of Computer Science, DePaul University

Montaner M, Lopez B, de la Rosa JP (2003) A taxonomy of recommender agents on the internet. Artificial Intelligence Review 19: 285-330

Newman WM, Lamming MG (1996) Interactive system design. Addison-Wesley, Harlow, UK

Nguyen NT (2001) Conflict profiles' susceptibility to consensus in consensus systems. Bulletin of International Rough Sets Society 5(1/2): 217-224

Nguyen NT, Sobecki J (2003) Using consensus methods to construct adaptive interfaces in multimodal web-based systems. Universal Access in Information Society 2(4): 342-358

Sobecki J (2003) XML-based interface model for socially adaptive web-based systems user interfaces. Lecture Notes in Computer Science 2660: 592-598

Chapter 13

Transforming Musical Notations for Universal Access

S.S. Brown and P. Robinson

13.1 Introduction

Some disabilities can be assisted by using alternative notations and alternative input methods. This chapter describes a system for transforming between different musical notations, which can be customised to an individual's requirements, hence supporting many unusual needs that did not specifically have to be accounted for in the initial design. The customisation is brief, which encourages experimentation because new ideas can be explored more quickly.

Musical notations are coded instructions for musicians to perform music. They represent co-ordinated events in a stream of time. Internationally, several written notations are in widespread use, such as Western staff notation, Chinese Jianpu notation, sol-fa, many instrument-specific notations such as guitar tablature and Japanese koto notation, and Braille music for the blind, which has numerous different versions across the world. See Figure 13.4 for examples. It is often possible to transcribe a piece of music from one notation into another in order to make it accessible to a greater number of musicians. Software exists to effect such transcriptions, such as the music-to-Braille projects MFB (Langolff *et al.*, 2000) and Goodfeel (McCann, 1997). Such software works by obtaining a semantic (symbol-based) computer representation of the source notation, and algorithmically transforming this into a representation of the desired notation which is then realised by a suitable output device. However, existing systems are limited to dealing with a few specific notations; if a highly unusual or customised notation is required, this will often call for specialist programming or manual intervention.

13.1.1 Customised Notations

All of these notations can be customised for training purposes, or for particular tasks such as rapid overview (this is particularly useful in Braille music). Printed notations can further be customised to address print disabilities such as low vision or dyslexia, by using a modified set of symbols or a modified layout – for example, a person with tunnel vision benefits if musical directions are moved closer to the notes to which they apply, especially if the print is large. Ideally, software should support such customisation in an open-ended way, to facilitate needs that the designer did not originally anticipate.

13.1.2 Input

Musical composition and input presents another challenge. It is possible to enter music into a computer by playing it on an electronic keyboard or other instrument, but the results do not always match the user's intentions due to quantisation errors, and many disabled users are excluded because of the dexterity required. A music notation editor is frequently more appropriate. However, notations that are optimal for reading are not necessarily optimal for writing or editing – conceptual similarity between reading and writing is useful, but this can be overshadowed by a disabled person's accessibility needs. For example, someone with typing difficulties might prefer a terse input notation even if it means more training. People with print disabilities often find direct manipulation music publishing systems such as Sibelius (Finn and Finn, 2001) difficult to use, and prefer character-based music languages that can be written in any text editor, including any specialist or customised text editing environments they may have.

Several different character-based notations are in use by music typesetting systems and online repositories, and it is possible to design new ones. The ideal notation will vary with the style of music and the individual's method of composing or editing, as well as their disability and input device. For this reason it is useful to support flexibility in input ("write only") as well as output ("read only") notations when supporting musical activities with software.

13.2 Related Work

Besides the specialist Braille transcription software that has already been mentioned, and numerous music typesetting tools and other software that is capable of dealing with more than one notation (e.g. recent versions of Sibelius can convert between Western staff and guitar tablature), there are also some efforts to generalise the problem of transcribing between musical notations so that new or rarely-used notations can be supported as needed. In an earlier project (Brown, 2000), the first author represented musical scores as databases with each record corresponding to an event in the music; a special reporting language was used to generate various forms of Braille as well as data for music typesetting software. The main limitations were the difficulty of supporting new input formats and the verbosity of the languages used.

The problem can also be addressed by considering musical data as an example of general structured data, and utilising a generalised transformation framework such as XSLT, the XML transformation system (W3C, 1999) or TXL (Cordy *et al.*, 1988) to effect the transcriptions. These languages are verbose, so customising them involves considerable work, particularly for print-disabled people – those with blindness, low vision, dyslexia or another impairment that restricts the use of print.

There is no built-in support for multi-dimensional data, but music is inherently multi-dimensional, and forcing it into a hierarchical structure introduces arbitrary assumptions about its processing order and introduces difficulties when there are exceptions to the structure (Castan *et al.*, 2000). This increases verbosity.

13.3 Implementation

The authors' transformation framework 4DML (Brown and Robinson, 2002) has been used as the basis of a transformation system for musical notations. The 4DML framework consists of four main components:

1. an internal representation of structured data with multi-dimensional structures;
2. matrix mark-up language (MML), a generalised mark-up language designed to facilitate the input of multi-dimensional data;
3. a transformation tool that takes XML or MML as input, uses the above internal representation, and produces output in any text-based language by following a model of the desired structure;
4. compact model language (CML) for representing the model (models may also be represented using XML).

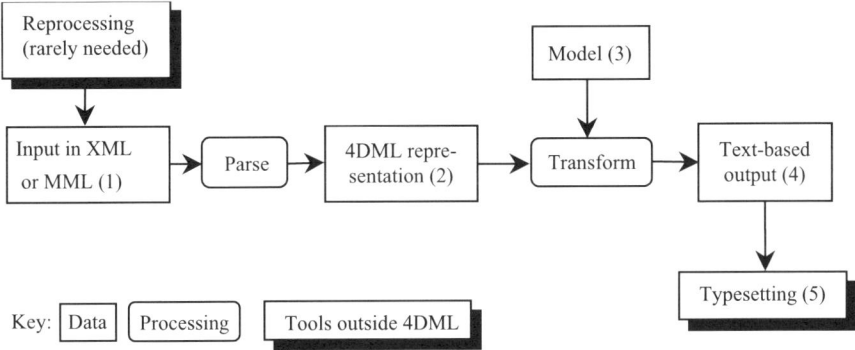

Figure 13.1. Overview of the 4DML transformation framework.

As shown in Figure 13.1, data in XML or MML (1) is first converted into 4DML (2)—a process which needs no external information as XML and MML are both self-describing formats – and then transformed into any text-based output language (4) under the direction of a model (3). The entire process may be surrounded by other transformations, such as the passing of the output through a typesetting system (5).

13.3.1 Matrix Markup Language (MML)

It can be cumbersome to hand-code multi-dimensional data in a hierarchical markup language like XML, since the markup is very verbose and repetitive.

For example, in coding the lyrics of a song, one might have to enclose each syllable in a <SYLLABLE>...</SYLLABLE> pair, whereas it would be easier to define a separator (for example, hyphen) to stand for "next syllable" (other separators can advance the word, verse number or translation).

In the general case, one can construct a parser for an arbitrary input language, but this can be a significant amount of effort for an end-user. There is scope for a markup language that provides for some simple re-definitions (such as "whitespace means next syllable") while not being as complex as a complete parser generator tool.

Matrix Markup Language (MML) is a text-based language that can represent structure in several ways. It consists of a mixture of directives and data. For example, the !block directive begins a matrix-like block of data that starts with directives such as

```
Have paragraph 1 newline 2 whitespace 3 - 4
    as system 1 verse 2 word 3 syllable 4
```

which defines how the text is to be parsed – paragraphs represent "systems", lines represent "verses", whitespace separates "words" and hyphens separate "syllables" (the numbers are for illustrative purposes only and are not part of MML). The have directive takes a list of input tokens, the word as and then a list of the corresponding components in the structure being described. These tokens are then referred to by the model (see below) during output. If desired, the lists may be built up from several have...as directives. Punctuation and other arbitrary strings may also be defined as separators, and there are facilities for representing overlapping sets of independent markup via multiple have directives separated by the word also. The data is also checked for consistency as it is processed, so any errors such as missing data are reported.

A "system" is a unit of physical layout, and the layout will probably change with the transformation. Nevertheless, representing the original layout (if any) often facilitates error correction and cross-referencing.

13.3.2 Compact Model Language (CML)

4DML uses a "model" to outline the structure of the desired output, which facilitates adjusting the output notation as needed. The data is automatically rearranged into the structure given by the model – the model guides a complex sorting operation, and also specifies any extra typesetting instructions in the language of whatever typesetting system is to be used. This means there is very weak coupling between the design of the input and that of the output; each can be customised independently of the other.

CML is a text-based language designed to facilitate the brief coding of models. It consists of literal text to be output directly, interspersed with code that generates output from the 4DML representation. In practice, most models have a repetitive structure; they express such things as "for each song, for each verse, for each syllable, …" which is expressed as song/verse/syllable. CML also has other operators and can represent any hierarchical document, but its syntax is designed for representing typical models concisely.

13.4 Evaluation

People with print disabilities should be able to program this transformation system by themselves, to assist with their musical work. To demonstrate this, an individual with low vision has used the system for the tasks described in this section. We hope to find other interested individuals in the future.

```
!block hand
have whitespace , character . as bar beat note string

r,r,r,Bd e,dB,e,dB A,B,D,EF GB,AG,E,ED E,r,r,Bd e,dB,e,dB
A,B,D,EE GB,AG,E,ED E,r,r,EF G,GB,d,cB A,A,B,GA B,g,ed,Bd
e,r,r,Bd e,dB,e,dB A,B,D,EF GB,AG,E,ED E,r,r,Bd etc
!endblock

!block hand
have whitespace , / character as bar beat note string

r,r,r,r EG,r,EA,r D,r,r,r E,r,r,r r,r,E,r EG,r,EA,r
D,r,r,r E,r,r,r r,r,r,r E,r,EGB,r DE,r,EG,r EG,r,EG,r
EG,r,EG,r EG,r,EG,r E,r,r,r E,r,r,r B/G,EB/G,EGB,r etc
!endblock
```

Figure 13.2. Input in MML using a syntax designed by the user.

The individual arranged some music for the Japanese Koto and encoded in a text editor using a notation that was invented for the purpose and appropriate to the music.

This was achieved by means of MML and is shown in Figure 13.2 – notice that the notation changes half way through the figure. Koto tablature was then produced by using 4DML to drive the layout engine Lout (Kingston, 1993), which is a general document preparation system that takes a description of page layout and typesets it as PostScript or PDF. The Japanese characters were implemented as images, as Lout does not support Unicode.

@Include{koto.setup} @Doc @Text @Begin
@Display clines @Break { @Heading 18p @Font {The Foggy Dew}
(Irish) }   *(alternatively, the titles could be kept in the MML)*
Tuning: Nogijoshi @PP   *(Now follows a preparatory translation table)*
[[cml chord export-code /
 string begin="@OneCol {" **end=**"}" **/ (**   *(for each string,)*
  note value=D/"@IncludeGraphic kanji2.ps",
  note value=E/"@IncludeGraphic kanji3.ps",
  note value=F/"@IncludeGraphic kanji3.ps",   *(re-writing F as E)*
... *(more notes follow)*
)]]   *(End of translation table; start of layout proper)*
@RightDisplay -90d @Rotate   *(because Koto is read in columns from right to left)*
21c @Wide {ragged 1.5vx}@Break {
[[cml bar group-size=20 group="} @RightDisplay -90d @Rotate 24c @Wide {ragged
  1.5vx}@Break {" **/(**   *(for each bar, with new page every 20 bars)*
  ]]# Bar **[[cml bar count]]**   *(comment the bar number—useful in debugging)*
3.9c @Wide @Box {   *(each bar is a 3.9cm-wide box before rotating downward)*
    [[cml hand between="//0.1c @FullWidthRule //0.1c"**/(]]** *(for each hand)*
       90d @Rotate 2c @Wide {   *(each hand is a 2cm box rotated left)*
         [[cml beat between="//0.1c 1.3c @Wide @LocalWidthRule //0.1c"**/(]]**
           @Centre {   *(two cases—1 or 2 notes in the beat*
                —handle differently because it affects scaling)
              [[cml note total=1 no-strip call=chord]]   *(call the*
              [[cml note total=2 no-strip call=chord   *translation table)*
                 begin="{0.8 0.5} @Scale " **between=**" // "**]]**
           }
         [[cml)]]   *(end of code for each beat)*
            //0.1c   *(this Lout code means 0.1cm vertical gap)*
       }
    [[cml)]]   *(end of code for each hand)*
  }
[[cml)]]   *(end of code for each bar)*
} @End @Text

Figure 13.3. 4DML model as CML embedded in Lout. The literal text is shown in roman type, the code in bold sans serif type, and the comments in italics are added here for explanatory purposes only and are not part of CML.

The model is shown in Figure 13.3, which is less "cluttered" when the comments are removed. It consists of a translation table of notes to symbols, and then nested loops over bars, hands, beats and notes – notice that the nesting order is different from that of the input and its transposition is automatic. Other 4DML models allowed the same music to be sent to Western music typesetting systems, Braille printers using multiple versions of Braille, and other formats as shown in Figure 13.4. It is possible to implement models for new types of output as needed.

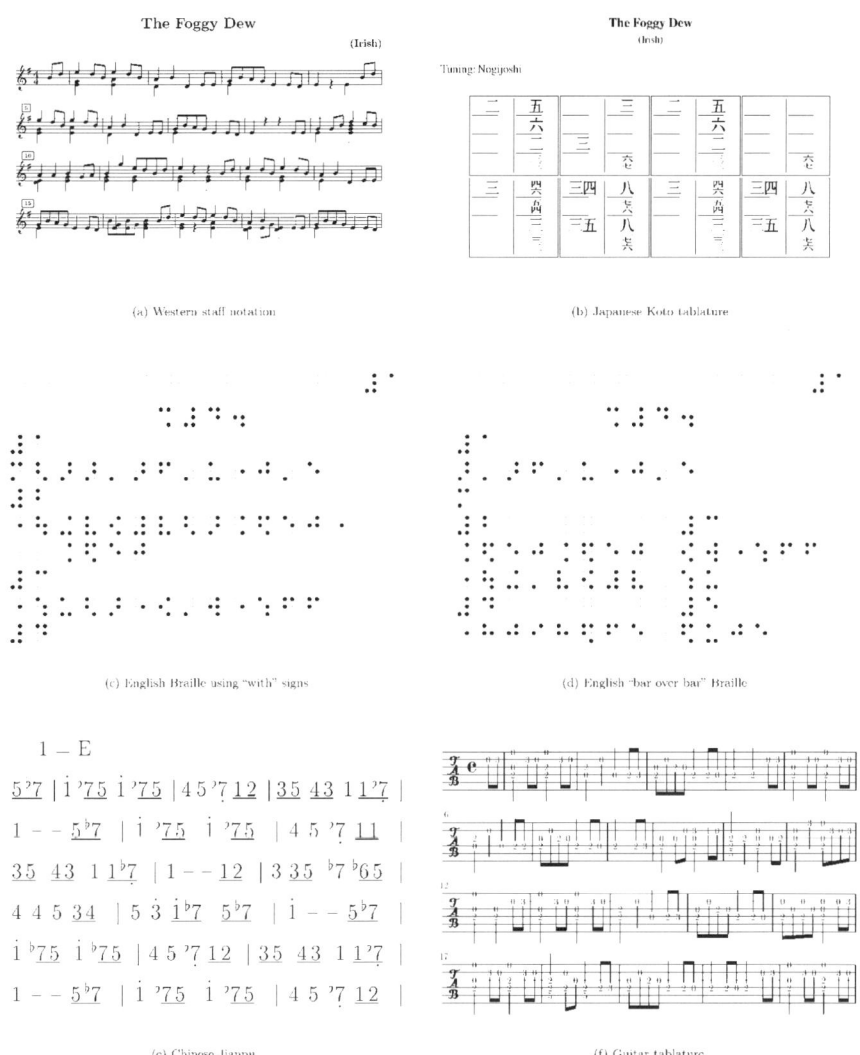

Figure 13.4. Output in various notations.

Another experiment involved the use of "aspect-oriented" music encodings, in imitation of aspect-oriented programming (Elrad *et al.*, 2001). Different aspects of the music, such as note letters, octaves, durations, enharmonics, ornaments, etc, were coded on separate passes through the score (Figure 13.5), and the model interleaved them when producing the typesetting instructions (Figure 13.6). This facilitated the transcription of already-written music because the user need consider only one aspect at a time, avoiding the need to switch rapidly between many different features of a complex input language; the user was able to encode a complex score that he had been unwilling to attempt using conventional methods.

```
begin music
begin part

!block pitch
have whitespace character as bar note

r rrrd ddddfca aarrd ddddfca aadce gfcdfeca gfcddfeeg
gfbagffg dcfffg feaabb ddcc bbaa gfgaabaadfa ddcbbdf
baggbdgfe egfee gfeebdrad daffaaaad drdcbbdf baggbdgfe egfee
etc
!endblock

!block duration
have whitespace character as bar note

0 2488 8881144 28888
8881144 28114 11481148
114111148 11481148 114848
114848 4882 4882 88888883333
etc
!endblock
```

Figure 13.5. Part of a piece in an aspect-oriented encoding. Other aspects (not shown) are octaves, enharmonics, dots, tuplets, phrasing, articulation, ornaments, dynamics, text, time and key changes and typographic adjustments.

```
bar between="&#10;&#10;" / part between="&#10;" (
  uptext begin="U: " end="&#10;",
  keychange/posn number=1 after=" ",
  note between=" " / (
    tie/posn number=1 end=" ",
    pitch, accidental, dot, duration,
    octave, shift, tuplet, articulation,
    tie/posn start-at=2 begin=" ",
    dynamics begin=" "
  ),
  keychange/posn number=2 before=" "
)
```

Figure 13.6. CML code to interleave Figure 13.5 into the format of M-Tx (a music typesetter).

Another experiment involved the use of "aspect-oriented" music encodings, in imitation of aspect-oriented programming (Elrad *et al.*, 2001). Different aspects of the music, such as note letters, octaves, durations, enharmonics, ornaments, etc, were coded on separate passes through the score (Figure 13.5), and the model interleaved them when producing the typesetting instructions (Figure 13.6). This facilitated the transcription of already-written music because the user need consider only one aspect at a time, avoiding the need to switch rapidly between many different features of a complex input language; the user was able to encode a complex score which he had been unwilling to attempt using conventional methods.

Aspect-oriented encoding also proved beneficial for original composition, the different aspects of the composition being added at different times. In this case the "aspects" were not always aspects of musical notation; they also included aspects of the compositional framework defined by the user (such as "arpeggio type" and "time distortion") which were converted into musical notation by the user's model.

The system was also used to typeset a large number of Chinese songs in various formats including an invented sol-fa like notation; in this case most of the work was in arranging for the model to produce and typeset pronunciation aids in an accessible form, and this is discussed elsewhere (Brown and Robinson, 2003).

13.5 Conclusion

A transformation system for musical notations has been constructed using the 4DML framework. This allows people with unusual accessibility needs to customise both the presentation of musical notations and the means of inputting them to their individual requirements, and allows music to be transformed between different presentations for different people. This should increase the accessibility of music as an educational subject, a vocation and an avocation. The aspect-oriented method of encoding music that was introduced also holds potential for music publishers and repositories, because it could be used to divide encoding skills among several people.

4DML's primary contribution is the brief-but-readable nature of its models, which aids in the rapid prototyping of transformations. It encourages a consideration of the notations themselves rather than the algorithmic methods for their transformation, hence allowing new notations to be experimented with more easily. In future it could be used to assist in experimenting with completely new ways of presenting music, such as via sign language, pictorially, or in tactile forms other than Braille (some physical conditions preclude good Braille reading but allow other tactile forms of communication). This would make music accessible to an even greater number of individuals.

4DML has also been used for the transformation of other notations; a forthcoming thesis will demonstrate its applicability to mathematics, diagrams, web-sites, experimental data and personal notes. Virtually all information-society applications involve notations, and the transformation of these between different versions is a component part of universal access, since it can help to cater for special needs and for differing tasks and environments. Tools that support the programming of such transformations, such as 4DML, can make it easier to create new notations on demand and to implement universal design.

13.6 References

Brown SS (2000) An extensible system for conversion of musical-notation data to Braille musical notation. Computing in Musicology 12: 45-74

Brown SS, Robinson P (2002) Automatically rearranging structured data for customised special-needs presentations. In: Universal Access and Assistive Technology, Springer-Verlag, London, UK

Brown SS, Robinson P (2003) Addressing print disabilities in adult foreign-language acquisition. In: HCI 2003, Vol.4: Universal Access in HCI, Lawrence Erlbaum Associates, Mahwah, NJ

Castan G, Good M, Roland P (2000) Extensible markup language (XML) for music applications: An introduction. Computing in Musicology 12: 95-102

Cordy JR, Halpern CD, Promislow E (1988) TXL: A rapid prototyping system for programming language dialects. In: Proceedings of the International Conference of Computer Languages, Loyola University Chicago, USA

Elrad T, Filman RE, Bader A (2001) Aspect-oriented programming: Introduction. Communications of the ACM 44(10): 29-32

Finn B, Finn J (2001) Sibelius: The Music Notation Software. Sibelius Software Ltd, Cambridge. Available at: http://www.sibelius-software.com/

Kingston JH (1993) The design and implementation of the Lout document formatting language. Software – Practice and Experience, 23: 1001-1041

Langolff D, Jessel N, Levy D (2000) MFB (music for the blind): A software able to transcribe and create musical scores into Braille and to be used by blind persons. In: Proceedings of the 6th ERCIM Workshop on "User Interfaces for All", Florence, Italy

McCann B (1997) GOODFEEL Braille music translator. Dancing dots Braille music technology. Available at: http://www.dancingdots.com/

World Wide Web Consortium (1999) XSL Transformations (XSLT) Version 1.0, W3C Recommendation. Available at: http://www.w3.org/TR/1999/REC-xslt-19991116

Chapter 14

Evaluation of Multimodal Techniques for Blind People to Track Moving Objects

W. Yu, J. McStay, G. Dodds and S. Ferguson

14.1 Introduction

This chapter describes the evaluation of an accessible computer game for blind and visually impaired people. Unlike other accessible computer games, this game uses force feedback and stereo sound to provide players with an interactive environment in which they can engage with dynamic objects. The evaluation is conducted to assess the techniques developed to help blind people to catch the moving objects in the game. The evaluation results are useful for developers to develop interactive environments with dynamic objects for blind people. This game is our first attempt to apply multimodal interaction technology to accessible entertainment software. The accessible game is introduced in this chapter as well as the evaluation process and results.

Sighted people are spoiled by having access to thousands of computer games which are comprise of elaborate 3D graphics, digital surround sounds and sometimes good storylines. However, blind people have very limited access because the majority of computer games are not designed with them in mind. Most of the specially designed accessible games are simply direct transfers of card games or board games which are less attractive to blind people. The traditionally accessible games are term-based and relatively static. Game information is read out to the player by using synthesised speech. Players use a keyboard to enter commands. Recently, there have been some improvements in the accessible games. Companies like GMA Games, ESP software and Bavisoft have produced some interactive and dynamic games for blind people. In these games, i.e. Lone Wolf, Shades of Doom, Dynaman, players have to complete the task in real-time. 3D sounds are produced in the game to guide and inform players about the events in the games. These games are thus more entertaining than the traditional games.

With recent developments in tactile and force feedback based gaming devices, i.e. game pads, joysticks and mice, as well as in supporting software i.e. the Immersion TouchSense SDK and Microsoft DirectX, computer games with haptic interaction can be developed for blind people. Instead of using complex computer graphics, games for blind people can utilise haptic feedback and 3D sounds to create an interactive entertaining environment. Following the same principle, an accessible game for blind people has been developed in the GRAB project (Wood *et al.*, 2003). In this game, players need to search and collect items in a 3D virtual environment. Audio and haptic feedback are provided to the players. To explore the virtual environment, a custom-built haptic device is used. A similar approach is used in another game developed in the TIM project (Archambault *et al.*, 2001). Instead of using 3D force feedback device, Braille display and tactile boards are used to present information to blind people's sense of touch.

A research project is being conducted at the Virtual Engineering Centre (VEC), Queen's University of Belfast to investigate the use of commercially available haptic gaming devices and 3 D sound in accessible computer games for blind people. The haptic device used is the low cost Logitech WingMan Force Feedback mouse (Figure 14.1) which is specifically designed for playing games.

The main objective of the project is to produce a dynamic game in which players can engage in the game play and interact with moving objects through audio and haptic feedback. The game is developed by using Macromedia Flash, JavaScript and Immersion TouchSense Studio. The game is thus web-based and blind people can access the game via a standard web-browser with Flash and Immersion Web plug-ins installed. The game will be published on the VEC web-site shortly.

14.2. Game Implementation

The interactive accessible computer game is called Duck-Hunt. It is similar to the shooting games that can be found in a video game arcade. The player needs to shoot the flying ducks by using the mouse cursor as the aim. A screen shot of the game is given in Figure 14.1.

The game has a graphical display, and presents information to the player through audio and force feedback. The display is irrelevant for the blind players but is useful for game development and to allow sighted players or people with low vision to enjoy the game too. The main input device is the WingMan Force Feedback mouse. A keyboard will also be used to start the game and get the speech read-out of the cursor location. To hear the sound speakers can be used but a pair of headphones is recommended for better stereo sound quality.

The main graphical display of the game consists of a background picture of a field. Ducks fly across the screen from the right to the left. The mouse cursor has been changed into a crosshair to represent an aiming device. Two pieces of information are shown on the screen. On the top left corner is the score achieved by the player while the time remaining on the game is shown on the top right corner. The flight paths of the duck are predefined and 6 different paths are created. They are randomly used for every duck appears on the screen. Therefore each duck appears to have a different flight pattern. The speed of the duck is also randomly assigned for each duck. In average, 12 ducks will fly across the screen in 1 minute.

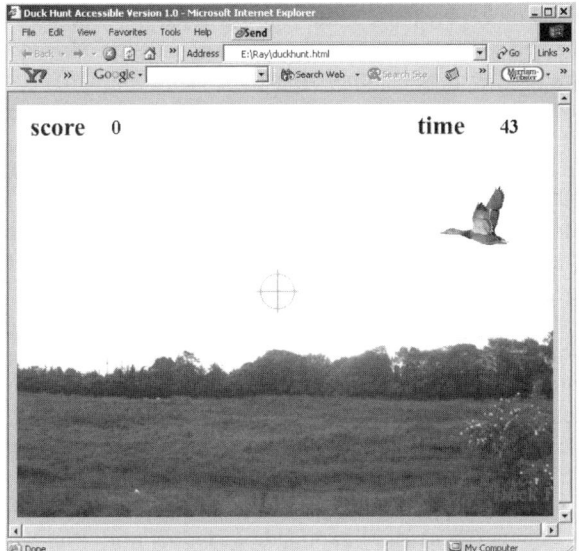
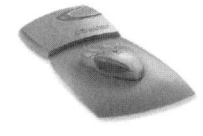

Figure 14.1. Duck Hunt Screenshot, and the Logitech WingMan Force Feedback mouse

The ducks are moving objects and thus create a challenge to blind people. It is uncommon in an accessible game that blind people need to catch a moving object. To present the location of the duck to the player, we use both audio and haptic representations. A 'ping' sound is associated with the duck. It pans from the right headphone to the left headphone according to the duck's position on the screen (assuming the listener's position is in the middle of the screen). It gives an indication of where the duck is however it does not give the altitude of the duck. This is due to the limitation of the sound rendering capability of Flash. A true 3D sound cannot be created.

To compensate the limitation in sound, a force feedback feature is used to give the indication of the exact location of the duck. Whenever the mouse cursor moves onto the duck, the force feedback mouse will vibrate and thus inform the player that she is on target. Therefore, the stereo sound provides horizontal location of the duck and the force feedback allows the player detect the presence of the duck in the vertical direction. Once the player is on target, she can shoot the duck by pressing the left mouse button. A force feedback routine is implemented so that once the shot is fired, the mouse is pulled back automatically to the centre of the screen in preparation for the next duck. In so doing, the player can re-orient herself quickly.

The stereo sound rendering of the duck described above is based on the listener's position in the middle of the screen. This would give a good indication of the duck position with respect to the whole screen. It also maintains the player's overall perspective of the screen. This kind of stereo panning has been found useful in exploring static objects (Yu and Brewster, 2002). However, there is little information about the current location of the mouse and its distance to the duck. Players' proprioception should give some hints about this information from the mouse because the WingMan Force Feedback mouse is restricted in a fixed area (the mouse is physically attached to the based by a linking mechanism). However due to the small work space of the mouse (approximately 2cm x 1.5cm), it is difficult to tell how far the mouse is from the centre or the edge of the screen. Therefore help is given here. The whole screen is evenly divided into 9 sectors. Once the player press the space bar on the keyboard, the game will speak out the ID of the current sector in which the mouse is located.

Unfortunately, this still does not give players the information about the distance between the mouse and the duck. In an attempt to address this problem, a second stereo sound rendering has been implemented. In this case, the listener's position is attached to the mouse cursor. The sound is rendered according to the position of the mouse. If a duck is on the left of the mouse, players will hear the sound from the left headphone. The panning position and the volume of the sound depend on the distance between the duck and the mouse. When the mouse comes closer to the duck, the sound will become nearer and louder. If the mouse is at the same horizontal position of the duck, the sound will appear on both headphones. If the mouse continues to the left and moves pass the duck, the sound will appear on the right headphone as the duck is now on the right hand side of the mouse. This kind of dynamic sound rendering enables players to judge the distance between the mouse and the duck.

In order to determine the effectiveness of these two types of sound rendering techniques, a comparative study has been conducted. The results of this experiment gives us some information about which sound rendering technique would be more useful in helping blind people to catch moving objects.

14.3. Evaluation

14.3.1. Experiment Set-up

A series of experiments were conducted to evaluate the Duck Hunt accessible computer game. The issues to be investigated in the experiments are listed below:

- comparing the two different sound rendering techniques;
- investigating the effectiveness of the force feedback features;
- acquiring players' comments on the game.

The experiments were divided into two parts: (1) with sighted people, (2) with blind and visually impaired people. Conducting experiments with sighted people had several advantages. It was used as a pilot study so that bugs and problems of the game could be revealed and experimental procedure could be verified. Moreover, the results obtained from sighted people could act as a reference when analysing blind people's results.

In the experiment with sighted people, a between group test was conducted. 12 sighted people were recruited and divided evenly into two groups. The first group played the game with static sound rendering and the second group played the game with dynamic sound rendering. The screen was not shown to them so that they had to rely on their sense of hearing and touch just like blind people. With blind people, a within-group test was conducted. 6 blind and visually impaired people were invited to take part in our experiment. They first played the game in static sound condition and then in dynamic sound conditions. Table 14.1 shows the demographics of the blind participants.

Table 14.1. Demographics of blind participants

Player number	Age	Gender	Blindness	Computer Experience	Education
1	58	female	registered blind	Very low	secondary school
2	52	female	blind	medium	secondary school
3	23	male	blind	medium	secondary school
4	16	female	blind	high	secondary school
5	27	male	blind	medium	secondary school
6	22	male	blind	high	higher education

During the experiment, players were asked to shoot as many ducks as they could. There was a one-minute time limit. Before the experiment, they were given a training session in which they could become familiar with the game and the control interface. The training usually lasted about 10-15 minutes. In the experiment, they were asked to play the game three times in each sound condition. The score of each game was recorded. Afterwards, the players filled in a questionnaire. The questionnaire asked players about 3 aspects: (1) usefulness of the sound rendering, (2) effectiveness of the force feedback, (3) areas for improvement. After players finished the experiment, they undertook a NASA TLX assessment to show the workload they experienced. The TLX asked players to give a rating between 0-20 to indicate their workload experienced during the experiment (Hart & Wicken, 1990). It is a subjective test as ratings are all depend on players experience in the experiment. The workload consists of the following categories: mental demand, physical demand, temporal demand, effort, performance, and frustration level. An overall workload index was calculated based on the ratings on the six categories.

14.3.2. Experiment Results (Sighted Players)

The results of the experiment with 6 sighted people in the static sound rendering condition are listed in Table 14.2. The average score of the three attempts is calculated for each player. The overall average score of the 6 players is 1.94 which means that players managed to shoot 2 ducks in the game with static sound rendering.

Table 14.2. Results of sighted people in static and dynamic sound conditions

Player no.	Static sound rendering				Dynamic sound rendering			
	1st Score	2nd Score	3rd Score	Average	1st Score	2nd Score	3rd Score	Average
1	1	3	2	2	3	5	4	4
2	3	3	4	3.33	2	2	4	2.67
3	0	2	2	1.33	3	4	6	4.33
4	1	1	4	2	5	6	4	5
5	2	1	4	2.33	6	8	9	7.67
6	1	0	1	0.67	4	4	7	5
	Overall Average			1.94	Overall Average			4.78

The results of 6 sighted people in the dynamic sound rendering condition are also listed in Table 14.1. The overall average score of 6 players is 4.78 which is higher than the group which undertook the static sound condition.

The simplified version of NASA TLX assessment was performed to obtain the workload of each player. A summary of the results are given in Figure 14.2. The overall average workload in the static and dynamic sound condition is 16.93 and 14.8 respectively. (The ratings of the performance have been removed from the data set because some blind players misunderstood its definition. The new workload index is calculated based on the ratings of the other categories.)

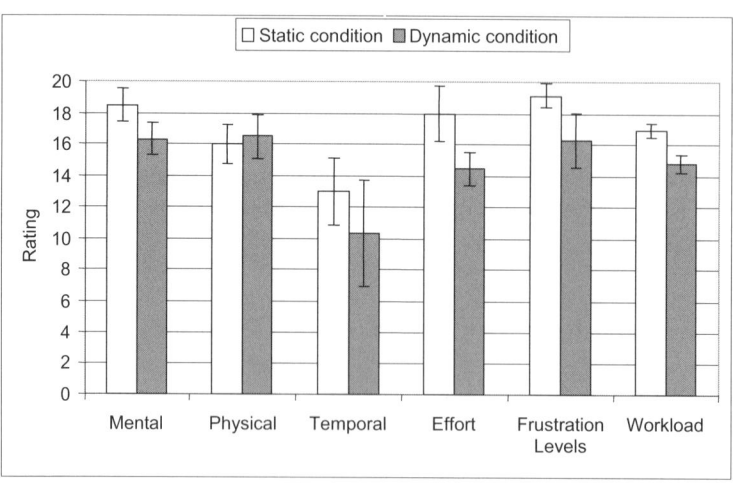

Figure 14.2. Sighted players' workload index in the static and dynamic sound conditions

14.3.2. Experiment Results (Blind Players)

Six blind people played the game in both static and dynamic sound rendering conditions. Their scores of the games are listed in Table 14.3. The overall average score of the players in the static and dynamic conditions was 3.28 and 4.28 respectively.

The blind players also undertook the NASA TLX assessment. The results show that the overall average workload experienced by the players in the static and dynamic sound condition is 10.2 and 9 respectively. The average distribution of the workload index is given in Figure 14.3.

Table 14.3. Results of blind people in static and dynamic sound condition

Player number	Static sound rendering				Dynamic sound rendering			
	1ˢᵗ Score	2ⁿᵈ Score	3ʳᵈ Score	Average	1ˢᵗ Score	2ⁿᵈ Score	3ʳᵈ Score	Average
1	3	2	2	2.33	3	2	4	3
2	2	2	1	1.67	2	0	1	1
3	5	5	2	4	3	2	2	2.33
4	4	3	2	3	7	4	5	5.33
5	2	5	2	3	8	8	7	7.67
6	5	7	5	5.67	6	7	6	6.33
	Overall Average			3.28	Overall Average			4.28

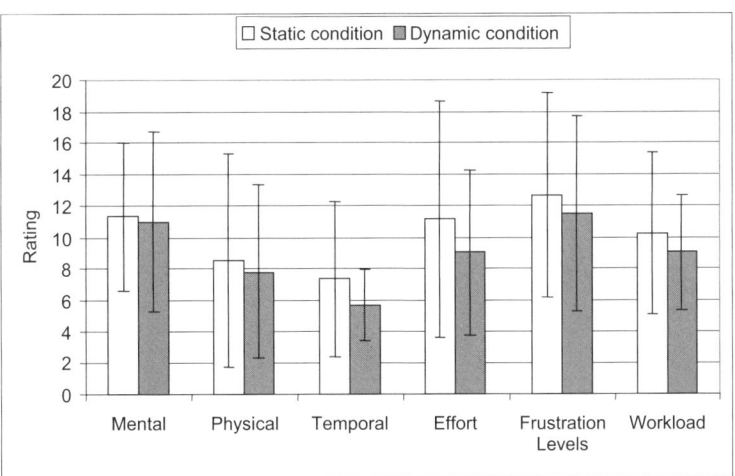

Figure 14.3. Blind players' workload index in the static and dynamic sound conditions

14.3.3. Discussion

Sighted players' performance shows the advantages of dynamic sound rendering technique even though there are not enough data to conduct the significance test. The group who played the game in the dynamic sound condition could shoot a minimum of 2 ducks and maximum of 9 ducks whereas the other group could only get from 0 to 4 ducks in the static sound condition. The players' comments on the sound rendering confirm the results. Comments from the dynamic group overwhelmingly praise the usefulness of the sound compared with the comments from the other group. Comments like the following confirm the usefulness of the sound:

> *"You could notice the clear difference in sounds if you were far away from the duck, or if you were near to it. All you had to do from here was to move the mouse up and down to try to find the duck on the Y-axis."*

The workload index shows that the first group of sighted players (static condition) also needs to work slightly harder than the second group (dynamic condition). There is an exception on the physical demand where the second group gave higher ratings. This may be due to players being able to move the mouse more in the dynamic sound condition in order to pin point the duck. Overall, the dynamic sound rendering does provide a means for players to locate the duck more effectively.

Blind players did the experiments in both static and dynamic conditions. The difference in scores in these two conditions is not as obvious as in the sighted people's case. In average, there is only 1 duck difference and this may due to the learning effect. More exposure to the game may improve players' performance. However, as the sound rendering is very different between the two conditions, the players need some time to adapt to it. Improvement in some players' score may not entirely due to the learning effect. The workload index shows the same trend as the scores.

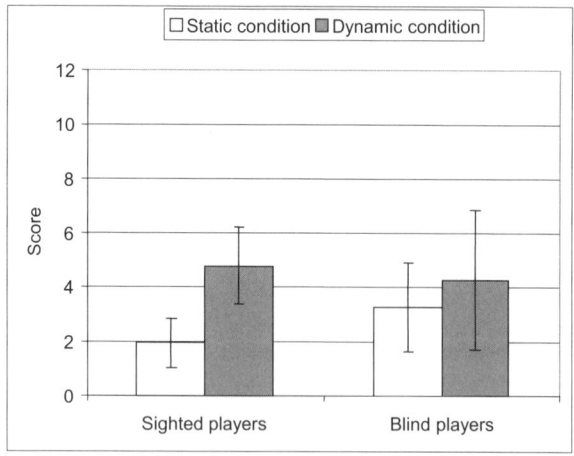

Figure 14.4. Overall scores of sighted and blind players

The results of sighted and blind players are not directly comparable. However it gave us some indication about the difference between these two groups of people (Figure 14.4). In sighted player group, the results are more consistent (small standard deviation), whereas in the blind player group, large values can be seen in the standard deviation. The standard deviation in the workload also exhibits the same trend. It shows that blind people are unique individuals with different levels of visual impairment, computer experience and skills. Quantitative experiments may not be suitable for such evaluation. Individual case study may give evaluators more information about the system.

The comments from blind players on both sound rendering techniques are very positive. They all think that the sounds are useful for them to tell the location of the duck. Only player 5 preferred the static sound over the dynamic sound. However, he shot more ducks in the dynamic sound condition. One player's comments is like "*Sound made the game more fun, easier to line-up the duck, made it more enjoyable, and feel more like a game*". Players also pointed out that there is no altitude information about the duck in the sound. The 'ping' sound sometimes becomes too monotonous. One player liked that there was no background noise in the game while another player prefers to have different sounds to indicate different parts of the screen.

Players gave very good comments on the force feedback features in the game. One player said "*excellent force feedback, enabled me to move around the screen without losing too much position*". Another player said "*first time experienced force feedback. I could get used to it. I liked it compared to other games for the blind which didn't have force feedback*". Force feedback feature is some players' favourite part of the game. With force feedback they definitely know when they are on target.

There are also some interesting findings discovered during the observation of the blind players in the experiment. It is noticed that younger people performed better than older people. They were quicker to grasp the idea of the dynamic sound. In the dynamic condition, players had more interaction than in the static condition. They were able to aim at the duck rather than just shooting around like using a machine gun in the static condition. Force feedback features received much praise from the players but the WingMan Force Feedback mouse actually hindered players' performance due to its very small workspace. A small movement on the mouse would cause a big jump of the cursor on the screen. Therefore, it increased the difficulty when players were searching for the duck.

14.4. Conclusion

The dynamic sound rendering technique allows players to perform better according to the scores achieved by the players and their comments. This sound rendering technique provides more information to the player who can then have more interaction in the game. Blind players enjoyed the game and they like the force feedback features. Combining force feedback and audio allows them to perform the task more easily. They would also like to find that more computer games incorporating force feedback.

The sound needs to be improved so that the altitude information of the duck can be presented to players. This can be done by using Microsoft DirectX 3D sound approach or by simply varying the pitch of the sound. At the current design, global information about the duck is given in the static sound rendering while relative position between the mouse and the duck is presented in the dynamic sound rendering. Actually both of these types of information are useful to assist players to locate moving objects. Therefore, investigation on the methods to combine different sound rendering techniques is required. Moreover, an alternate input device will be used to replace the WingMan Force Feedback mouse due to its limitations. We will experiment with the force feedback joysticks and a P5 gloves with custom-built tactile feedback device because of their larger workspace which can possibly improve players' performance.

Multimodal techniques will be further developed to represent multiple moving objects and movements in 3D. As a result, animated computer graphics, and interactive computer games will become accessible to blind and visually impaired people.

14.5. Acknowledgements

Authors would like to thank the blind people who participated in the experiment as well as Royal National Institute of the Blind (RNIB, NI), The Blind Centre for Northern Ireland (BCNI), Craigavon and Banbridge Community Health and Social Services Trust for recruiting experiment volunteers. Gratitude also goes to Prof. Stephen Brewster at the University of Glasgow for the loan of the Logitech WingMan Force Feedback mouse.

14.6. References

Archambault D, Burger D, Sablé S (2001) The TIM project: Tactile Interactive Multimedia computer games for blind and visually impaired children. In: Proceedings of the AAATE'01 conference, Ljubljana, Slovenia

Hart SG, Wicken SC (1990) Workload assessment and predication, in MANPRINT, an approach to systemsintegration. Van Nostrand Reinhold, New York, USA

Wood J, Magennis M, Francisca E, Arias C, Graupp H, Gutierrez T, Bergamasco M (2003) The design and evaluation of a computer game for the blind in the GRAB haptic audio virtual environment. In: EuroHaptics 2003, Dublin, Ireland

Yu W, Brewster SA (2002) Multimodal virtual reality versus printed medium in visualization for blind people. In: Proceedings of the 5th International ACM SIGCAPH Conference on Assistive Technologies, Edinburgh, Scotland, UK

Chapter 15

Movement Time Prediction for Tasks Assisted by Force-feedback

F. Hwang, S. Keates, P.M. Langdon and
P.J. Clarkson

15.1 Introduction

Movement plays an integral role in human-computer interaction. In particular, mouse movements can occupy as much as 65% of the time spent interacting with a graphical user interface (Johnson *et al.*, 1993). However, for users with impaired motion, symptoms such as tremor, spasm, and co-ordination difficulties can make it often difficult, and sometimes impossible, to perform the movements required to control a mouse accurately (Trewin and Pain, 1999).

Haptic computer interfaces, interfaces that provide users with feedback through the sense of touch, have been investigated as means of improving human-computer interaction. Force feedback gravity wells, i.e. attractive basins that pull the cursor to the centre of an on-screen target, have widely been shown to help users perform "point and click" tasks faster and more accurately (e.g. Hasser *et al.*, 1998; Oakley *et al.*, 2001)

For motion-impaired users, "point and click" times could be reduced by as much as 50% with gravity well assistance (Keates *et al.*, 2000). These studies typically involve the comparison of a "force feedback" and a "no force feedback" condition, with parameters such as target distance, target width, and gravity well width remaining constant.

However, an understanding of how the limits and capabilities of human movement vary when these parameters change and interact can facilitate the design of improved interfaces and interaction methods.

This chapter investigates the performance of motion-impaired computer users in "point and click" tasks across a range of target distances, target widths, and gravity well widths.

Performance is compared with the predictions of Fitts' Law, which has proven to be a powerful means of predicting movement time in computer interaction, and of evaluating interface designs (e.g. MacKenzie, 1995; McGuffin and Balakrishnan, 2002).

15.2 Fitts' Law

Fitts' Law (Fitts, 1954) is an equation predicting movement time from the relationship between target distance and target width. Since the original law was published in 1954, it has undergone a number of refinements. A version commonly used in human-computer interaction research today is the Shannon formulation (MacKenzie, 1995):

$$MT = a + b \times ID \tag{15.1}$$

where a and b are constants, MT is the movement time, and ID is the index of difficulty:

$$ID = \log_2\left(\frac{A}{W} + 1\right) \tag{15.2}$$

where A is the distance or amplitude of the movement and W is the target width.

According to Fitts' Law, different combinations of A and W giving the same ID should result in similar task completion times.

For example, reducing the distance to the target by half should give the same performance increase as doubling the width of the target. At a given ID, only random effects should differentiate the times, and there should be no systematic effects of A nor W (MacKenzie, 1991).

15.3 Experiment

An experiment was conducted to investigate the performance of motion-impaired computer users in "point and click" tasks across a range of target distances, target widths, and gravity well widths.

The questions to be addressed are as follows:

- How well are movements for non-force feedback tasks described by Fitts' Law?
- Are the effects of distance and target width equivalent?
- If the movements for non-force feedback tasks can be predicted with Fitts' Law, can the effect of gravity wells be described using the same paradigm?
- When gravity wells are active, a spring force pulls the cursor to the centre of the target. Does the target width then become irrelevant?
- If the movements for non-force feedback tasks can be predicted with Fitts' Law, how do performance improvements obtained by increasing target width compare with improvements obtained by using gravity wells?

15.3.1 Method

Participants. Six volunteers with motion-impairments participated in the study. The group represented a wide range of capabilities, exhibiting symptoms including tremor, co-ordination difficulties, stiffness, numbness, and reduced dexterity in the dominant hand and arm. The users were affected by Cerebral Palsy (3), Friedrich's ataxia (1), head injury (1), and spinal infection (1).

Task. Users performed a discrete, "point and click" task using a Logitech Wingman force feedback mouse for input. This device can generate a wide range of haptic effects, including vibro-tactile sensations and directional forces. Users were presented with a black "X" ("radius" = 20 pixels) on the screen and asked to move the cursor to it (Figure 15.1). When the cursor came within 20 pixels of the centre of the "X", the target appeared to the right of the "X" at the same height, represented as a white circle with a black outline. Users had to hold the cursor over the "X" for two seconds in order for the trial to begin. If the cursor moved farther than 20 pixels from the centre of the "X" before the two second dwell period was over, the target disappeared and the task began again. To assist the user during this "dwelling" portion of the task, the "X" sat at the centre of a gravity well with a radius twice that of the "X". The extent of the gravity well was indicated with a grey circle.

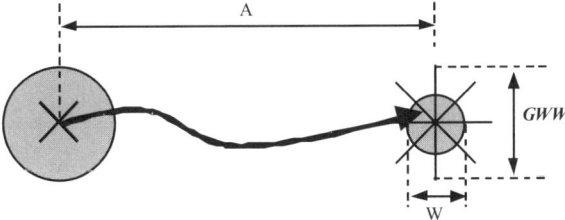

Figure 15.1. The display for the "point and click" task.

Once the cursor had successfully dwelt over the start point for the two second period, the colour of the target changed from white to red. When target selection was assisted with a gravity well, the extent of the gravity well was also indicated with eight "spokes" that radiated out from the centre of the target. Users had to move the cursor to the target and select it by clicking the left mouse button.

A trial was defined to begin after the dwell period had passed, i.e. once the target became "active", and to end after the target had been successfully selected. The time to complete each trial, the number of mouse clicks in each trial, and the cursor position throughout the trial were automatically logged.

Design. The experiment was a 4×3×5 factorial within-subjects design. The factors and levels were as follows:

- distance to target, *A*   {125, 250, 500, 750} pixels;

- target width, W {20, 40, 80} pixels;
- gravity well width, GWW {0, 20, 40, 80, 160} pixels.

The distance, A, was defined to be the distance between the centres of the "X" and the target (Figure 15.1). As the start point was the same for every trial, A was varied by moving the target closer and farther from the "X". Trials with $GWW = 0$ were not assisted by any force feedback at all. For trials where $GWW > 0$, when the cursor entered the gravity well, a spring force pulled the cursor toward the centre of the target. The resolution of the 14.1" display used was 1024 by 768.

Trials were carried out in blocks, each block consisting of the 20 A-GWW combinations appearing in random order as W remained constant. The presentation of W values between blocks was varied to counter order effects.

15.3.2 Results

The No-force Feedback Condition. Considering first the conditions in which tasks are performed without any force feedback, i.e. all A-W combinations with $GWW = 0$, Figure 15.2 shows the average task completion time for the users plotted against the index of difficulty, ID, as defined in Equation 15.2. The data yield a regression line (Equation 15.1) with movement time in seconds predicted as

$$MT = 0.558 + 0.887 \times ID \tag{15.3}$$

with a correlation of r = 0.896 (F = 40.7, p < 0.01). Correlations above 0.900 are considered very high for experiments involving measurements on human subjects (MacKenzie, 1995), so Fitts' Law gives a good description of how overall times observed for these motion-impaired users relate to the index of difficulty, when all A-W combinations are considered together as a group.

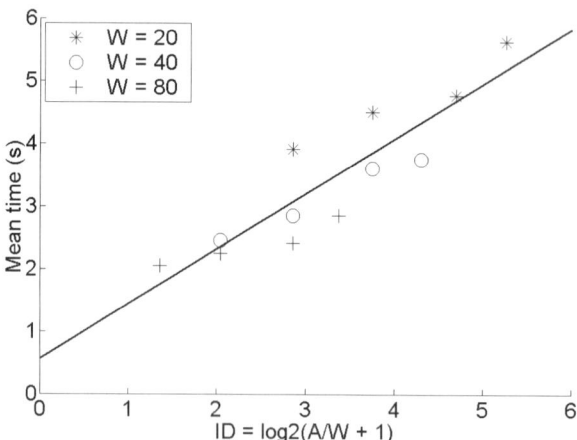

Figure 15.2. A Fitts' Law regression line for conditions where GWW=0.

However, contrary to the behaviour predicted by Fitts' Law, the data within the group also give evidence of a systematic effect of A and W. At a given ID, bigger targets are selected faster than smaller targets.

The relative impact of these two variables are further illustrated in Figure 15.3, which shows how time increases with A and the reciprocal of W, where A and W are plotted on logarithmic scales. The trends indicated by the tops of the bars suggest that changes in W have roughly twice the effect on times than changes in A. For example, doubling the target width gives twice the time improvement compared with halving the distance to the target. In contrast, Fitts' Law predicts that doubling the target width and halving the distance should have an equivalent effect on movement time.

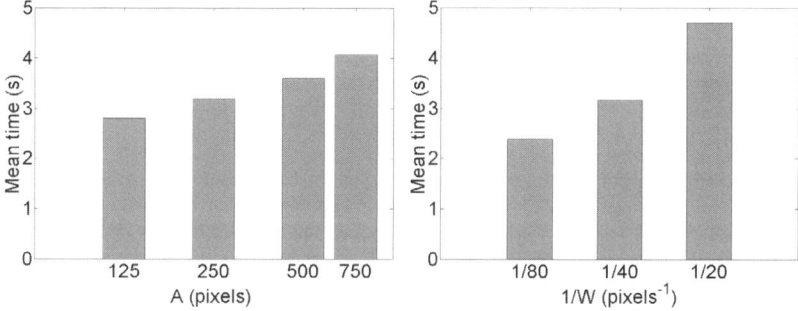

Figure 15.3. Time increases with A and the reciprocal of W (x-axes are logarithmic).

Despite the unequal scaling of amplitude and width effects, Fitts' Law gives a good description of behaviour when all A-W combinations are considered together, and thereby provides a useful means for evaluating the effects of force feedback gravity wells. Comparisons of performance across different sizes of gravity wells are reported in the next section.

The Force Feedback Condition. Study participants performed all A-W combinations of the task with different gravity well widths, GWW. Figure 15.4 shows the Fitts' Law regression lines for the five values of GWW, where $GWW = 0$ represents the condition performed without any force-feedback assistance. For clarity, only the data points for $GWW = 0$ and $GWW = 160$ are shown. Figure 15.4 shows the following:

- For ID greater than approximately 1.6, the lines for $GWW > 0$ all fall below that of $GWW = 0$. In other words, at a given ID in this range, a gravity well of any of the sizes studied here will reduce the task completion time.
- There is a general trend for the slopes of the regression lines to decrease with increasing GWW. In other words, as the gravity well size increases, task difficulty has a lesser impact on performance.
- The distance between $GWW = 0$ and the other regression lines increases with ID. In other words, the more difficult the task, the more benefit is received from the gravity wells.

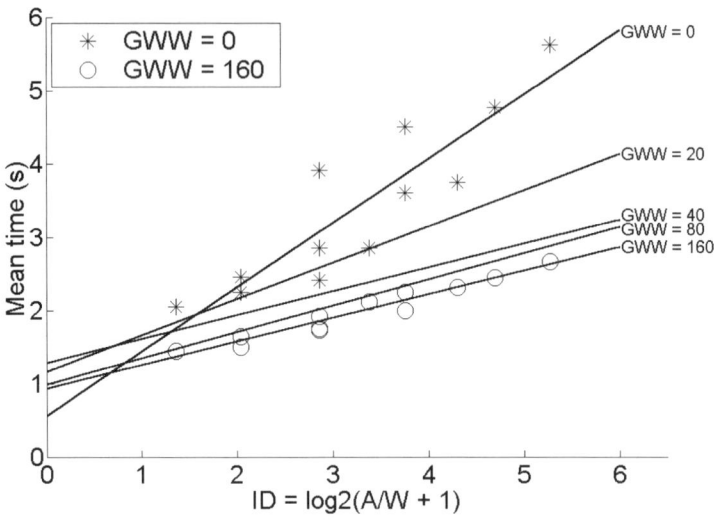

Figure 15.4. Fitts' Law regression lines for five gravity well sizes.

Further insights can be gained by studying the interaction between target width, W, and gravity well width, GWW, at a single value of distance, A. Figure 15.5 shows the W by GWW interaction when $A = 500$. There is a clear separation between the three lines representing the different W values, indicating that the presence of a gravity well does not *eliminate* the effect of W on performance. However, as the separation between the lines decreases in the presence of a gravity well, the force feedback effect does *reduce* the effect of W. This is consistent with the decreasing slopes shown in Figure 15.4.

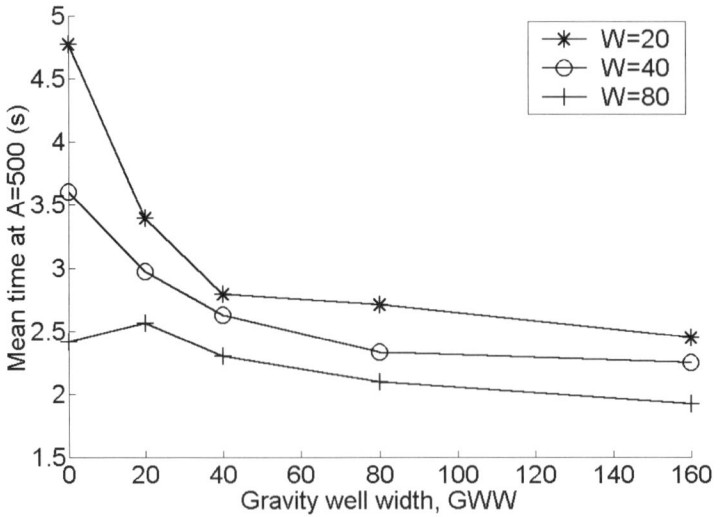

Figure 15.5. The interaction between target width, W, and gravity well width, GWW, at a distance of $A = 500$.

Figure 15.5 also provides a means of comparing the benefits of increasing the target width against the benefits of using a force feedback gravity well. This can help answer questions such as, "Is having a gravity well twice the width of the target equivalent to doubling the target width?"

The plot shows that for a *GWW-W* combination of 40-20, performance is approximately 0.8s faster than for a *GWW-W* combination of 0-40. In this case, having a gravity well twice the width of the target is considerably *better* than doubling the target width. However, for a *GWW-W* combination of 80-40, performance is just 0.08s faster than for a *GWW-W* combination of 0-80. Again, we see that the degree of benefit provided by the gravity wells varies with the task difficulty.

15.3.3 Modifying Fitts' Law

The preceding sections have shown that for tasks assisted by force feedback gravity wells, movement time is affected not only by *A* and *W*, but also by *GWW*. However, a model of the relationship among time and these three factors remains to be defined. In this section, a potential method of modifying Fitts' Law to include *GWW* is proposed.

Figure 15.4 illustrates that the data are described by a series of Fitts' Law regression lines, one for each value of *GWW*. Movement time may then be represented as:

$$MT = a' + b' \times ID \tag{15.4}$$

where *ID* is the index of difficulty unchanged from Equation 15.2, but the slope and intercept, a' and b', are now also dependent on the value of *GWW*. If the relationships between a' and *GWW* and between b' and *GWW* (Figure 15.6) can be modelled, Equation 15.4 may then be rewritten to express movement time as a function of *A, W*, and *GWW*. This approach to reformulating Fitts' Law is currently being investigated.

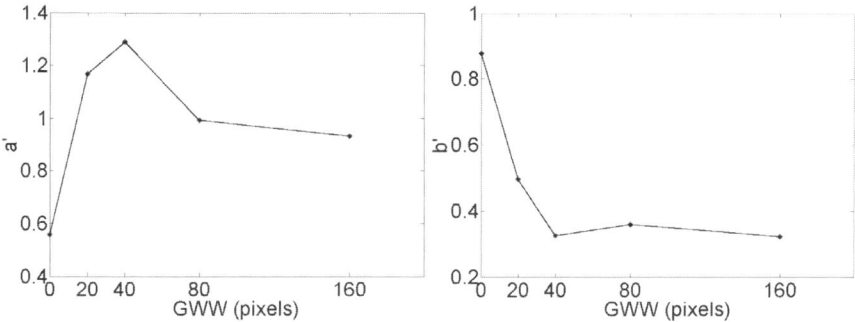

Figure 15.6. This figure illustrates how the intercepts and the slopes, a' and b' of the Fitts' Law regression lines shown in Figure 15.4 vary with gravity well width, *GWW*.

15.3.4 Discussion

For tasks performed without any force feedback, this study has shown that Fitts'
Law gives a good description of the overall times observed in this group of motion-
impaired users when all A-W combinations are considered together. However, this
is not to say that the underlying process responsible for generating these times is
the same for motion-impaired users as it is for non-impaired users. On the contrary,
cursor trajectory analysis has shown that the cursor movements of these two groups
of users differ in a number of ways, including more target re-entries, sub-
movements, and high curvature segments observed for the motion-impaired group
(Hwang et al., 2002).

The values of a and b in Equation 15.1 obtained from the experimental data
also suggest that the underlying movement process for motion-impaired users is
different from that of able-bodied users. Values for a for b in this study were 0.558
s and 0.887 s respectively, whereas values reported in the literature for studies
involving non-impaired users are around 0.5 s and 0.104 s (MacKenzie, 2003).
This indicates that motion-impaired users are affected by increasing task difficulty
roughly $0.887/0.104 = 8.5$ times more than able-bodied users. However, a theory to
explain this behaviour predicted by Fitts' Law is a topic that requires further
investigation.

Results of this study have also indicated that changes in W have roughly twice
the effect on times than changes in A. Studies of cursor behaviours can help
explain this. Motion-impaired users can sometimes navigate the cursor more or less
directly to the target, then experience a great deal of difficulty stabilising the cursor
inside the target for a successful selection (Hwang, 2002). The total task
completion time can consequently be dominated by the latter, which in turn is
directly affected by the target width.

For tasks performed with force feedback gravity wells, at any given ID greater
than approximately 1.6, a gravity well of any of the sizes used in this study will
reduce the task completion time. The regression lines in Figure 15.4 also predict
that for ID less than 1.6, performance with gravity wells can be worse than
performance without any force feedback. This may be partially explained by
considering the mechanical properties of the force feedback mouse. Take, for
example, the case where $A = W/2$ and $ID = \log_2(1.5) = 0.6$. In this case, the starting
point of the task lies at the edge of the target. With the spring force of a gravity
well acting on the mouse, the mouse gathers a certain amount of momentum, and
has a tendency to "ricochet" for a period of time before the cursor settles at the
target's centre and is sufficiently steady for the selection to be performed. This
"ricochet" period may be longer than the time required to select the target from a
point just inside the target's edge.

An improved understanding of the effects of target distance, target width,
gravity well width, and their interactions can lead to the development of tools to
assist interface designers. From Figure 15.5 for example, a designer is able to
predict the outcome of a decision to use a certain GWW-W combination.
Alternatively, faced with a constraint, for example that average movement times
should be faster than 2.5s, certain GWW-W combinations can be ruled out, leaving
the designer to choose only from viable alternatives. By defining a mathematical

relationship among *A*, *W*, and *GWW*, for example through a modification of Fitts' Law, one can provide designers with a means of evaluating novel interfaces based on predicted performance.

The benefit of such a model lies also the fact that it can be calibrated, for example, for a particular level of capability or for a particular input device. Although the current analysis has focussed on identifying general performance trends across participants, important differences among the users were also observed. For example, although Fitts' Law provided a good description of the performance of each of the study participants, the slopes of the individual regression lines ranged from 0.280 to 2.376 when *GWW*= 0.

Also, although the slope of the Fitts' Law regression line was generally observed to decrease with increasing *GWW*, the degree of benefit was observed to be greatest for the most impaired users. Similarly, performance differences can exist between input devices. The current study involved using a Logitech Wingman force feedback mouse, whose limited workspace and transfer function will have a particular effect on performance.

Although the trends shown in Figure 15.4 would be expected for gravity wells implemented on an alternative force feedback device, the parameters of the regression lines may differ. With parameters that can be adjusted to match the characteristics of a particular user and of a particular input device, a model relating performance to *A*, *W*, and *GWW* may form the basis for the development of perceptive user interfaces that can respond automatically to user needs.

15.4 Conclusion

This chapter has described an experiment to investigate the performance of motion-impaired computer users in "point and click" tasks across a range of target distances, target widths, and gravity well widths. To conclude, the questions posed at the start of the experiment are re-addressed:

- Fitts' Law gives a good description of the *overall* behaviour observed for these motion-impaired users performing the task with no force feedback.
- However, contrary to Fitts' Law, changes in target width have roughly twice the effect of changes in distance. For a given index of difficulty, bigger targets are better, even though they are located farther away.
- Force feedback gravity wells reduce the slope of the Fitts' Law regression line, thereby increasing performance and reducing the effect of task difficulty on time.
- A gravity well does not *eliminate* the effect of *W* but does *reduce* the effect of *W* on performance.
- For difficult tasks, performance improvements gained from using gravity wells are *better* than performance improvements gained from using larger targets. However, the difference between the two methods is reduced as the task becomes easier.

15.5 Acknowledgements

The authors thank the volunteers and staff of the Papworth Trust. This work is funded by the Canadian Cambridge Trust, NSERC, and the EPSRC.

15.6 References

Fitts PM (1954) The information capacity of the human motor system in controlling the amplitude of movement. Journal of Experimental Psychology 47: 381-391

Hasser C, Goldenberg A, Martin K, Rosenberg L (1998) User performance in a GUI pointing task with a low-cost force feedback computer mouse. In: Proceedings of the ASME Dynamic Systems and Control Division. American Society of Mechanical Engineers, USA

Hwang F (2002) A study of cursor trajectories of motion-impaired users. In: Extended Abstracts of CHI 2002 (Minneapolis, MN). ACM, New York, NY

Hwang F, Langdon P, Keates S, Clarkson PJ, Robinson P (2002) Cursor characterisation and haptic interfaces for motion-impaired users. In: Universal Access and Assistive Technology. Springer-Verlag, London, UK

Johnson, PW, Hewes J, Dropkin J, Rempel DM (1993) Office ergonomics: motion analysis of computer mouse usage. In: Proceedings of the American Industrial Hygiene Association. Fairfax, VA

Keates S, Langdon P, Clarkson J, Robinson P (2000) Investigating the use of force feedback for motion-impaired users. In: Proceedings of the 6th ERCIM Workshop, Florence, Italy

MacKenzie, IS (1991) Fitts' law as a performance model in human-computer interaction. Doctoral dissertation. University of Toronto: Toronto, Ontario, Canada

MacKenzie, IS (1995) Movement time prediction in human-computer interfaces. In: Readings in human-computer interaction, Kaufmann, Los Altos, CA, pp 483-493

MacKenzie IS, Soukoreff RW (2003) Card, English, and Burr (1978) – 25 years later. In: Extended Abstracts of CHI 2003 (Ft. Lauderdale, FL). ACM, New York, NY, pp 760-761

McGuffin M, Balakrishnan R (2002) Acquisition of expanding targets. In: Proceedings of CHI 2002, Minneapolis, MN. ACM, New York, NY

Oakley I, McGee MR, Brewster SA, Gray PD (2000) Putting the feel in look and feel. In: Proceedings of CHI 2000, The Hague. ACM, New York, NY

Trewin S, Pain H (1999) Keyboard and mouse errors due to motor disabilities. International Journal of Human-Computer Studies 50(2): 109-144

Chapter 16

Recognising Expression in Speech for Human Computer Interaction

T.S. Shikler and P. Robinson

16.1 Introduction

Human-computer interaction and human-human communication via computer interfaces have become a major part of our lives, but still lack the basic means of recognising and responding to non-verbal cues of attitudes, emotions and mental states, that we take for granted in human communication. They fail to appreciate the users' reactions and intentions. This problem is more acute in speech interfaces, used by the general population and specifically by people with degraded motor abilities. In these systems speech is used to convey commands and data, while natural behaviour also uses speech for thinking out loud, expressions of frustration, misunderstanding, discomfort, and more. Most of these functions relate to nuances of expressions, and some of them are obvious only in speech.

Several studies have considered social aspects of computer use. Nass (1996) found that people interact with computers the same way they interact with each other. Picard (2001; 2002) surveyed human emotional needs and recommended the development of human computer interface (HCI) applications that support these needs, both in human-computer interfaces and in computer-mediated interfaces (human-machine-human interactions). The performance of computer interfaces can be improved by recognising human emotions and mental states.

There have been considerable advances in the field of automated affective speech analysis recently. Most research in this field is analysis of basic and extreme emotions like joy, anger, sadness, fear, disgust and surprise (Lisetti, 2000; Oudeyer, 2003; Yacoob, 1994). A few other mental states like stress, frustration and depression have also been investigated in the context of automated systems (Cohn, 1998; Fernandez, 2003; Guojun, 1998; Klein, 2002). Several projects have tried to map additional emotions according to their prosody and articulation characteristics (Cornelius, 2003; Cowie, 2001; Scherer, 2000).

However, expressions in general, mental states, behavioural patterns, attitudes and personality traits have not been thoroughly investigated. Indeed the only expressions and emotions related to HCI tasks and environments that have been studied is frustration.

In this work we examine part of the large variety of expressions evoked by HCI tasks. We show that these expressions are separable by analysis of non-verbal speech cues. These expressions relate to subtle emotions, attitudes, and mental states, such as uncertainty and enthusiasm, that have not been investigated before.

The inference of such expressions may contribute not only to better dictation and other speech-dependent computer interaction systems, but also to the development of a large variety of aids such as feedback systems that allow people to learn, improve, or practice communication skills, for example people with hearing disorders, people who have communication deficiencies, and even interview skills, negotiation or lecturing skills. Other applications include remote diagnosis of extreme situations and mental states, and voice activated remote controls for people who have limited speech ability.

The investigation of such expressions requires a body of test data. Section 16.2 describes the recording set-up for the Doors database, a multi-modal database of naturally evoked data in an HCI task. Section 16.3 outlines the speech analysis and focuses on feature extraction. Some experimental results are presented in Section 16.4, and Section 16.5 concludes with a discussion and suggestions for future work.

16.2 Reference Data

A major challenge in this research area is the lack of conventional, public databases of naturally evoked, labelled expressions databases, both for single mode and for multi-modal analysis. This shortage requires each group or researcher to construct a new database. Therefore, the findings are not easily translated from one work to another, and it does not allow comparison among the performances of different systems.

Many works are based on staged expressions or read paragraphs, using actors (Petrushin, 1999). Another approach is to collect emotional episodes from films (Polzin, 2000; Yan Li, 2001). Several speech databases include nonsense speech, trying to eliminate the effect of text. Most of these databases focus on Ekman's 'basic emotions' (Ekman, 1999), or on other small sets of extreme emotions.

The problem is that extreme emotions are rare in everyday life; nuances are common, everyday expressions may include a mixture of intentions, mental states and emotions. In addition, staged expressions are different from real expressions; an example is the difference between a facial expression of smile and an expression of happiness.

Several approaches for eliciting natural or natural-like emotions have been developed. The first method, and the most natural is to use recordings of people in real situations, for example during telephone dialogues, or pilots during flight. A different method is to use photographs, film episodes or music that elicit certain emotions, and record people while watching or hearing them (Cohn, 1998). This method is used mainly for facial expression recordings. Another method is to give people a certain task and record them while doing it. For example a frustrating computer game (Klein, 2002), solving mathematical problems while driving for stress investigation (Fernandez, 2003) or asking young mothers to perform a certain task with their babies (Moore, 1994). This method provides the researchers with more control on the content and the setting.

A common problem to all these methods is the association of names or labels to the recorded expressions. In many cases, under one definition of an expression, many sub expressions may be defined (Wierzbicka, 2000), for example, different types of anger. Mixtures of expressions and emotions and different valence also pose a problem. In addition, most of the databases include only one modality, elicit a small variety of expressions, consider time-discrete events, and are proprietary.

The first stage of this research was to define and record a new database of naturally invoked expressions.

16.2.1 The Doors Database:

The Doors database was constructed in collaboration with the Psychology and Bio-Engineering Departments in Tel Aviv University. Our aim was to record a multi-modal database of naturally evoked expressions in a controlled set-up, to facilitate the analysis of each modality and of the combination of modalities. The database consists of recordings of people engaged in a human-computer task. The task is a computer game designed to evoke emotions and expressions, based of Damasio's cards experiment (Bechara, 1997). The participants group included 15 Hebrew speakers, both male and female; the range of ages was 24 to over 50. The recording system set-up is described in Figure 16.1.

The video records of facial expressions include painted dots on the participants faces to avoid the problem of tracking pose changes during analysis. The speech consists of two repeated sentences, forming a corpus of 200 sentences for each participant, in addition to free speech sessions. The same sentence was repeated in order to allow extraction of features that are only related to expressions, eliminating differences due to textual content. The electrocardiogram (ECG), galvanic skin response (GSR) and blood volume in the periphery were also measured. In addition, the database includes the number and rate of mouse movements, calculated by the game program, and the records of the participants' actions and the corresponding results. These measurements and recordings allow comparison among modalities; it gives a measure of arousal and explanation to the recorded expressions.

The database was labelled manually to include the names of the emotions, attitudes or mental states that are associated with the expressions. However, the various kinds of information reveal significant events and expressions. In addition, we plan to undertake a psycho-acoustic test to confirm the labelling. This database does not reflect the whole spectrum of human expressions. It includes a small set of expressions, in a specific kind of HCI application. It focuses on nuances and on temporal changes, which have not been thoroughly investigated yet. Another drawback, from the processing point of view, is the large amount of information; the raw data requires a lot of pre-processing before any analysis can be run on it.

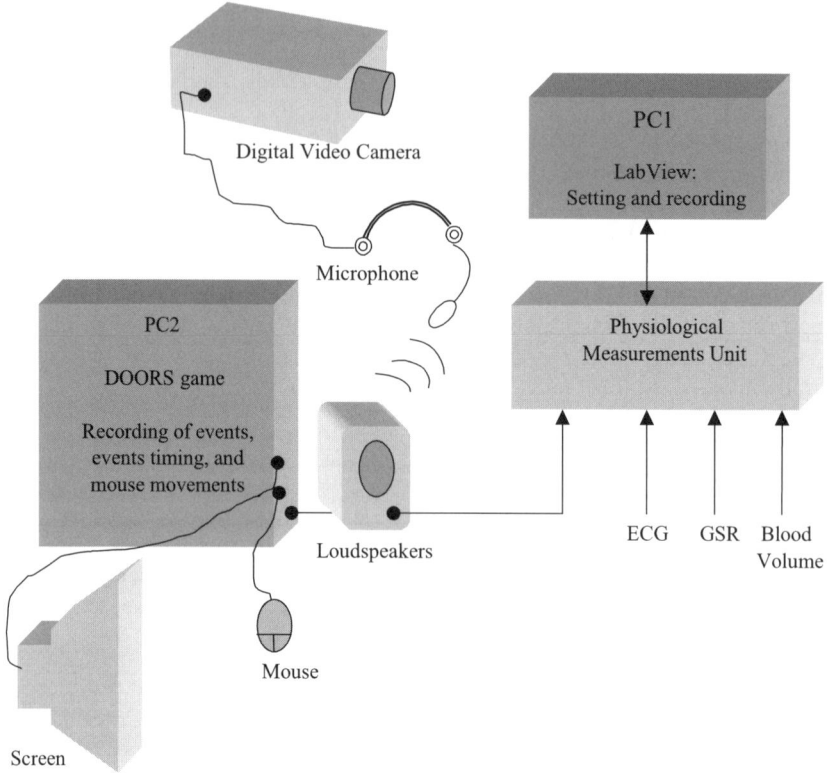

Figure 16.1. Database Set-up: video camera, microphone, a system for measurements of physiological cues, together with a PC running the computer game, which controls the loudspeakers, used for synchronisation.

For example, the video recordings of facial expressions run continuously for 15 minutes, while many vision research groups still struggle with discrete streams of 2-3 seconds.

The method chosen for segmentation of the speech signals into sentences was based on the modified Entropy-based Endpoint Detection for noisy environments, described by Shen (1998). In order to include end-points we used zero-crossing rate calculation (Deller, 1993) at the edges of the identified sentences. This method yielded very good results, recognising most speech segments (95%) for male participants and eliminating most of the noise segments, but it requires different parameters for men and for women.

16.3 Feature Extraction

One of the goals of our research is to identify the features that differentiate expressions, nuances of expressions, and specify temporal changes in expressions, for both analysis and synthesis applications. Unfortunately, the features for speech analysis and especially for prosody analysis are not well defined. For every feature there are multiple definitions and several calculation methods, not all of them yielding the same results. Any classification attempt relies heavily on these results and therefore choosing the features is crucial for the rest of the research.

The central feature for automated recognition of expressions in speech is the intonation (Deller, 1993; Mozziconacci, 2001; Murray, 1993). Intonation refers to patterns of the fundamental frequency, the rate of vocal chord vibrations, usually referred to as pitch.

The analysis of intonation is performed by considering pitch patterns, for which pitch range, height and direction of change are characterized. This relates to the speech rate, i.e. the variations in duration of pronunciation. Other features that signify expressions in speech are the energy, also referred to as intensity, and the spectral content of speech.

Recent research has tried to locate the most significant features in emotional speech, using the characteristics mentioned above and deriving statistical features from them, for further statistical pattern recognition and clustering. For example, Dellaert (1996), found that the most important features were *maximum, minimum,* and *mean* of the pitch, and the *maximum* and the *median* of the smoothed pitch and the *mean positive derivative*. Oudeyer (2003) used another set of 200 features, and later a sub-set of 15, including statistical features of pitch and of intensity of filtered signals.

However, the specific contribution of each feature to expression is still unclear. The determination of features is not well defined and there is no uniform way or a single algorithm to extract each feature. Definitions of time dependencies are still missing.

There are many ways to calculate the pitch (Deller, 1993; Moore, 1994; Zhao, 1999). However, none of these methods is robust. All the methods either generate outliers or fit only a certain range of frequencies. In addition, speaker dependency is a major problem in automatic speech processing. The pitch ranges for different speakers can vary dramatically. It is often necessary to clarify the pitch manually after extraction. In this work, we have used the method described by Boersma (1993). We have adapted the extraction algorithm to extract the pitch automatically for different speakers, using a search limit of twice the mean pitch value of the speech signal.

The calculation of speech rate, which seems to be an intuitive feature, is usually also a derivative of the pitch. There are many different definitions of speech rate in the speech analysis literature; for example: the average length of the voiced part of speech (Dellaert, 1996), or the sum of voiced frames in which the energy is above a threshold, divided by the number of words in the utterance. In this work, we calculate the speech rate as the voiced part of the speech signal divided by the length of the signal. Voiced speech is where the principal pitch is higher than zero and unvoiced is where it equals zero.

Another feature is the intensity of the speech signal, or its energy. Energy in time was calculated as the square of the signal at each point. A smoothed curve of the energy, using average of the energy over a 40 ms time frame, was also calculated.

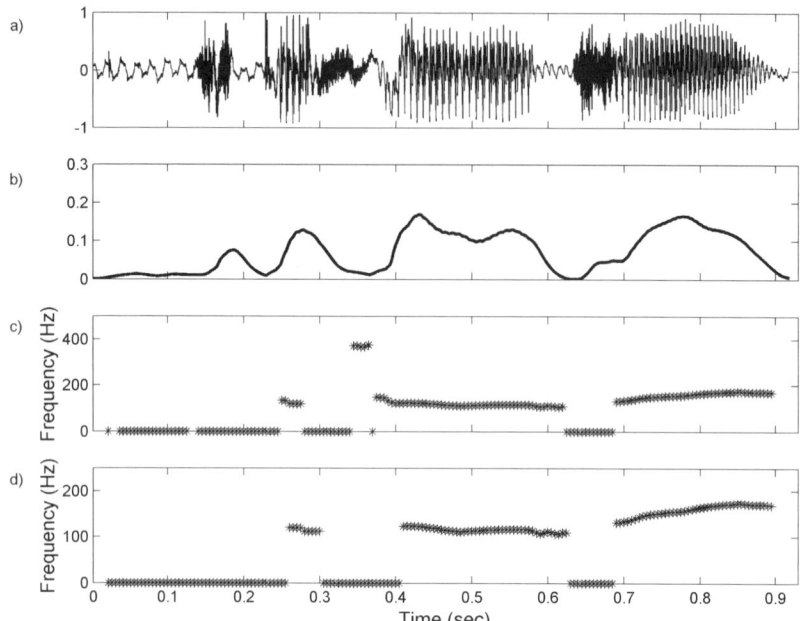

Figure 16.2. Features of a speech signal: a) the speech signal, b) smoothed energy, c) pitch, the frequency bounded to 600 Hz, d) pitch, the frequency bounded to 200 Hz

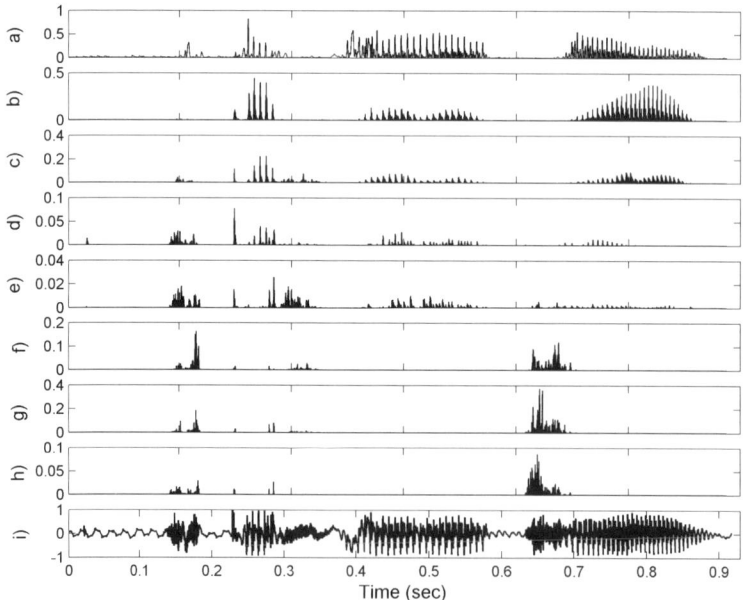

Figure 16.3. Energy in frequency bands 0-500Hz (a), 500-1000Hz, (b) , 1-2KHz (c), 2-3KHz (d), 3-4KHz (e), 4-5KHz (f), 5-7KHz (g), 7-9KHz (h), and the speech signal (i)

Figure 16.2 shows plots of a speech signal uttered by a male speaker, the related smoothed energy curves, and two calculations of the pitch. The first pitch curve was calculated in the range of 75-600 Hz and is not as smooth as the second contour which was calculated in the range of 75-200 Hz. It can also be seen that the energy and pitch events' boundaries occur at different times.

In addition, the energy in eight frequency ranges was extracted using band-pass filters. The ranges of the filters vary with the frequency, narrow windows for low frequencies and wider windows for higher frequencies. We also calculated the relative energy in these bands in comparison with the total energy of the speech signal.

Figure 16.3 shows how the energy is divided among these different frequency bands for the same speech signal.

For each of the extracted features we also calculated statistical features like maximum, range, mean, standard deviation, median, and range, in addition to time related features like distances among extreme points. A set of 80 features was extracted using a MATLAB tool written for this purpose.

16.4 Results

The first stage of analysis is to find significant features that distinguish among different expressions. We have successfully visualised differences among task dependent expressions, in a speaker dependent mode, from the Doors database.

Out of the 6320 possible graphs of all the 80 calculated features coupled with all the other features, we have examined manually over 600 graphs, in order to verify the existence of relevant information in the data. Some of the results can be seen in Figure 16.4

Figure 16.4(a) demonstrates how nuances of expressions from human-computer interactions are separable using non-verbal speech cues. Figure 16.4(b) shows that speech segments related to the same expressions are grouped together, but the distinction among the groups is not always simple because they may be located on continuous scales.

The expressions were labelled by listening to the consecutive sentences. The given labels are: uncertain, testing, cheered (or encouraged), down (meaning remote due to thinking, misunderstanding and maybe disappointment), and vital (or enthusiastic). These labels define subtleties of expressions that have not been examined before.

The labels were found to be highly related to the recorded events. The most significant features found until now are the relative part of the energy in the frequency band of 500-1000 Hz, and the rising slope of the smoothed energy curve, i.e. the length of energy increasing curve relative to the length of the sentence.

Other features are the mean energy in the frequency band of 1-2 kHz and the median of the time intervals among energy maxima points.

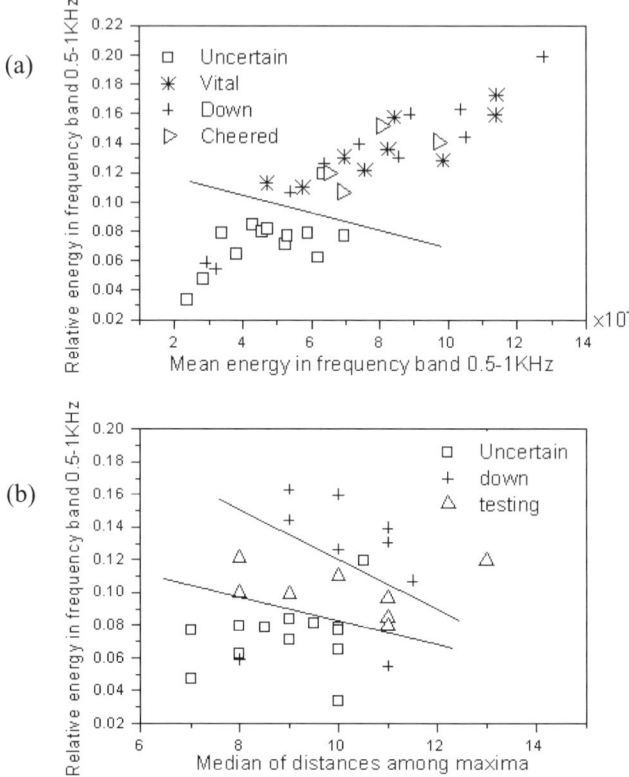

Figure 16.4. (a) The expression of uncertainty separated from the expressions of cheered, down (remote due to thinking, misunderstanding or disappointed) and vital or enthusiastic, by the median of the energy in the frequency band of 500-1000 Hz, and the relative energy in this band. (b) The speech expressions of down, uncertain and testing, divided by the mean energy in the frequency band of 1-2 kHz

16.5 Discussion

We have demonstrated that the situation of human computer interaction evokes a variety of expressions. These expressions are related not only to emotions in the narrow definition of the word, but also to mental states and attitudes. We also showed that these expressions are distinguishable using the non-verbal cues of speech, and in particular energy related features in different frequency ranges. Speech based applications that can recognise these mental states and emotions, and respond to them, by ignoring periods of 'thinking out loud' or speaking with another person while the application is active, can be very helpful. These lower the stress that may arise from the use of insensitive systems, and the lack of other means of interaction, while keeping the cost of the system low, and the set-up simple.

Further investigation should include data mining and learning methods for feature selection. However, these features can give us only the basic idea of where the main information exists. Other speech related features which relay on behaviour in time should also be investigated for better understanding and probably for improved recognition. The recognition of speaker independent expressions using subtle expressions and nuances of expression still poses many problems, both in regard to databases, expressions labelling and analysis. Multimodal analysis is a further step in that direction.

16.6 References

Bechara A, Damasio H, Tranel D, Damasio AR (1997) Deciding advantageously before knowing the advantageous strategy. Science 275(5304): 1293-1295

Boersma P (1993) Accurate short-term analysis of the fundamental frequency and the harmonics-to- noise ratio of a sampled sound. In: Proceedings of the Institute of Phonetic Sciences, Amsterdam

Cohn JF, Katz GS (1998) Bimodal expression of emotion by face and voice. In: Workshop on Face / Gesture Recognition and Their Applications, The Sixth ACM International Multimedia Conference, Bristol, UK

Cornelius R, Cowie R (2003) Describing the emotional states that are expressed in speech. Speech Communication, 59

Cowie R, Douglas-Cowie E, Tsapatsoulis N, Votsis G, Kollias S, Fellenz W, Taylor JG (2001) Emotion recognition in human-computer interaction. IEEE Signal Processing Magazine 18(1): 32-80

Dellaert F, Polzin Th,Waibel A (1996) Recognizing emotions in speech. ICSLP 96

Deller JRJ, Proakis JG, Hansen JHL (1993) Discrete-time processing of speech signals. New York: Macmillan Publishing Company

Ekman P (1999) Basic emotion. In: Handbook of cognition and emotion, Wiley, Chichester, UK

Fernandez R, Picard RW (2003) Modeling drivers' speech under stress. Speech Communication 40: 145-159

Guojun Z, Hansen JHL, Kaiser JF (1998) Classification of speech under stress based on features derived from the nonlinear Teager energy operator. In: Proceedings of the ICASSP '98, New York, USA

Klein J, Moon Y, Picard RW (2002) This computer responds to user frustration: theory, design, and results. Interacting with Computers, 14(2): 119-140

Lisetti CL, Schiano DJ (2000) Automatic facial expression interpretation: Where human-computer interaction, artificial intelligence and cognitive sciences intersect. Pragmatics & cognition, 8(1)

Moore CA, Cohn JF, Katz GS (1994) Quantitative description and differentiation of fundamental frequency contours. Computer Speech & Language, 8(4): 385-404

Mozziconacci SJL (2001) Modeling emotion and attitude in speech by means of perceptually based parameter values. User Modeling & User-Adapted Interaction, 11(4): 297-326

Murray IR, Arnott JL (1993) Toward the simulation of emotion in synthetic speech: a review of the literature on human vocal emotion. Journal of the Acoustical Society of America, 93(2): 1097-1108

Nass B, Reeves C (1996) The media equation. Cambridge University Press, Cambridge, UK

Oudeyer PY, (2003) The production and recognition of emotions in speech: features and algorithms. International Journal of Human Computer Interaction 59(1-2): 157-183

Petrushin V (1999) Emotion in speech: Recognition and application to call centers. Intelligent Engineering Systems Through Artificial Neural Networks, ASME Press

Picard RW, Klein J (2002) Computers that recognise and respond to user emotion: theoretical and practical implications. Interacting with Computers, 14(2): 141-169

Picard RW, Vyzas E, Healey J (2001) Toward machine emotional intelligence: analysis of affective physiological state. IEEE Transactions on Pattern Analysis & Machine Intelligence, 23(10): 1175-1191

Polzin T, Waibel A (2000) Emotion-sensitive human-computer interfaces. In: ISCA Workshop on Speech and Emotion, Belfast, UK

Scherer KR (2000) Emotion effects on voice and speech: Paradigms and approaches to evaluation. In: ISCA Workshop on Speech and Emotion, Belfast, UK

Shen JL, Hung JW, Lee LS (1998) Robust entropy-based endpoint detection for speech recognition in noisy environments. International Conference on Spoken Language Processing, Sydney, Australia

Wierzbicka A (2000) The semantics of human facial expressions. Pragmatics & cognition, 8(1)

Yacoob Y, Davis LS (1994) Recognizing human facial expressions. Image Understanding Workshop. In: Proceedings. San Francisco, CA, USA

Yan Li FY, Ying-Qing X, Chang E, Heung-Yeung S (2001) Speech driven cartoon animation with emotions. In: ACM Multimedia 2001, Ottawa, Canada

Zhao WW, Ogunfunmi T (1999) Formant and pitch detection using time-frequency distribution. International Journal of Speech Technology 3(1): 35-49

Chapter 17

Emotional Hearing Aid: An Assistive Tool for Children with Asperger's Syndrome

R. El Kaliouby and P. Robinson

17.1 Introduction

Children diagnosed with autism, and its milder cousin- Asperger's Syndrome-often have difficulties operating in the highly complex social environment in which we live and are, for the most part, unable to read or understand other people's emotions (e.g. Baron-Cohen, 1995; O'Connell, 1998). Consequently, they need to be taught explicitly how to read other people's minds from non-verbal communication channels such as the face. This chapter reports work in progress on the emotional hearing aid, a portable assistive computer designed to help children with Asperger's Syndrome read and react to facial expressions of the people they interact with.

The chapter starts with a survey of key therapeutic technologies used for autism, and draws attention to the lack of assistive tools for this disorder. Motivated by the need for this type of technology, the emotional hearing aid draws inspiration from the "emotional indexing" method, an approach for teaching children with autism how to read and respond to emotions. This teaching method is introduced in section 17.1.2. An overview of the tool, including typical use-case scenarios, is discussed in Section 17.2, while section 17.3 details the architecture and design of each of the modules. Section 17.4 presents results obtained so far, before section 17.5 concludes this chapter.

17.1.1 Therapeutic Tools for Autism

An increasing number of studies show that computer-aided learning and therapy are well accepted by individuals with Autistic Spectrum Disorders (Moore *et al.*, 2000). Consequently, computing technology is increasingly being used in therapeutic contexts of autism. Mind reading (Baron-Cohen and Tead, 2003) is an interactive guide to learning about emotions, which provides children with a library of over 400 videos and games to test their progress on reading those emotions. Kidtalk (Cheng *et al.*, 2003) is a therapist-moderated online chatting environment, where children work through common social situations, such as going to the movies by chatting online. The virtual sand box (Hirose, 1997) and the environment developed by Strickland (1996) enables children to interact in a virtual setting modelled around real-life social scenarios. The AURORA project (Werry *et al.*, 2001; Dautenhahn and Billard, 2002) utilises an autonomous robot as an interactive toy that can engage children in a therapeutically relevant environment.

The toy is meant to encourage pro-active social behaviours towards the robot, elicit robot-child eye contact, and teach the child the basics of turn-taking and interaction games. Different embodiments of this toy have been investigated including a doll, and a four-wheeled vehicle-like toy.

The affective social quotient project (Blocher, 1999) consists of short digital videos that embody one of several basic emotions and a set of physical "dolls" linked by infrared to the system. The system knows which dolls correspond to which clips, so that the child can explore emotional situations by picking up dolls with certain emotions, or the system can prompt the child to pick up dolls that go with certain clips. Finally, Kozima and Yano (2001) investigate the possibilities of using humanoid robots in therapy.

Those technologies are mostly remedial tools aimed at providing a learning environment to teach children the fundamentals of social behaviour. They do not provide assistance to individuals with autism beyond that gained through teaching. In addition, as they do not operate in a natural human-human interaction environment, they risk failing to generalise (Howlin *et al.*, 1999).

In contrast to existing work, our proposed portable assistive device is designed to assist people diagnosed with autism in real life situations. In a sense, our tool is analogous to a hearing aid, which allows people with hearing problems to communicate with the rest of the world.

17.1.2 Emotional Indexing in Autism

A number of approaches to teaching emotion understanding to children with autism exist. The methods may differ in the amount of structure involved (highly-structured methods use carefully planned teaching material deployed in a relatively controlled environment), the setting in which the teaching takes place (ranges from being hypothetical to being natural), and whether it is interactive or not. One approach, especially suitable for use with children, involves emotional indexing of the child's surrounding environment (Fling, 2000). Typically the child's carer indexes the emotional content of situations as they arise, and suggests possible actions that can be taken by the child. For example "Oh, Mary got hurt. She is crying. Can you tell Mary, 'I am sorry'?" This approach to teaching emotions has been shown to improve the social competence of some children (Fling, 2000; Howlin *et al.*, 1999). In contrary to most other teaching approaches, social indexing works in the child's natural interaction environment reinforcing appropriate social behaviour in a spontaneous setting.

Unfortunately, this method is not always available for the child, as it requires the physical presence of the carer, which in some cases (e.g. school) might be impractical. Also, unlike highly structured approaches, with this method it is almost impossible to recreate events once they have occurred.

17.2 Overview

The emotional hearing aid aims at providing real time assistance with reading facial expressions of other people, and reacting to it in a child's natural social environment. It is designed as a portable assistive device, which consists of a digital camcorder, a personal digital assistant (PDA), and an earpiece speaker.

Figure 17.1 illustrates how the emotional hearing aid provides assistance in a typical interaction scenario between a child with Asperger's Syndrome (character A in the figure) and another person (shown as B). Video sequences of B are sent to the PDA. The PDA is responsible for analysing the incoming video, and any available context cues for mental state information. It also indexes this event for further retrieval, and uses it, along with a repertoire of situations to suggest a course of action. This advice is sent back to the wearer in real time, but continuous feedback is avoided to minimise the number of distractions. Also depending on the level of engagement, the output can be visual or audio, and varies in the degree of detail presented.

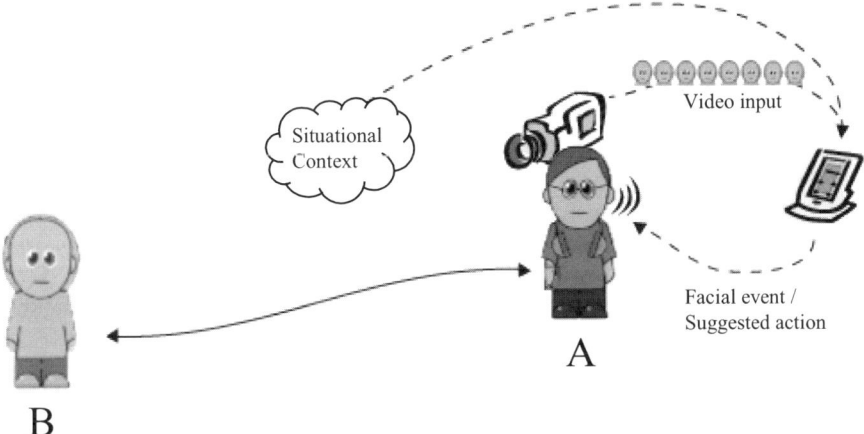

Figure 17.1. A typical interaction scenario

Humans make considerable use of the contexts in which expressions occur to assist interpretation (Bruce and Young, 1998; Edwards, 1998), including situational context. Howlin *et al.* (1999) define situation-based emotions as those that involve inferring a person's emotional state from a particular sequence of events. We thus define several profiles (very much like those used on mobile phones) to indicate the various situations the child is in. Profile information is used along with the input video to boost the reliability of the inference process.

Currently, only simple profiles, such as "in school", or "in playground" are supported, and are explicitly selected. As the tool gets more sophisticated, more detailed profile information would be deduced automatically.

The emotional hearing aid is also designed to work in tandem with the child's carer as shown in Figure 17.2. The carer can define the emotional states the tool can address, can review and update the archived events, and can engage in discussions about past events with the child.

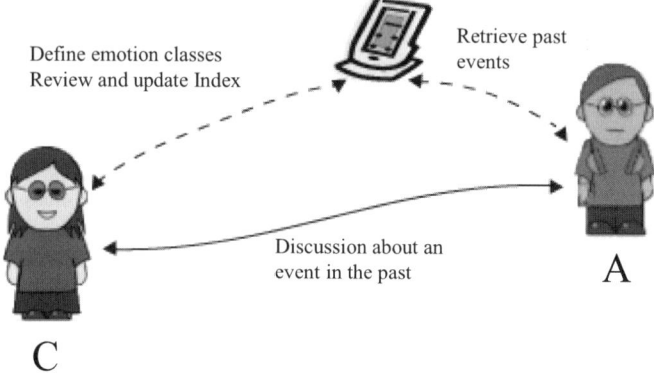

Define emotion classes
Review and update Index

Retrieve past
events

Discussion about an
event in the past

A

C

Figure 17.2. Another interaction scenario

17.3 Architecture and Detailed Design

The main modules of the emotional hearing aid (shown in Figure 17.3) parallel that of the child's carer in emotional indexing. For every incoming video frame, the facial affect analyser identifies facial feature points, and uses their displacements to infer facial actions and head gestures. Those displays are then combined temporally to form micro expressions, a sequence of which portrays a mental state. A representative frame of the mental state, its label, intensity, valence (whether is a positive or negative state), and accompanying context cues are input to the emotional indexer and re-action advisor.

The emotional indexer, responsible for keeping an archive of past events, appends that event to an index, while the re-action advisor appraises the current situation and suggests appropriate courses of actions to take when a similar one arises. The emotional indexing approach also allows events to be re-played. The interface manages the communication between the user and the other modules, namely the action advisor and emotional indexer.

17.3.1 The Facial Affect Analyser

The facial affect analyser extracts facial feature points on the face, and uses that along with colour information to determine facial actions (Figure 17.4).

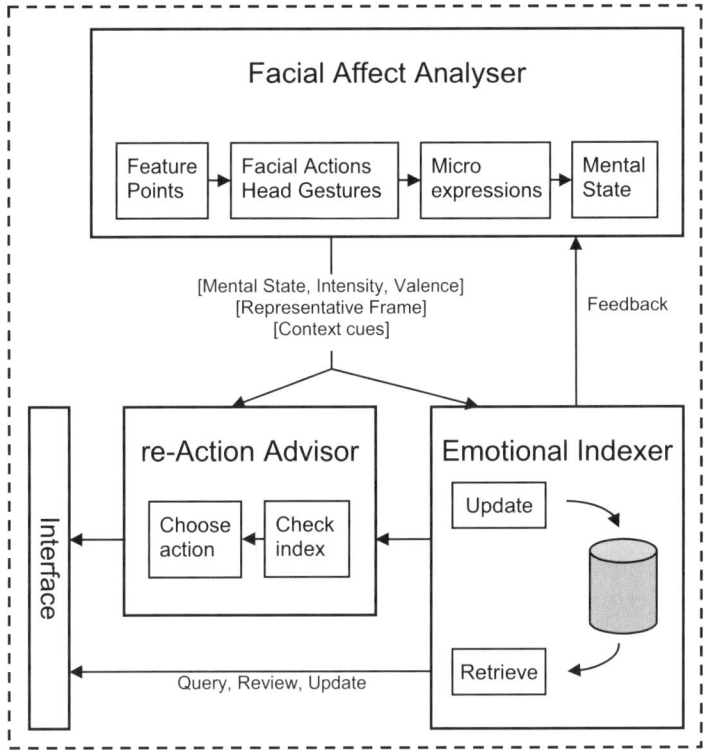

Figure 17.3. The main modules defining the emotional hearing aid

A close up of the mouth feature points, the inner and outer lip contours, and additional colour information (teeth, aperture) is also shown in Figure 17.4. The pose estimation points (e.g. nose tip and nose root) are tracked to recognise head gestures.

For every frame extracted from the incoming video sequence, twenty-two points are identified on the face using prior knowledge of face shapes. The points include pose estimation ones (such as nose tips, nose root, and nostrils), and feature points used for emotion classification (such as inner and outer eyebrow, upper and lower lips, and pupils). Feature point displacements are calculated between consecutive frames. In addition, two head translation parameters indicate the head's movement and three rotation ones are calculated to indicate the head's rotation along three axes: horizontal, vertical and planar.

Feature point displacements and head motion parameters (calculated every hundredth of a second) are tracked over time to identify head and facial gestures. Those in turn typically last between one to two seconds, emphasizing the fact that facial expressions are inherently dynamic processes. Head gestures in particular follow some pattern of temporal regularity (Davis and Vaks, 2001). For instance, a head nod is a series of vertical up and down movement of the head used to show agreement, excitement, or comprehension while listening. Head gestures vary in duration as well as in intensity. Such variations often signify different user intents. For example, a quick and strong nod tends to indicate more agreement than a weaker and slower one. In El Kaliouby and Robinson (2003), we define a number of parameters that are used to estimate the strength of a head gesture, and present a state machine that processes accumulated head motions (such as move-up or move-down) to recognize a number of head gestures in real time.

Upper (eyes and eyebrows) and lower (mouth) facial action analysis is performed simultaneously with head gesture recognition. We extend the approach used in Tian et al. (2000), which combines both shape (geometric) and colour information to determine the different states of the mouth. As shown in Figure 1.4, the mouth area is represented by eight feature points. In addition, an origin is defined as the intersection between the lines joining the two lip corners, and the two central ones. The distance between the two corners is used to determine the width of the mouth, while the distance from the upper centre point to the origin, and lower centre point to origin depicts two height parameters. The angle of orientation of the mouth is also calculated. A total of four hyperbolic arcs approximate the lip contours. The two arcs representing the outer contours pass through the upper and lower mouth feature points, whereas the inner two require further colour information to approximate. Colour information is mainly used to determine if teeth are present or not (aperture) indicated by the luminance of the pixels. Once shape and colour information are calculated, mouth states (open, open with teeth, closed, tightly closed) are determined. Mouth states are tracked over time to infer the underlying lower facial action. For example, if the mouth progresses from being closed, to being open, with lip corners pulled outward, and teeth present, then this would indicate a smile.

A similar approach is used in determining the states of the eye (open, shut, wide open, squinting). With regards to the eyebrows, the displacements of the feature points are tracked over time to find out if the eyebrows have been raised, and if the two inner points have moved closer (as in a frown).

Finally, concurrent facial and head gestures combine to form a micro-expression, a sequence of which constitutes an emotion (Edwards, 1998). This typically lasts between six to eight seconds. The analyser also extracts a number of parameters on the mental state level such as intensity and valence (positive or negative), and a representative clip of that mental state. This is all then sent to the emotional indexer and the re-action advisor.

17.3.2 The Emotional Indexer

The primary function of the emotional indexer is to archive facial events as they occur. The archive is accessible to the facial affect analyser and re-action advisor modules to improve inference results. The archive is also made available (through the interface layer) to the child and carer for discussion, learning and reviewing purposes. The latter is particularly important if the stored events are going to affect future inference results. Every event is stored as a tuple in the index containing the representative frames of the facial expression, a label, any additional parameters and context cues available.

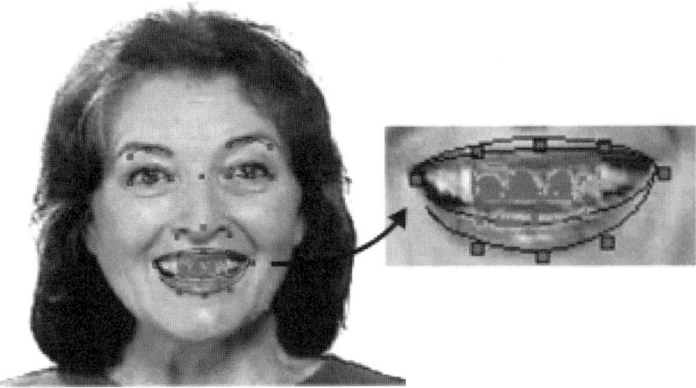

Figure 17.4. The facial affect analyser (Video courtesy of the Autism Research Centre, Cambridge).

17.3.3 The Re-Action Advisor

This module's primary function is to appraise the current facial input, making use of profile information and archived events, in order to suggest a number of possible courses of action to take. We identify several issues that are fundamental to the design of this module. The most obvious one is associated with the timing of a suggestion: when and how often should a reaction be suggested, and how soon after a change of emotional state is detected should an action be suggested. Needless to say, while the analyser module emits an inference every 6 seconds on average, it would only cognitively overload (and indeed frustrate!) the child if an action is suggested with every inference.

Deciding on the function of a suggested reaction is also important. Reactions to facial expression can be for the purposes of feedback, empathy (Surakka and Hietanen, 1998), or communicative (e.g. signal turn-taking).

Finally, determining the intensity of a reaction also needs to be considered. Intensity is a function of the facial event, its valence and intensity, the current situation and the degree of approachability of the other person.

17.3.4 The Interface Layer

The interface layer manages communication between the child (or carer) and the other modules of the emotional hearing aid. To start with, the interface informs the wearer whenever a facial event occurs, and returns the possible courses of actions suggested by the advisor module. The interface also decides on the modality and format of the output depending on the active profile and level of engagement of the child with the current social scenario. A summary-mode is adopted when the user is actively taking part in an interaction, and only needs assistance with the suggested course of action. In this case, the output is unobtrusive to avoid interrupting the interaction, and can be visual (coded-coded characters) or audio (ambient sounds). In the detailed output mode, all available information pertaining to the event is presented to the user visually.

In query mode, the interface allows the index to be queried by both the child and carer using a number of different parameters such as emotion labels, intensity, valence, and date of event. In the update mode, the carer is able to retrieve event entries, and update them. Finally, the carer can also define the emotion classes the analyser deals with, activating and de-activating classes as needed.

17.4 Preliminary Results

The prototype currently in place, utilises a commercial digital camcorder connected to a standard PC. Our system operates in real time (30 fps) and does not impose a frontal position on the user. In contrast to other existing systems, which operate on short clips (1-3 seconds), we place no constraints on the duration of the input because the facial affect analyser keeps a rotating buffer of the input.

Table 17.1. List of mental states supported, their characteristic head gesture and facial actions

Mental State	Head Gesture	Lower actions	Upper actions
Agreeing	Nod	(Nothing specific)	(Nothing specific)
Comprehending	Nod	(Nothing specific)	Drawn inwards
Confused	Tilt in one direction	Tightly closed	Frown
Convinced	Medium nod	Subtle smile	Eyebrow raise
Decided	Strong, quick nod	(Nothing specific)	(Nothing specific)
Delighted	(Nothing specific)	Smile	Eyebrow raise
Disagreeing	Headshake	(Nothing specific)	Frown
Disbelieving	Quick headshake	Open	Drawn inwards
Grieving	Slow headshake	Tightly closed	(Nothing specific)
Undecided	Alternate head tilts	Pulled sideways	Squint

Preliminary tests were carried out on subjects from within the Computer Laboratory at the University of Cambridge, asking them to act out basic emotions (e.g. happy, disgusted) and various head gestures (e.g. head nods, head shakes). In addition, further tests were carried out using videos from the mind reading DVD (Baron-Cohen and Tead, 2003). Videos and emotional labels from that database were verified by a panel of judges to ensure that they correctly match. So far, we are able to distinguish between a number of prominent head gestures: head nod, headshakes, and head tilts, and facial actions: smile, mouth open, mouth closed, eyebrow raise, and frown. Table 17.1 lists the mental states that our system supports so far, and the characteristics of each state exploited by the analyser.

Finally, the only action advice supported so far is in the form of real time feedback, acknowledging a facial event, its class and intensity. The feedback also provides information as to when the emotional state started and ended.

17.5 Conclusion

This paper reports work in progress on the emotional hearing aid, a portable assistive computer intended to help children diagnosed with Asperger's Syndrome read, understand and react to facial expressions in a socially-appropriate way. The architecture and detailed design of the modules were presented, drawing inspiration from the "emotional indexing" approach to teaching emotions to children with autism. We believe that such a tool offers children with Asperger's Syndrome more opportunities to engage in natural social interactions, beyond the hypothetical scenarios used in a teaching environment. The emotional hearing aid provides assistance even when the child's carer is not available, whereas the indexer ensures that events are accessible even after their occurrence for discussion and learning purposes. Future work includes completing the prototype and deploying the tool in a number of user studies to gain feedback on usability.

17.6 References

Baron-Cohen S (1995) Mindblindness: an essay on autism and theory of mind. MIT Press

Baron-Cohen S, Tead THE (2003) Mind reading: The interactive guide to emotion. Technical report. Autism Research Centre, Cambridge, UK

Blocher K (1999) Affective Social Quotient (ASQ): Teaching emotion recognition with interactive media and wireless expressive toys. S.M. Thesis, MIT, Cambridge, MA

Bruce V, Young A (1998) In the eye of the beholder: The science of face perception. Oxford University Press, UK

Cheng L, Kimberly G, Orlich F (2003) KidTalk: Online therapy for asperger's syndrome. Technical Report, Social Computing Group, Microsoft Research

Dautenhahn K, Billard A (2002) Games children with autism can play with robota, a humanoid robotic doll. Proceedings of CWUAAT In: Universal Access and Assistive Technology, Springer-Verlag London, UK

Davis J, Vaks S (2001) A perceptual user interface for recognising head gesture acknowledgements. In: Workshop on Perceptive User Interfaces

Edwards, K (1998) The face of time: Temporal cues in facial expression of emotion. Psychological Science 9: 270-276

El Kaliouby R, Robinson P (2003) Real time head gesture recognition in affective interfaces. In: Human Computer Interaction Interact'03, IOS Press

Fling E (2000) Eating an artichoke: A mother's perspective on asperger syndrome. Jessica Kingsley Publishers Ltd

Hirose M, Kijima R, Shirakawa K, Nihei K (1997) Development of a virtual sand box: An application of virtual environment for psychological treatment. In: Virtual Reality in

Neuro-Psycho-Physiology: Cognitive, Clinical and Methodological Issues in Assessment and Treatment, IOS Press

Howlin P, Baron-Cohen S, Hadwin J (1999) Teaching children with autism to mind-read: A practical guide for teachers and parents. John Wiley and Sons

Kozima H, Yano H (2001) Designing a robot for contingency-detection game. Working Notes - Workshop Robotic & Virtual Interactive Systems in Autism Therapy. University of Hertfordshire, Technical Report No 364

Moore D, McGrath P, Thorpe J (2000) Computer-aided learning for people with autism-a framework for research and development. Innovations in Education and Training International 37(3): 218-228

O' Connell S (1998) Mindreading: How we learn to love and lie. Arrow Books

Strickland D (1996) A virtual reality application with autistic children. Presence: Teleoperators and Virtual Environments 5(3): 319-329

Surakka E, Hietanen JK (1998) Facial and emotional reactions to duchenne and nonduchenne smiles. International Journal of Psychophysiology 29(1): 23–33

Tian Y, Kanade T, Cohn J (2000) Robust lip tracking by combining shape, colour and motion. In: Proceedings of ACCV'00, Taipei, Taiwan

Werry I, Dautenhahn K, Ogden B, Harwin W (2001) Can social interaction skills be taught by a social agent? The role of a robotic mediator in autism therapy. In: Proceedings CT2001, Springer-Verlag London, UK

Chapter 18

Fostering Universal Access: Lessons from Telecommunications and Disability

C. Newell, G. Goggin, G. Astbrink and H. Raiche

18.1 Introduction

Universal design is fundamentally important in fostering not just access but participation in the goods of life. In this chapter we explore an Australian model for including people with disabilities in processes of planning and evaluation which goes beyond inclusion to participation as experts in industry processes. This evaluated model of participation in a co-regulatory system is seen to have significant implications for not just the global telecommunications community but how to undertake universal design as a process.

In many respects the emerging and complex arena of telecommunications is providing new and exciting opportunities for inclusion and equally disheartening occasions of exclusion through design. Information technology and telephony are not just converging but creating new technologies in themselves, with emerging challenges for regulatory models and standard setting. We propose that rather than a special needs approach to disability, the needs of people with disability can provide a cutting edge opportunity for fostering universal design which is of benefit to the entire population.

18.2 The International Context

Telecommunications networks provide the foundations for digital interactive communications, supporting a wide variety of contemporary communications and media. We know these technologies under a variety of once exotic, now familiar names: Internet, audio and video streaming, digital music in the form of MP3s, digital broadcasting, and new modes of voice and text communications. For the last twenty-five years we have seen the endless "revolution" of communication and media shaped by these digital technologies in the process of convergence. As the computer, telephone, television, radio, book, and newspaper blend together, many in the Western world, if fewer elsewhere, find that their information and entertainment, goods and services, education and health, travel and recreation reach them through a stream of ones and zeros transmitted via phone lines and radio waves.

Telecommunications has an ongoing critical role in the exercise of power and governance within post-modern society. Telecommunications has significantly facilitated and shaped the multifaceted phenomenon we know as globalisation at the beginning of the twentieth-first century, something presaged by theorists of post-industrial societies (Bell, 1973).

Yet the participation of people with disabilities in telecommunications has been chequered, defined in terms of the dominant discourses and power relations outlined by such writers as Goggin and Newell (2003). Disability in such technological systems has been governed by narrow norms, left to the state in a world where, increasingly, the market rules, and "light-touch" regulation has been critiqued as offering inadequate specific beneficial effects to people with disability. The benefits of globalisation, such as they are, have not flowed evenly to people with disabilities. Of course, there have been the restricted forms of access enthusiastically offered by computer software and hardware manufacturers in accordance with charitable discourse. As we have globalised, we have also built in disability based upon ableist norms. Critical scholarship informed by those who live with disability invites us to reflect upon settings, locations, discourses, and power relations, which are tacit but actually constitute a paradoxical world: one that is constantly changing, but in certain respects remains the same.

18.3 The Australian Context

In many respects the Australian environment provides a unique and particularly useful case study, because of the co-regulatory approach adopted. As with many other countries, people with disability constitute some 20% of the Australian population. Research in the area dates back to a seminal study, commissioned by then Telecom Australia, published in 1981, the International Year of Disabled Persons (see Goggin and Newell, 2000). Much of the research into telecommunications and disability has tended to follow the biomedical model but in the last few years there has been emphasis on the social nature of disability within telecommunications.

In Australia, accessibility for people with disabilities was not recognised in legislation until the 1992 *Disability Discrimination Act*. The legislation establishing the framework for the introduction of limited competition in Australian telecommunications, the 1991 *Telecommunications Act*, featured a definition of universal service that mandated the delivery of standard voice telephony service throughout Australia that is "reasonably accessible" to all Australians, but implicitly separated the universal geographical availability issues from universal accessibility ones. Universal accessibility, such as ensuring access for people with disabilities, was not to be required under the Universal Service Obligation. Instead, the government undertook to provide funding as one of its "community service obligations". In a time of stringent fiscal management, no such funding eventuated for a number of years (Goggin, 1998). Note that "Community service obligations" was part of a rhetoric that developed through the late 1980s and early 1990s as a way of separating social aspects of service provision from narrowly commercial ones. The concept was deployed in a number of industries, especially utilities, where governments were seeking to privatise, corporatise, or commercialise service delivery.

The 1991 legislation allowed Telecom Australia (now Telstra), the government-owned former monopoly carrier, to continue operating its own "concession" scheme to provide people with disabilities some limited equipment for connecting to the telecommunications network. Telstra did not make telecommunications generally accessible, however, for Deaf people and people with speech disabilities who required text telephony equipment (known in Australia as teletypewriters or TTYs). A long and at times acrimonious battle to get Telstra to provide TTY equipment and relay services at affordable rates for Deaf and people with hearing and speech disabilities was required before this aspect of universal service was given any attention.

Telecommunications was explicitly left out of areas named as being important and worthy of disability standards in the Australian *Disability Discrimination Act 1992*. However, the overarching universal nature of this piece of legislation meant that when negotiations failed, a Deaf man, followed shortly after by Disabled Peoples' International (DPI) (Australia), the then umbrella organisation for people with disabilities and their organisations, successfully launched an action against the then Telecom Australia in 1995 in the Human Rights and Equal Opportunity Commission (HREOC) (*Geoffrey Scott & DPI v Telstra*). This decision (available at: www.hreoc.gov.au) found that Telstra's USO obligation to provide a standard telephone service that is "reasonably accessible" to all Australians, combined with the non-discrimination requirements of the *Disability Discrimination Act 1992*, meant Telstra had to provide accessible teletypewriters to those requiring them, and at the same cost as providing a standard telephone service handset to all Australians. The decision eventually resulted in a change to government policy which recognised the import of the Scott decision and included a requirement in the *Telecommunication Act 1997* that the functional requirements of people with disabilities be included in universal service provision. This Act broadens the definition of the standard telephone service to include another form of voice communication that is equivalent to voice telephony, if voice telephony is not practical for a person with a disability.

In telecommunications, people with disabilities have very much been asked to be active agents in regulation in a range of macro- and micro-arenas. To take one example, the introduction of competition in telecommunications has been accompanied by a language of "customer-focus", calling for consultation with consumers, inviting consumer representatives to sit on advisory boards or panels. These consultative forums have assumed greater importance because they have taken up some of the regulatory and policy-formulation roles previously played by the state and its agencies. In Australia, for instance, an industry self-regulatory body has been established by the telecommunications industry, the Australian Communication Industry Forum, which is responsible for developing regulation in areas previously governed by the government and industry, and also for initiating regulation in areas not previously subject to any state or self-regulation. This is an interesting example of the manner in which governmentality is being extended, under the guise of a discourse of deregulation and self-regulation.

18.4 The Australian Communications Industry Forum

The Australian Communications Industry Forum Ltd (ACIF) is an industry owned, resourced and operated company established by the telecommunications industry in 1997 to implement and manage communications self-regulation within Australia. ACIF's role is to develop and administer technical and operating arrangements that promote both the long-term interests of end-users and the efficiency and international competitiveness of the Australian communications industry. This primarily involves developing Standards, Codes and other documents to support competition and protect consumers; driving widespread compliance; and facilitating/co-ordinating the co-operative resolution of strategic and operational industry issues. ACIF comprises a Board, an Advisory Assembly, seven standing Reference Panels, various task-specific Working Committees, a number of Industry Facilitation/Co-ordination Groups, and a small Executive.

18.4.1 The ACIF Disability Advisory Body

In many respects the ACIF Disability Advisory Body (DAB) provides a unique model which has been tested in several ways. In particular it is a model of using people with disabilities as experts who work in a collaborative sense with those who are designing guidelines and regulations which shape not just Australian telecommunications but how those communication systems interface with other technologies. In this way ACIF has moved beyond a rhetoric and practice of inclusion to full partnership. The ACIF DAB, with the vast majority of members drawn from broadly represented organisations, and chaired by a person with disability respected in industry, consumer and academic circles, provides a key meeting place for consideration of not just current but future telecommunications issues.

The ACIF Disability Advisory Body (DAB) was established following a proposal by participants of an ACIF Disability Forum, held in February 1998. The DAB meets quarterly to review ACIF's works program and provides advice to ACIF regarding the implications for people with disabilities of ACIF's proposed Codes and Standards and other publications. The membership of the DAB is detailed in Table 18.1. ACIF Standards, Codes and other documents are prepared by Working Committees made up of experts from industry, consumer, government and other bodies. The requirements or recommendations contained in ACIF published documents are a consensus of views of representative interests, and also take into account comments received from other stakeholders.

Table 18.1. Membership of the ACIF Disability Advisory Body

Representative	Organisation
Dr Christopher Newell, AM (Chair)	Australian Federation of Disability Organisations
Hank Wyllie	Communications Aid Users Society
Gunela Astbrink	TEDICORE (Telecommunications Disability and Consumer Representation)
Jo-An M. Partridge	Women with Disabilities Australia
Rob Garrett	Australian Rehabilitation and Assistive Technology Association
Phil Harper	Australian Association of the Deaf
Harold Hartfield	Physical Disability Council of Australia
Tony Starkey	Blind Citizens Australia
Andrew Stewart	Deafness Forum of Australia
Holly Raiche	ACIF project management

18.4.2 Guidelines

There have been significant trialled outcomes from the ACIF DAB. In September 2001 the Australian Communications Industry Forum (ACIF) released a publication entitled ACIF G586: 2001 *Access to Telecommunications for People with Disabilities Industry Guidelines*, authored by the DAB (ACIF G586, 2001). These draw upon the considerable developments both in Australia and internationally in improving access to and equity in telecommunications for people with disabilities. Current Australian and international legislation (TA, 1996; ADA, 1990; RAA, 1998) and practical guidelines (COST, 1997; UN, 1993) and research (Trace, 2003; UD, 2003; DIEL, 2003) were used in developing this document.

The Guidelines aim to:

- assist ACIF and its Reference Panels and Working Committees to meet their responsibilities under the *Disability Discrimination Act 1992* and the *Telecommunications (Consumer Protection and Service Standards) Act 1999*; and
- assist ACIF and its Reference Panels and Working Committees to provide equity in access to telecommunications for people with disabilities.

The Guidelines are being applied in the development of all ACIF Codes and Standards, recognising that ACIF is the Australian member of the Global Standards Collaboration, although this is only relevant in relation to setting technical standards. The majority of the items in the Guidelines are based on issues that have already been raised during the development of draft ACIF Codes and Standards. The Guidelines do not preclude the inclusion of other specific accessibility requirements as needed.

In developing its approach, the DAB endorsed the Telecommunications Charter (Table 18.2) from the European Union's COST 219 bis (COST, 1997) as a statement of principles for the Guidelines and as a means of improving access and equity in Australian telecommunications for people with disabilities.

Table 18.2. The Telecommunications Charter:

1.1.1 Telecommunication facilities and services should be accessible to all.
1.1.2 The needs of older people and people with disabilities should be taken into account in the design of any new telecommunication equipment or service. Terminal equipment should be designed for the widest possible market.Network services should adequately support relevant special terminal functions so that all users experience equivalent end-to-end service.
1.1.3 Where inclusive design is not possible, provision should be made for people with disabilities to access the service by means of additional equipment and services.
1.1.4 People with disabilities should, as far as possible, be able to use telecommunication services at prices equivalent to those without disabilities. Most of the additional costs of providing access to all should be met by dedicated funds or absorbed within general operating costs.
1.1.5 Providers of telecommunication equipment and services and regulatory authorities should consult regularly with disabled and older users about their access requirements and take appropriate action. Equally, organisations representing older people and people with disabilities should be prepared to contribute their knowledge and experience.
1.1.6 Telecommunication products and services that improve and increase access for older and disabled people should be actively advertised and promoted, with information also available in accessible formats.

18.4.3 Specific Provisions

The Guidelines uphold the principles of universal design, plain English (Eagleson, 1997) explanation of the Code or Standard, and documents being available in alternative formats upon request; for example, large print and Braille and electronic format. Further, international web accessibility guidelines are endorsed.

Likewise the availability of a TTY (Telephone Typewriter) line for people who are Deaf, or speech or hearing impaired is advocated where customer enquiry or assistance lines are provided, and it is suggested that customer service staff should receive regular training in communicating with people with a range of communication needs, including speech impairments.

Other provisions include availability of sign interpretation on request for Deaf people, language assistance for community languages and communication facilitators, and a counter loop for the hearing impaired at customer enquiry or assistance service counters. The importance of the function of an advocate or attendant care worker to assist some customers is also noted, as is a recognition that when the Emergency '000' number is mentioned in codes, the TTY Emergency number '106' should also be mentioned.

18.4.4 Validating the Work

Such a document is important for driving positive developments in the Australian scene (Goggin and Newell, 2000), drawing upon Australian legislation and best overseas practice. Perhaps most importantly, this is an example of the type of work which is necessary; where the expertise of people with disability is utilised in drawing up guidelines about disability, and in fostering win-win coalitions between the disability community and the telecommunications industry.

The work of the DAB may be seen to be validated and subject to peer scrutiny in several ways. This is exemplified by the process adopted with the guideline referred to above. Subject to consultation and circulation within industry and consumer circles, the guideline was also the subject of professional scrutiny by the telecommunications industry through ACIF working parties and, finally, subject to approval by the ACIF board which has industry and consumer representatives as part of it.

18.4.5 Partnerships at Work

No better example of partnerships at work, using disability expertise, proving to yield important opportunities for partnerships in mainstream work can be found than in current work by ACIF with regard to telecommunications futures. In particular, two projects managed by ACIF on behalf of the industry incorporate experts from the Disability Advisory Body on the mainstream working group. These are representatives who live with disability. These projects are the ACIF Any-to-Any Connectivity and the Next Generation Networks projects. In many respects, both of these cutting edge futures projects have been partially defined by early work from the DAB defining the problems.

18.4.6 ACIF Any-To-Any Text Connectivity Project

Following the ACIF Any-to-Any Text Connectivity Seminar held on 17 February 2003, an Any-to-Any Text Connectivity Options Working Group was established.

The Working Group has a membership including representatives from consumer and people with disability groups, carriers, the national relay service provider and the ACA. The Working Group is looking at short term and long term real-time text communication issues, with particular attention to the support of Text Telephony for people who are deaf or who have hearing or speech impairment. The Working Group also recognises the communication needs of people with other disabilities, such as those with an intellectual impairment or people with physical impairments.

The issues relating to evolving telecommunication technologies are of particular interest, as some of these technologies cannot effectively carry the traditional TTY signals. The initial activity is concentrating on the short term, but with likely future needs in mind. The longer-term aim, however, is for any-to-any connectivity for all using text and/or video available at home, at the workplace and on the move.

18.4.7 ACIF Next Generations Network Project

The ACIF Next Generations Network (NGN) project was launched at an ACIF seminar in May 2002, at which it was agreed that ACIF should provide a mechanism for all the industry stakeholders (including policy makers, regulators, carriers and service providers, equipment providers and consumers) to consider the options and develop appropriate arrangements for migration to the Next Generation Networks.

It is most likely that Next Generation Networks will develop from the current circuit switched public telecommunications networks, and be largely packet based. Various sub-groups will be established under the NGN project to discuss and make recommendations on issues from the NGN, including support for current and new services, implications for network architecture and inter-carrier network arrangements, and the policy and regulatory issues that will need to be developed.

The challenge in a Next Generation Network environment will be to support both current and new services to the public, while ensuring current consumer protections are carried forward in the new network environment.

18.4.8 Fostering Professional Development

In addition, the ACIF DAB work has provided an opportunity for professional development workshops with ACIF staff and key industry participants on disability needs and incorporating disability into the life of telecommunications from research and development through to policy. All of this work is subject to yearly review by a formal process, which includes the opportunity for anonymous input.

In this way, we would suggest that the model adopted by ACIF moves beyond inclusion, where so often non-disabled structures and norms may be left unchallenged, to fundamentally incorporating disability as expert knowledge within industry processes. Goggin and Newell (2003) however, provide a significant unmet challenge when they call for such expertise to be present on boards of management as well.

18.5 Conclusion

Hence, it is argued that the fostering of universal access is not just vital but also has important practical dimensions. This has certainly been shown in the Australian environment recently where GSM technology was adopted in mobile telephony, and after the mediation of legal settlement through the Human Rights and Equal Opportunity Commission a later fix with many additional costs to industry was adopted. Incorporation of the skills and life experience of people with disabilities from the research and development stage onwards is vital for win-win outcomes.

In particular, we would suggest that the following points may be seen as key aspects to fostering universal design which truly embraces people with disability. This is based upon our peer-reviewed work within ACIF and the wider telecommunications arena:

- affirming the expertise of people with disability in structures which support participation and input into the mainstream;
- facilitating participation by establishing structures to support and encourage representative and accountable participation by people with disability;
- the adoption of universal design principles in industry guidelines;
- the use of disability considerations in industry and regulatory structures as Key Performance Indicators;
- utilising disability as a litmus test for universal access and design;
- evaluating initiatives with peers which include professionals, industry and disability representatives.

Accordingly, we propose that rather than being difficult and expensive, the incorporation of disability into mainstream telecommunications is an essential dimension to fostering universal access and design.

18.6 References

ACIF G586 (2001) Access to telecommunications for people with disabilities. Industry Guidelines, Australian Communications Industry Forum, Sydney.
  Available at: http://www.acif.org.au
ADA (1990) Americans with Disabilities Act of 1990. US Public Law, pp 101-336
Bell D (1973) The coming of post-industry society: A venture in social forecasting. Basic, New York, USA
COST (1997) COST 219 bis – Telecommunications: Access for disabled and elderly people. The COST 219 bis charter. Available at: http://www.stakes.fi/cost219/charter.htm
DIEL (2003) UK disability and elderly advisory group. Available at:
  http://www.acts.org.uk/diel
Eagleson R (1997) Writing in plain English, AGPS, Canberra
Goggin G and Newell C (2003) Digital disability: The social construction of disability in new media. Rowman & Littlefield, Boulder, Colorado, USA

Goggin G, Newell C (2000) Twenty-five years of disabling technology: The case of telecommunications. In: Clear, M. (ed.), Promises Promises: Disability and Terms of Inclusion. Federation Press, Sydney, Australia

Goggin G (1998) Universal service: Voice telephony and beyond. In: Bruce Langtry (ed.), All Connected: Universal Service in Telecommunications, Melbourne University Press, Melbourne, Australia

RAA (1998) Rehabilitation Act Amendments of 1998 – Electronic and information technology (particularly section 508)

TA (1996) Telecommunications Act of 1996. The federal communications commission. Available at: http://www.fcc.gov/Reports/tcom1996.txt

Trace (2003) The Trace Center. Details available at:
http://www.trace.wisc.edu/world/tool_nav.html

UD (2003) The center for universal design. Details available at:
http://www.design.ncsu.edu:8120/cud/

UN (1993) The UN standard rules on the equalisation of opportunities for persons with disabilities. United Nations, New York, USA

Chapter 19

Assessing the Accessibility of Digital Television Set-Top Boxes

S. Keates and P.J. Clarkson

19.1 Introduction

The aim of this study was to investigate the accessibility of DTV technology, focussing on the current generation of set-top boxes (STB) which provide 'free to view' services (DTI, 2003).

The objective of the study was to identify specific causes of concern with regard to user interaction with DTV that might lead to exclusion, i.e. situations where users may be unable to use the new technology. In particular, it was important to identify challenges presented to users by DTV that are not found when using the current analogue equivalent.

The number of STBs is increasing rapidly, but for the purposes of this study, efforts were focused on looking at just two set-top boxes that will be referred to throughout the report as STB1 and STB2. STB1 was selected because it was being marketed as 'easy-to-use', while STB2 was chosen because it was the market leader at the time.

Note: the assessments described in this report were performed over the period April to June, 2003, and thus all comments expressed within this chapter are derived from the services available during that time period. With the continually evolving nature of DTV, some of the interaction details will have changed by the time that this chapter is published.

19.2 Background

The objective of this study was to identify specific causes of potential user exclusion with regard to current DTV. The STB, satellite or cable box and its remote control form only a part of a larger system, which also includes the television itself and the service providers (see Figure 19.1 for an example).

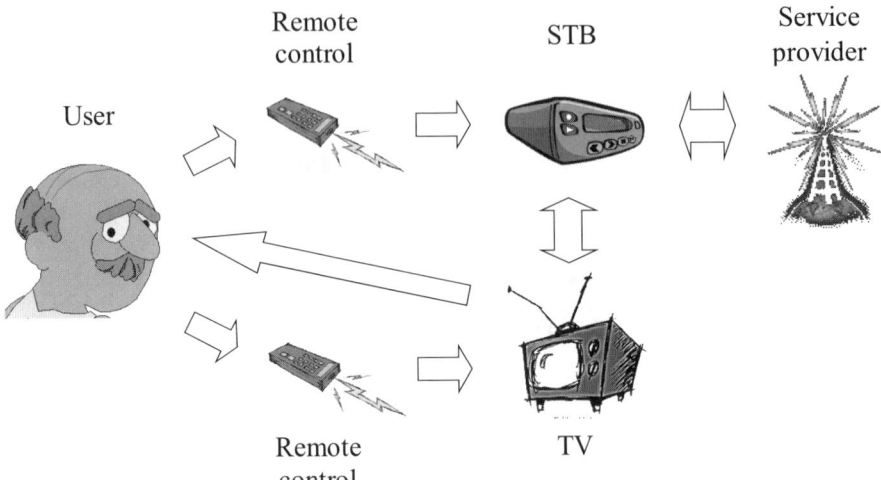

Figure 19.1. The system components involved in the delivery of terrestrial, Free-to-View digital television

In assessing DTV it is important to understand the contribution of each of the elements to the potential for exclusion. The system must be tested as a whole and in a way that represents 'normal' use. As a result, a number of use scenarios were used to investigate the accessibility of DTV focusing on the purchasing, installation and use of STBs. These included:

- choosing which STB to buy in a shop or from a web-site (e.g. how to tell the difference between them; which one is easier to use? etc.);
- identifying the set-up requirements (e.g. what cables do I need?);
- installing the STB;
- tuning the STB (or re-tuning, if after installation);
- re-ordering the TV channels (setting up a list of favourites);
- finding out what's on and selecting the desired channel (using either the interactive electronic programme guide (EPG), or by random surfing);
- using subtitles, accessing additional settings, navigating the menu structure;
- accessing interactive content (e.g. Teletext, BBCi).

The investigation needed to focus on identifying the broad steps involved in the interaction between the user and the STBs. The aim was to establish the potential causes of exclusion that may prevent users from interacting with the STBs effectively.

19.3 User Observation Sessions

The accessibility of DTV systems was analysed by a series of user observation sessions. User observations are an invaluable tool when assessing both the usability and accessibility of a product (Nielsen, 1993).

19.3.1 Sampling Users

Ideally, the users sampled for participation in product assessments should represent the full range of end-user capabilities that can reasonably be expected to be found in the intended target population. However, to achieve statistical significance at all possible levels of capability across the target users would require a large number of participants. So, methods of reducing the number of users are needed.

The most popular approaches to sampling issues are to either find users that represent a spread across the target population (Grundy *et al.*, 1999), or else to find users that sit at the extremes of that population (Keates and Clarkson, 2003). The advantage of working with users that represent a spread across the population is that they ensure that the assessment takes the broadest range of needs into account. The disadvantage, though, is that there is not much depth of coverage of users who may experience difficulties in accessing the product.

The advantage of working with the extreme users is that the user observation sessions will almost certainly discover difficulties and problems with the interaction. However, the disadvantage is that there is a real danger of discovering that particular users cannot use the product, and little else beyond that. For example, giving an instruction book to a user with complete sight loss yields the obvious difficulty arising from the inability to read the text.

Further, subsequent questions about the content of the instructions are not possible because of the over-riding difficulty of reading. This is of only limited value in an assessment such as this, as the difficulties encountered by the extreme users are comparatively predictable and provide little information about how many other users may or may not be able to use the product. It could also be argued that such users may reasonably be expected to make use of assistive technology to help access particular products.

Of more use is to identify users who are more likely to be 'edge-cases', those who are on the borderline of being able to use the product, and who would commonly be accepted as should be able to use the product.

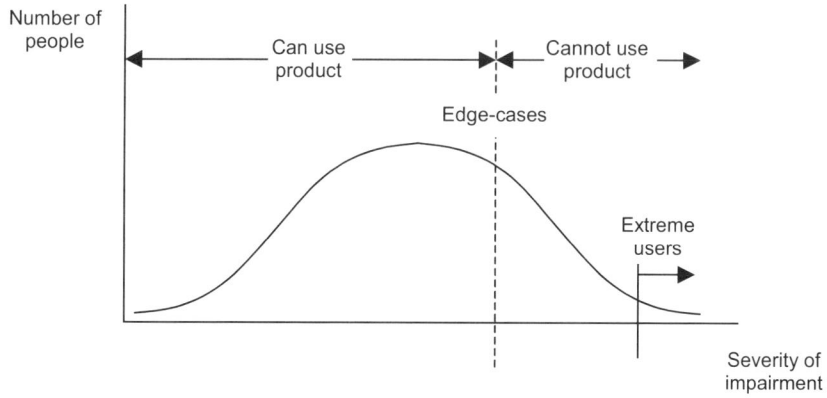

Figure 19.2 The different approaches to sampling the users

Going back to the example of someone with a visual impairment attempting to read an instruction book, while someone with complete vision loss would certainly not be able to use the instructions, someone with only partial sight loss may be able to do so. Even more interestingly, that person might be able to read some bits and not others and thus it is possible to begin to infer a wide range of very useful data from such a user.

On top of that, if the user cannot read the instructions, then it may be inferred that any user with that level of sight loss or worse will not be able to use them, automatically encompassing the users with complete sight loss in the assessment of product exclusion.

Figure 19.2 summarises the different approaches to sampling the users. The implication of this is that whichever group of users participates in the assessment, it is important that their capability profiles are known so that it is known how many users share the same characteristics.

19.3.2 Working with Users

When dealing with users with more severe impairments, it is especially important to be sensitive to their needs. For example, such users will often tire more easily than the person supervising the assessment may normally expect.

One of the other major issues to consider when working with users, especially for assessments, is the presence of coping strategies (DTI, 2000). Many people with functional impairments find strategies for compensating for their impairments - sliding heavy objects that were designed to be lifted, using two hands instead of one, making customised alterations to products to make them easier to use.

Identifying coping strategies can be difficult for someone who is not familiar with the nature of functional impairments. Users will often perform the coping strategy as if it was second nature to do so (through practice) or alternatively may actively disguise any such strategies to avoid drawing attention to any functional restrictions that they may have. However, even when coping strategies have been identified, finding the cause of them is not always straightforward. For example, performing a one-handed operation with two hands may be a coping strategy for manoeuvring an object that is too heavy, but it is also a strategy for increasing accuracy.

19.3.3 User Selection

Thirteen users were recruited for the observation sessions. The users were identified based on a number of criteria, primarily focused around whether they were strong candidates for being edge-cases in terms of their ability to interact with STBs. Based on the results of the earlier assessments, it was decided to focus on recruiting older adults not living in residential care. As discussed in the Sampling Users section above, more extreme users could have been selected for the user group, however, the level of information that can be obtained is then limited.

Older adults typically exhibit a range of different kinds of capability loss and are more likely to show multiple minor impairments. This is important because most assistive technology is predominantly aimed at single major impairments and thus users with multiple minor impairments are less likely to be able to find assistive technology to aid them should they encounter severe difficulty interacting with a product. Older adults as a whole are also more numerous than younger disabled ones. Thus if it was shown that older users generally experienced difficulty interacting with the STBs, irrespective of their capability losses, then this equates to a much higher level of exclusion within the general population.

The decision to select users still living in private homes, rather than residential care was based on the desire to have users who still have enough functional capability to support independent living to some degree. They should therefore be able to perform tasks such as operating a television on their own. If they experienced significant difficulty, then it could be argued that the STBs are causing undue exclusion. As a comparison, a younger user with a more severe impairment was also recruited to highlight whether a more extreme user would also encounter the difficulties experienced by the older adults.

During the recruitment process efforts were made to ensure that the users exhibited a range of capabilities. Care was taken not to skew the sample towards any particular capability loss, rather to provide a balanced representation of motion, sensory and cognitive losses. Table 19.1 shows the users selected to participate in the user observation sessions.

Table 19.1 The user observation participants

User	Age	Gender	DTV owner?	No. of hours TV watched per evening	PC user
1	85	M	No	<1	Yes
2	82	F	No	1 to 2	No
3	65-69	F	No	2 to 4	No
4	80-84	F	No – analogue cable	>4	No
5	69	M	Yes – STB	1 to 2	Yes
6	62	F	Yes – STB	1 to 2	Yes
7	65-69	M	Yes – satellite	>4	Yes
8	65-69	M	Yes – iDTV	1 to 2	Yes
9	60	F	No – analogue cable	2 to 4+	Yes
10	70-74	F	No	2 to 4	No
11	70-74	F	No	>4	No
12	70-74	F	No	>4	No
13	24	M	No	<1	Yes

It is worth noting that a range of user capabilities was observed. Two users showed no obvious impairment on the ONS data scales, four showed single impairments and the remaining seven exhibited multiple impairments. Three of the users reported a loss of dexterity at levels expected to cause difficulties using DTV. Five of the users reported a loss of intellectual functioning, of which three were at levels that might also be expected to cause difficulties.

A number of PC-literate and DTV users were recruited to investigate the effect of prior experience of DTV and PC-based menu systems on the use of otherwise unfamiliar STBs.

19.3.4 Methodology

The user observation sessions were organised to be a subset of the usage scenarios described earlier, focusing on the functional stgaes of common interaction, rather than issues such as installing an aerial.

Each user session was limited to 2 hours to ensure that user fatigue was kept to a minimum. Thus the user activities were restricted to those operations that could be considered fundamental to watching television, such as the ability to change channels, and also to those advanced features that could be explored within the available timeframe. 2 STBs were assessed (STB1 and STB2), to ensure a balance between breadth and depth of study. The STBs reflected different design approaches, with one focused more on ease-of-use and the other on functionality.

Initially the users were interviewed for 30 minutes to find out their capability profiles and also background information on their attitudes towards television use and exposure to DTV. Two or three observers attended each interview, each recording the user responses.

Following the interview, the users began an equipment trial. This began with a familiarisation exercise with the analogue television set being used. All users used the same television and remote control. They were asked to perform basic operations, such as changing channel and volume. They were also asked to use teletext services and to call up subtitles.

The users were then asked to choose which of the two STBs being assessed they would prefer to buy. This involved showing them the external packaging and then the STBs themselves. The next stage was to provide the users with the installation instructions for their chosen STB and to ask whether they would install the box themselves. Those users who felt up to doing so were encouraged to connect up the STB to the television. For those users who declined to do so, the STB was connected for them. This was followed by simple television operations such as changing channels and channel-hopping. Users were encouraged to use the on-screen electronic programme guide (EPG) for one of the channel hops.

The more advanced interaction activities included finding weather and television programme guide information from both Teletext and BBCi, as well as calling up subtitles. The equipment trial took an average of one hour to complete. Finally, a closing de-brief session was held, that lasted approximately 15 minutes. During this session, the users were asked what they thought of their experience with the STBs.

19.3.5 Observations

Throughout the assessment on accessibility of DTV set-top boxes, interaction was considered in terms of the sensory, cognitive and motor demands placed on the users. Table 19.2 provides a summary of the incidence of difficulties experienced..

Common sensory problems included finding/reading buttons on the remote controls, reading on-screen text, and swapping between the two (especially for users with distance and reading glasses). These problems are made worse in comparison to analogue television because of the increased functionality leading to the need for more (and hence smaller) buttons and also increased use of on-screen text displays. Users with hearing impairments would find the presence of an explicit subtitle button on the remote control for STB1 very useful, but would be disadvantaged by the on-screen menu approach of STB2, where the user had to navigate through several levels of menu to reach the subtitles option.

The most common source of motor difficulties was pressing the buttons on the remote control. Again, while this is a common task for both analogue television and the STBs, it is made more difficult for the latter by the need for more (and hence smaller) buttons and also increased levels of user interaction.

However, while there was an increase in both the vision and dexterity demands made upon the users, by far the biggest cause of exclusion noted during the user observation sessions was the cognitive demands. The inherent increase in user cognitive effort associated with having to use two remote controls (or a single remote control with multiple modes) rather than a single remote control is further exacerbated by the mismatch between the users' mental models of the interaction and the interaction paradigms adopted. For example, users are familiar with the concept that pressing a button on a television remote control has an immediate effect on what they see on the screen. For example, pressing a channel number button causes the television to immediately tune to that channel. Thus a strong link between cause and effect is observed, and a solid user mental model of the interaction is developed.

The STBs, though, present the users with numerous new interaction paradigms, such as pop-up menus, combined with weakened cause and effect. For example, nothing happens when an item is highlighted on a pop-up menu until the OK/SELECT button is pressed (another new concept). The situation is worsened further by the seemingly arbitrary inconsistencies in language and interaction between similar purpose entities of the interface. For example, in BBCi the 'menu' option is called 'menu', whereas in Teletext it is 'control'. On one remote control the SELECT button was called just that, whereas on the other it was denoted OK. To enter BBCi, the user has to press the RED button, while for Teletext it is the TEXT button. These inconsistencies present unnecessary usability hurdles to the users. These differences breach one of the central tenets of usability theory, namely that of the need for consistency.

The prevalence of the cognitive difficulties encountered by users with no discernible loss of cognitive capability reinforces the estimation made during the exclusion analyses, that the levels of population exclusion predicted using data from the 1996/7 Great Britain Disability Follow-up Survey (Grundy et al., 1999) alone are demonstrably conservative.

Table 19.2 The distribution of causes of difficulty

	Activity	Users having difficulty	Motion problems	Sensory problems	Cognitive problems	Number of problems
Analogue TV	Switching on	8	1	-	1	2
	Changing to a specified channel	1	1	-	-	1
	Channel-hopping	-	-	-	-	-
	Changing volume	-	-	-	-	-
	Using teletext	6	1	3	3	7
	Using subtitles	-	-	-	-	-
Digital TV STB	Connecting up the STBs	4	1	-	1	2
	Switching on the television	1	1	-	-	1
	Switching on the STB	6	-	1	2	3
	Changing DTV channels	3	-	1	2	3
	Changing volume	7	-	-	1	1
	Changing channel number	10	2	2	2	6
	Changing channel via the EPG	13	3	4	6	13
	Teletext	13	2	4	12	18
	Subtitles – button (STB1)	6	-	1	1	2
	Subtitles – menu (STB2)	13	-	1	4	5
	BBCi	13	2	1	6	9
	Switching off	5	-	-	2	2

Many of the cognitive difficulties experienced were not directly attributable to any kind of 'medical model' impairment. Instead, lack of experience with, and mental model of, the interaction paradigms used in digital television was the principal cause of the difficulties encountered.

Note: two of the users (5 and 8) went home after the user observation session and were able to find additional functionality on their digital television systems that they thought was previously missing.

19.3.6 Discussion

The user observations showed that interacting with the STBs was more difficult than interacting with traditional analogue television services. Indeed, the typical digital system is likely to exclude at least twice as many users as the typical analogue system for basic operations such as channel selection (DTI, 2003). Thus the STBs are excluding potential users who at the moment are able to access and use the available television services.

The additional exclusion arose from two principal causes. First, the basic operations, such as changing channel or volume, switching on or off, or calling up subtitles are all made fundamentally more complex by the presence of either two remote controls, or a single remote control with multiple modes of operation. Second, digital television offers increased functionality and thus places additional burdens on the user.

Looking at the basic operations, when changing channel, etc., on an analogue television, the user only has the option of using a single remote control. This limits the amount of cognitive effort required by the user, as no decision as to which remote control to use is required.

When an STB is present, the user is faced with the additional decision of which remote control to use. This presents a fundamental additional cognitive load on the user, as well as an additional motion requirement to keep swapping between the two remote controls. Some STB manufacturers have responded to this difficulty by supporting both television and STB operation into a single remote control that operates in dual modes. However, unless some kind of affordance is provided indicating which mode the remote control is in (STB or television), the user can only find out by pressing a button and then seeing and interpreting the response. If the response was not the desired one, then the user needs to undo the action, change the mode and then perform the desired action a second time.

Consequently, STBs will only cease to exclude more people than analogue televisions when their operation is completely transparent from the user's point of view. Integrated digital televisions, for example, appear to manage to achieve this level of transparency for basic functions by using only a single remote control with minimal need for mode changes.

However, even iDTVs exclude more people than analogue televisions when considering the full range of operation. Put simply, digital television offers more functionality, and thus requires more cognitive effort to learn and operate. For example, if a user wishes to use the full functionality of DTV, then there is a greater need to be able to read the on-screen display and to swap to reading the remote control (vision demand). Similarly, the users need to be able to operate the arrow buttons and SELECT/OK, rather than just the channel numbers. The increase in number of channels means that users have to enter more double-figure channel numbers, with the inherent time-out limitations increasing the dexterity demand still further.

Only if all of the additional functionality is as accessible and usable as interacting with an analogue television, will digital television not be more excluding than analogue. This is a tough target to aim for, but a necessary one unless it is to be accepted that not all users will have access to all of the digital services.

19.4 Conclusion

The predominance of exclusion arising from the differences between the users' mental models and the interaction paradigms within the interface affects far more users than those that would typically be classed as a stereotypical 'special needs user'. This is well illustrated by the comparative lack of difficulty with the interaction experienced by the youngest participant who had the most severe vision impairment of any of the users, but who nonetheless experienced little difficulty completing the tasks, most probably because of his wide experience with high-technology products.

Consequently, manufacturers should be encouraged to look beyond the stereotypes of young, severely, impaired people when considering who may have difficulty using their STBs and to also consider the needs of older adults and those who may not be familiar with the interaction paradigms used. There is also a clear need to standardise within those paradigms to minimise the cognitive demand placed on the users and to make interaction with the STBs as transparent as possible.

Ultimately, what is being advocated is not special purpose design for a small market sector, but rather good 'design for all'.

19.5 References

DTI (2000) A study on the difficulties disabled people have when using everyday consumer products. Government Consumer Safety Research, Department of Trade and Industry, London, UK

DTI (2003) Digital Television For All - A report on usability and accessible design. Department of Trade and Industry, London, UK. Available at: http://www.digitaltelevision.gov.uk/dtv_for_all.html

Grundy E, Ahlburg D, Ali M, Breeze E, Sloggett A (1999) Disability in Great Britain. Department of Social Security, Corporate Document Services, London, UK

Keates S, Clarkson PJ (2003) Countering Design Exclusion. Springer-Verlag, London, UK

Nielsen J (1993) Usability Engineering. Academic Press, London, UK

Part III

Assistive Technology and Rehabilitation Robotics

Chapter 20

Robot Technology in Rehabilitation and Support – State of the Art

J.A. van Woerden, G.J. Gelderblom and
B.J.F. Driessen

20.1 Introduction

20.1.1 General

Rehabilitation Robotics is the discipline that deals with applying robot technology to rehabilitation and the support of disabled persons. In the robotics world, that moved from the idea of robotics (1920) via the introduction in factories (1960), Rehabilitation Robotics can be characterised by the development of service robots (1990 onwards) and is still in an infant stadium.

Currently a new area is entered with the integration of (Rehabilitation) Robotics with environmental control systems and smart home technology in ambient intelligent environments. The name of this new dimension is 'Assistive Environments'.

20.1.2 Rehabilitation Robotics

Rehabilitation Robotics is about applying Robot Technology in Rehabilitation and Support (Assistive Devices) for functional limited persons. Thoughts of human like machines capable of assisting real humans have been around for a long time. In 1920 the Czech writer Karel Capek introduced the term Robot in his play 'Rossums Universal Robots'. Robots entered factories on a large scale in the 1960's.

However, it has only been for a few decades that researchers and developers around the world are able to develop reliable Robotic Systems that actually assist persons with a functional limitation. In many, mainly scientific, places in the world concepts of Rehabilitation Robotics were studied and prototyped. The European situation is presented earlier (Buehler *et al.*, 1997) as well as a product overview

(Mahoney *et al.*, 1997). As a follow up this chapter describes the state of the art in Rehabilitation Robotics in 2003.

Rehabilitation Robot research today includes applications of human-friendly robots to everyday activities such as care labour, study and leisure. The position of robots is shifting from 'replacing humans' to 'collaborating with humans'.

Most recently the developments are going in the direction of support of independent living. (Rehabilitation) Robots will be integrated in an ambient intelligent environment (e.g. a user aware house) with environmental control systems, smart home technology, etc.

This so-called 'Assistive Environment' needs to be researched in the years ahead. In this chapter the need for an architecture and a simulation environment is analysed and two existing examples of user aware ambient intelligence are described.

20.2 Robotics in Rehabilitation and Assistive Technology

Robot technology has grown up in an industrial environment and only recently the use of robots to serve humans has been analysed. The state of the art in service robots as well as a definition of service robots is described in literature (IEEE, Robotics and Automation Society).

In general, the development of Rehabilitation Robotics applications is motivated by the promise that people with severe impairments will benefit from this development.

Although, over the decades, there has been continuous progress in technological developments (Gelderblom *et al.*, 2003), only very few systems have become commercially available, and even fewer are accepted for provision. As a consequence, the disabled person, although mentioned as the motivation for each newly started technological development, only enjoys limited benefits of them.

The development of technology itself is obviously an essential element of progress in the domain Rehabilitation Robotics. It is interesting to gain insight into the state of the art in the domain of Rehabilitation Robotics and to monitor the state of development of various robotic applications. That is why a review has been carried out.

20.2.1 Review

The review covered a) technological developments as reported in conference proceedings, grey-literature, exhibitions and on the Internet and b) rehabilitation applications of robotics, searched for in scientific literature.

On the basis of the gathered material, categories were identified. To provide an illustration of the developments of Rehabilitation Robotics in time, these categorisations were subsequently applied to the papers published in the proceedings of three ICORR conferences (1999, 2001, and 2003).

20.2.2 Results

In total over 90 applications were found. In general, the target groups for robot applications mostly suffer from some form of motor impairment, in some cases in combination with sensory impairment. Examples of assistive robot devices for cognitive impairment were all related to an additional motor impairment.

20.2.3 Categories

The collection of applications has been categorised. It concerns the type of application, four fields of application have been identified. Technology applications aimed at:

- supporting fundamental research;
- applications aimed at supporting diagnosis of individuals;
- applications aimed at supporting therapy and training;
- applications constituting some sort of assistive device; and,
- non rehabilitation specific devices.

Fundamental Research. A limited number of reports (10) were found in which robotics are applied in research for the purpose of better understanding human motor behaviour, e.g. (Takahasi *et al.*, 2001). This limited number is surprising because the high level of control and reproducibility of movement provides excellent opportunities for research into better understanding of (impaired) human motor behaviour.

Diagnostics. A very small number of reports (4) were found showing the application of robotics for diagnosis in individuals. Most often these were motor behaviour related diagnostics; force excerption and movement ranges. The found applications, e.g. (Reinkensmeyer D.J. *et al.*, 2000), were all of recent date and under development. The potential advantages of applying robotics to diagnosing motor abilities of individuals are obvious.

The combination of, on the one hand, force and movements, and on the other hand, the accuracy, speed and repetition possibilities, make the application of robotics to diagnosis attractive. However, the potential use of diagnosis systems is likely to be the most limited of the four categories, since it raises questions concerning cost-effectiveness.

It is probably for this reason that found diagnosis systems are (still) closely related to fundamental research.

Therapy and/or Training. The second largest category (15) concerning systems supporting therapy and/or training of individuals with various motor impairment (resulting from spinal cord lesion (SCL) or Cerebro Vascular Accident (CVA). Therapy concerns both arm-hand function, e.g. (Krebs *et al.*, 2000) and mobility, e.g. (Hesse *et al.*, 2000).

In most cases the therapy or training is complementary to therapy provided by a therapist and aims providing additional therapy facilities. Some examples however, seem to aim at replacing the therapist.

Assistive Technology. By far the largest category (41) contains a diversity of applications that somehow support individual users. The assistive devices include wheelchair mounted manipulators (exact dynamics) and robotised environments (afma robots) to support arm-handed function, smart wheelchairs (ibot, 2002) and smart walkers (Wasson *et al.*, 2001) to support mobility and care-robots, e.g. (Graf *et al.*, 2002; Koyanna *et al.*, 2001).

In this category the definition of Rehabilitation Robotics seems to be stretched to its limits. To provide control over the environment systems are reported, featuring complex interfaces in which robotics constitutes only part of the system.

Non Rehabilitation Specific. A final category is filled with a number of systems (24) that either could function as basis for a Rehabilitation Robotics application but cannot be considered as such in itself or are mainstream systems aimed at functioning as social supporting systems i.e. companions. This category was not included in the subsequent analysis.

20.2.4 Development

To provide an indication of the development of Rehabilitation Robotics over time, the contributions of the ICORR conferences in 1999, 2001 and 2003 were categorised over the first four fields of application. The results suggest that the attention to each of the fields hardly shifts over the years. One noteworthy difference in this comparison is the emergence of diagnosis applications at the 2003 conference.

A second type of categorisation that was applied to the applications found concerns the level of development of the application. In light of the question raised in the introduction concerning the result for the end-user of robotics development, a distinction was made between a) the research and development (R&D) phase and b) the use/effect monitoring phase.

The results show that the vast majority of the applications are in an early phase, ranging from drawing board to prototype, and in some cases have been so for some time. An explanation for this may be that developers are mainly located at technical institutes and universities. As a consequence the aspects under development (as far as could be judged) were mainly technical, with little reference to user requirements, commercial production or implementation.

A small proportion of the reports on applications found deal with commercial available products or effects of applications when used by end-users in their daily life.

20.3 Assistive Environments

Stemming from the world of Ambient Intelligence (Aarts) with the introduction of robot like assistants we may arrive at Assistive Environments, the world of ubiquitous computing, ubiquitous communication and intuitive human interfaces.

Envisioned by Mark Weiser (Weiser 1991) in the early 1990s, ubiquitous or pervasive means that computation embedded in the environment is available everywhere to assist users in accomplishing their daily tasks. In the ubiquitous computing world, computing is embedded in physical objects such as clothing, coffee cups, tabletops, walls, floors, doorknobs, roadways, and so forth. For example, while reading a morning newspaper, our coffee placed on a tabletop is kept warm at our favourite temperature. A door opens automatically by sensing current running on our hand; more intelligently detecting our fingerprint, or sensing our approach. The computation is seamlessly and invisibly integrated into physical artefacts within the environment (ambient intelligence), and is always ready to serve us without distracting from our daily practices.

The vision in Assistive Environments is concentrated, but not restricted to, ubiquitous computing and ubiquitous communication and need to be extended to the integration of assistive devices for disabled and older adults. That is why an open architecture and simulation methods need to be chosen and tested. Finally two examples of components of an Assistive Environments are given.

20.3.1 Architecture

An architecture for Assistive Environments is needed. At this moment Smart-homes, environmental control systems, domotic systems, etc., are based on proprietary technology and are too fragmented to be adopted as architecture elements.

For pervasive space infrastructures as Assistive Environments the Open Service Gate way Initiative (OSGI), specifying an extensible framework for the interconnection of devices, is something to look at. An example of an application is 'OSGI based service Infrastructure for Context Aware Connected Homes (Zhang *et al.*, 2003). For home services Universal Plug and Play (UPnP) may be considered for the integration of devices.

20.3.2 Simulation Tools for Assistive Environments

Designing ambient intelligent living environments for handicapped and elderly people is far from straightforward. Questions like the optimal number of situational awareness sensors, their optimal location, the required communication bandwidth between objects, the functionality of the active objects can hardly be answered at design time. However, changing the structure of the ambient intelligent environment after initial implementation can result in high costs. That is why a simulation environment is needed, which can be used not only for designing different components present in ambient intelligent environments (e.g. robotic systems), but also for evaluating the entire (complex) ambient intelligent environment.

The development environment must have the following characteristics:

- support of 3D visualisations (for visual user feedback);
- interaction of objects in a realistic way (e.g. it must not be possible to drive through a wall with a wheelchair);
- simulation in real-time (allowing real-time evaluation by end-users).

A simulation environment is described in this chapter, useful as a design tool (by engineers) and an evaluation tool (by end-users) of ambient intelligent environments. First, the general architecture of the environment is given.

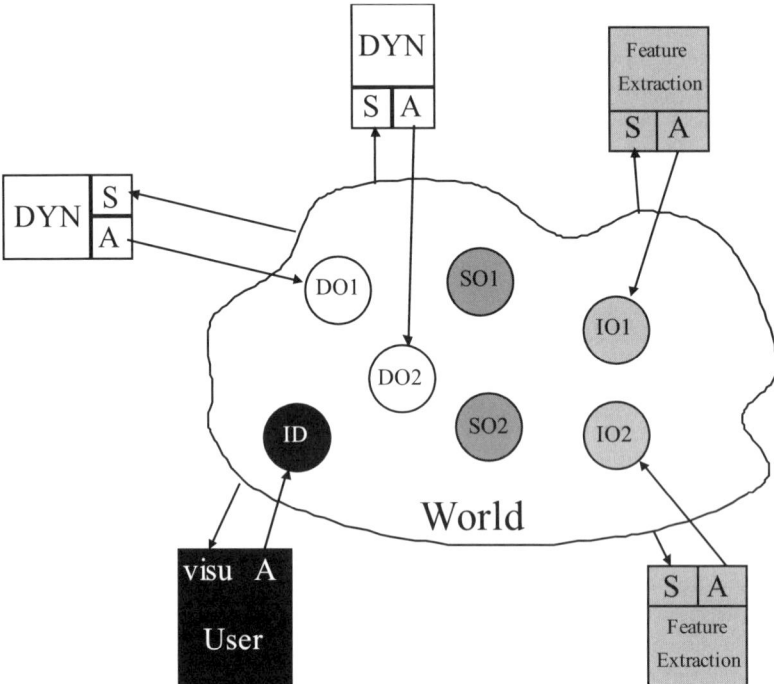

Figure 20.1. Simulating multiple objects.

Conceptually, the simulation environment is shown in Figure 20.1. In this environment, the world is composed of objects, which can be dynamic (DO)static (SO) or intelligent (IO).

Examples of DOs are wheelchairs or robotic systems, while SOs represent things like furniture. The situational awareness sensors are the IOs. The user is considered as a separate entity, which communicates with the environment via an input device (ID), such as a joystick, for direct controlling of devices (wheelchair). Necessary visual feedback to the user is taken care of by the visualisation, indicated by "visu".

Each DO has a dynamic simulation entity (DYN), responsible for calculating control actions, and simulating dynamics of the device. Sensory information used by the controllers can be retrieved via sensors (S). The (global) state of the DO is updated using actuators (A). The same principle applies for the situational awareness sensors (IOs), with the difference that an intelligent feature extraction algorithm replaces the dynamics of DOs. The actuator of situational awareness sensors communicates the extracted feature to the global world (Driessen *et al.*, 2003).

20.3.3 Component examples

Mathilda's House (Sumi Helal et al 2003)
Mathilda's Smart House project is an effort to innovate pervasive applications and environments specifically designed to support the older adults. The project is funded by the Rehabilitation Engineering Research Center *(RERC)* hosted at the *Pervasive Computing Laboratory* at the University of Florida (Helal *et al.*, 2003). The project research pervasive computing spaces that can particularly assist elder people live independently. The project explores the use of emerging smart homes, smart phones and other wireless technologies to create assistive environments and "magic wands" to enable elder persons with disabilities to interact with, monitor, and control their surroundings. By integrating the smart phone with Assistive Environments, older adults are able to turn appliances on and off, check and change the status of locks on doors and windows, and aid in grocery shopping. It also explores the use of smart phones as devices that can proactively provide advice such as reminders to take medications or call in prescription drug refills automatically.

Intelligent Bed Robot system as an example (Bien et al 2003)
The Intelligent Bed Robot system was developed as an active service agent to assist the older adults or disabled persons to live a convenient daily life. These persons usually spend much time in their beds and suffer of great inconvenience even for small movements. As shown in Figure 20.2, "Bed" + "Robotic Arm" is a motivation and a concept to give effective service. "Bed" is a suitable place for a long time service and "Robotic Arm" is proper as an active agent.

Figure 20.3 shows the prototype of the system consisting of three parts, an automatic bed, a robotic arm and a motion capture device. The bed is designed considering the of human body and can change its pose in various ways. The MANUS arm is attached to the side of the bed and is utilised to serve four kinds of tasks: pulling a book and putting it back on the bookshelf, transporting a newspaper, giving a massage, and pulling a quilt over and putting it away. To this end, the robotic arm needs the on-line position information of objects with high accuracy and the motion capture device is utilised to supply the position information in real time. The motion capture system is also used to control human-friendly motion trajectories of the robotic arm. The tasks can be extended by adjusting the motion trajectories of the robotic arm by applying effective position sensors.

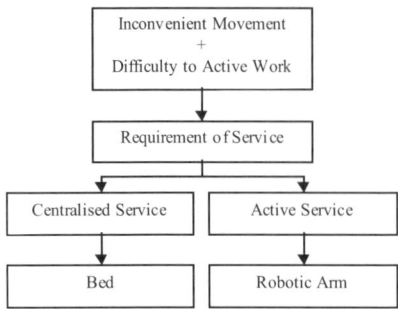
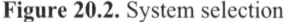

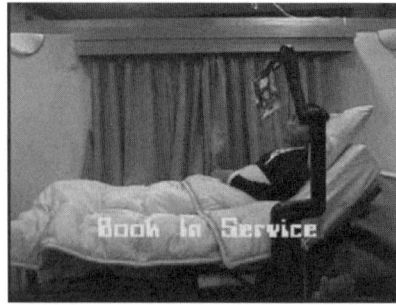

Figure 20.2. System selection   **Figure 20.3.** Intelligent Bed Robot

20.4. Conclusion

The domain of Rehabilitation Robotics has not been able yet to turn the underlying promises into reality. In Europe two small companies, Rehabilitation Robotics Ltd. and Exact Dynamics deliver products on a sizeable scale. Only in the Netherlands as far as known a Rehabilitation Robotics application has been accepted as a health care insurance provision. It is (almost) on the prescription list. Far too little information is available on the effects of usage of Rehabilitation Robotics on for instance care substitution, rehabilitation outcomes or quality of life. Albeit, the domain of Rehabilitation Robotics is still developing and in a positive sense.

Service Robots as a subject in general is gaining interest of larger companies and the research and development institutes world-wide. A convergence of entertainment and mainstream comfort robotics, with obvious potential for rehabilitation applications is evolving. Not only concerning the technical disciplines but also the science of cognition and intuitive user interfacing.

The world of Assistive Environments, where intuitive user interfacing, ambient intelligence and the integration of different domains of assistive technology are relevant, need to be considered by the research community to pursue benefit (in the end) for the disabled and older adults. Since this type of technology has a potential wide spread application, significant involvement of mainstream industries is likely, which could boost developments.

20.5. References

Aarts E, Ambient Intelligence. The paradigm Philips.

Bühler C (1997) Robotics for rehabilitation. A European (?) Perspective. In: Proceedings ICORR 1997, University of Bath, UK

Driessen BJF, van Woerden JA, ten Kate TK, Versluis AHG (2003) Developing and evaluating intelligent environments for disabled and elderly people. In: Proceedings of ICOST 2003, Paris, France

Gelderblom GJ, Cremers G, Soede M(2003) Rehabilitation robotics - The state of the art in 2003. CD-Rom, iRv, Hoensbroek, Netherlands

Graf B, Hans M, Kubacki J, Schraft R D (2002) Robotic home assistant - Care-O-Bot. In: IEEE Engineering in Medicine and Biology Society: Conference Proceedings 24th Annual International Conference of the Engineering in Medicine and Biology Society

Helal S et al. (2003) Assistive environments for successful ageing. In: ICOST 03, Paris, France

Helal S, Winkler B, Lee C, Kaddoura Y, Ran L, Giraldo C, Kuchibhota S, Mann W (2003) Enabling location aware pervasive computing applications for the elderly. In: Proceedings of the first IEEE International Conference on Pervasive Computing and Communications

Hesse S, Uhlenbrock D (2000) A mechanised gait trainer for restoration of gait. Journal of Rehabilitation Research and Development, 37(6)

Krebs HI, Hogan N, Volpe BT, Aisen ML, Edelstein L, Diels C (1999) Robot-aided neuro-rehabilitation in stroke: three year follow-up. In: Proceedings of ICORR 99, Stanford University, Palo Alto, California, USA

Mahoney R M (1977) Robotic products for rehabilitation: status and strategy. Proceedings ICORR 1997 pp 12-17. IEEE, Robotics and Automation Society. Available at: http://www.service-robots.org/IEEE-start.php

Park KH, Bien ZZ (2003) Intelligent sweet home for assisting the elderly and the handicapped. In: Proceedings of ICOST 2003, Paris, France

Reinkensmeyer DJ, Kahn LE, Averbuch M, McKenna-Cole AN, Schmit BD, Rymer WZ (2000) Understanding and treating arm movement impairment after chronic brain injury: Progress with the ARM Guide. Journal of Rehabilitation Research and Development 37 (6): 653-662

Takahashi CD, Scheidt RA, Reinkensmeyer DJ (2001) Impedance control and internal model formation when reaching in a randomly varying dynamical environment. Journal of Neurophysiogology 86: 1047-1051

Wason G, Gunderson J, Graves S, Felder R (2001) An assistive robotic agent for pedestrian mobility. International Conference on Autonomous Agents, Montreal, Canada

Weiser M (1991)The computer for the 21st century. Scientific American 256(3): 94-104

Zhang D, Whang X, Leman K, Huang W (2003) OSGI based service infrastructure for context aware connected homes. In: Proceedings of ICOST 2003, Paris, France

Afma Robots http://www.afma-robots.com/pages/afmaster.htm

Exact Dynamics http://www.exactdynamics.nl/

iBot (2002) http://www.independencenow.com/ibot/index.html

UpnP Forum. Homepage http://www.upnp.org

Chapter 21

Powered Lower Limb Orthosis for Assisting Standing Up and Sitting Down Movements

T. Raparelli, P. Beomonte Zobel and F. Durante

21.1 Introduction

For older and some classes of disabled people there is often the need for assistance in sitting down and standing up, although they may be able to walk. This is due to limited power in the muscles of the legs.

Some authors propose innovative armchairs with motorised folding seats which are able to hold the user's body weight during the sitting down and standing up operations (Sanada, 1999). Although these devices work well, there is the need for an environment with many of these units if they are to be truly effective, which is expensive to implement. Moreover, it is not possible to have many such environments outside of the domestic one.

Another strategy is to use a motorised orthosis for the lower limb, worn by the person, which is able to assist the user during these operations. In this case, the orthosis has to fulfil certain technical specifications such as acceptability, usability and safety. To satisfy all these constraints, the actuators play a major role in the development of the device. The Pneumatic Muscle actuators (PMs) provide good compliance and a high power-to-weight ratio. Furthermore, they are clean, low cost and similar to human muscles from the point of view of their force/contraction characteristics.

In this chapter the development of a lower limb orthosis is presented. The orthosis is designed to help older and disabled people to stand up and to sit down. The key requirements of the orthosis' design are psychological acceptability by the user, usability, safety and low cost. The knee joint is driven by two McKibben pneumatic muscle actuators working together.

With regard to the control system, two strategies are implemented for testing purposes: one based on an on/off logic and the other based on a proportional one. Both systems use a reference signal generated by a electro-pneumatic "user intention sensor", specifically developed by the authors, which measures muscle hardness. Some experimental tests were carried out with a healthy user, demonstrating that the device works well and suggesting further improvements.

21.2 The Mechanical Design of the Orthosis

The powered orthosis was required to meet the following general specifications (Raparelli *et al.*, 2002). The device had to be able to supply a sufficient level of force for assisting the sitting down and standing up movements, it had to be acceptable from the psychological point of view by the user, it had to be usable, it had to be safe and, if possible, cheap. These general specifications led to other more detailed specifications which may be presented as:

- *sufficient force to stand up and to sit down* → to lift a person of 70 kg;
- *acceptable from the psychological point of view* → small, anthropomorphic architecture, wearable under the clothes;
- *usable* → low weight, comfortable, easy to use, minimal training, to permit free movement whilst walking, sufficient energetic autonomy;
- *safe* → simple architecture, structural compliance;
- *cheap* → to use cheap technologies.

In Figure 21.1, all the steps encountered during the design process are presented. Starting from the technical specification it was possible to define all the practical solutions for the orthosis. The specifications suggested a concept which has an anthropomorphic exoskeleton structure with one motorised degree of freedom at knee level. Hence, the orthosis has a 'femur' and a 'tibia', connected together by means of a rotational joint, the 'knee', manufactured by two hinges with coincident axes.

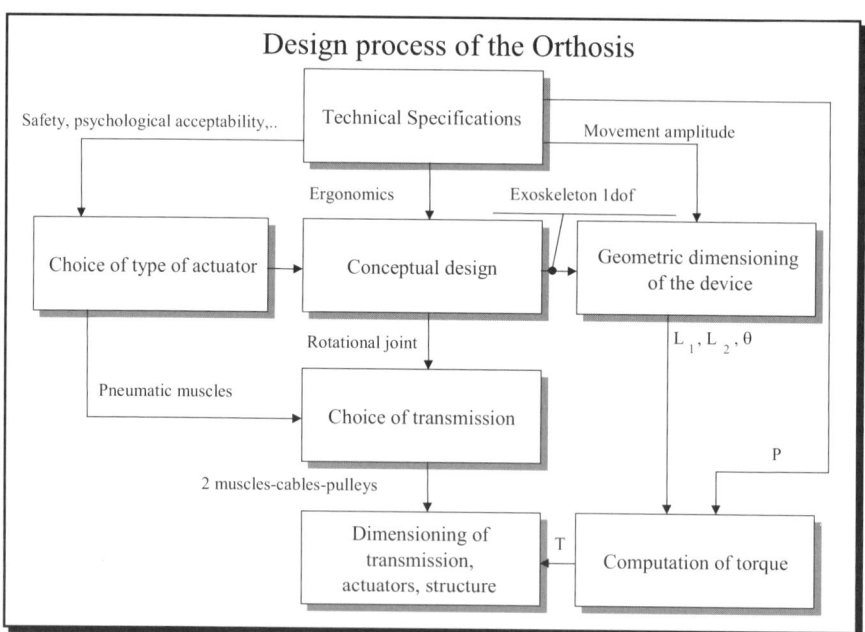

Figure 21.1. The mechanical design process of the orthosis

The next step was to define the lengths of the two links corresponding to the tibia (L_1) and the femur (L_2) and their relative angular excursion (θ). Using these values, the torque (T) that the orthosis had to provide at the joint was computed for a variety of different geometrical configurations.

With regard to the actuators, the safety and human likeness requirements pointed towards the use of McKibben type 'pneumatic muscles'. This kind of actuator can be manufactured without the need for special technology and, due to its shape, can be easily integrated into the orthosis, along the tibia or the femur, maintaining small overall dimensions. To initiate movement, a cable - pulley transmission was chosen.

Finally, it was possible to dimension, from a quantitative point of view, the actuators, the transmission and the layout of the device. In order to calculate the driving torque required from the orthosis, a mechanical model of the human body was used. It was a bi-dimensional model, in the sagittal plane, composed of three skeletal segments: the shank, the thigh and the part of the trunk between the hip and the centre of mass of the body.

The segments were joined together by frictionless hinge joints and the following two hypotheses considered: during movement the shank segment is always parallel to the trunk and the centre of mass of the human body remains directly above the ankle (Figure 21.2(a)).

The angle (θ) between the tibia and the femur changes from 70° (sitting position) to 180° (upright position). The length of the segments are assumed as follows: L_1= 418 mm, L_2= 428 mm, L_3= 214 mm. The model is useful to estimate the torque required at knee level (C) for a given weight of the human body (P). Movements were considered to be quasi-static, allowing inertial loads to be ignored.

Two actuators were symmetrically installed on opposing sides of the leg and, due to space considerations, were placed in correspondence with the tibia. Hence, the transmission was constructed by fixing a pulley to the upper part of the device, corresponding to the femur. The radius (R) of the pulley determined the pneumatic muscle characteristics, relating the angular excursion ($θ$) to the shortening of the pneumatic muscle (ΔL), and the torque (C) to the force (F) required by the actuator.

After several cycles of an iterative process, in which a value for the pulley radius was chosen, the characteristics of the muscles were defined. Then the muscle was dimensioned and verified, leading to a pulley radius of 45 mm and the following characteristics for the pneumatic muscles: resting diameter Φ = 20 mm, resting length L_0= 260 mm, maximum working pressure P_{max}= 0.5 MPa, maximum shortening ΔL_{max}= 85 mm. Some rules from Raparelli et al. (2000) were used to dimension the pneumatic muscles.

The pneumatic muscles were manufactured and experimentally tested. Figure 21.2(b) shows the result of the tests on the muscles compared with the desired force. The pneumatic muscles are fixed to the lower part of the orthosis, by one end of each muscle. The other end is linked to a cable, engaged on the pulley, which terminates on the upper part of the orthosis just above the knee joint.

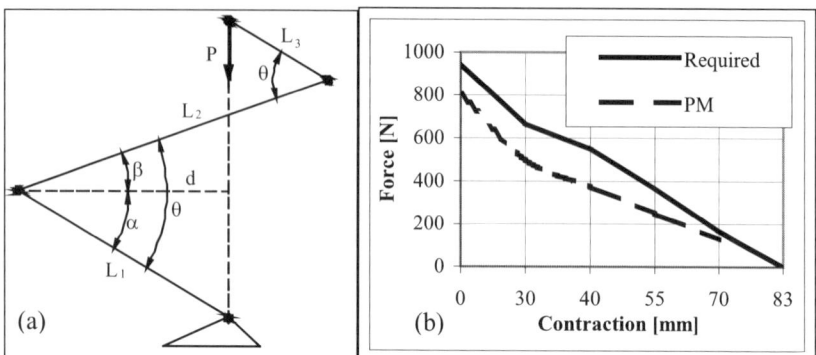

Figure 21.2. (a) three segments model of the human body; (b) force vs. contraction of the PM (for a 0.65 MPa pressure) and as the movements require.

The frame of the orthosis was made up of two lateral structures, each comprising 3 parts: a lower rod, an upper rod and a hinge joint. The rods were made of aluminium, while the hinge joint was made by steel. To permit application to the lower limb and to transmit the forces, two shells, made of a thermosetting material, were used. These also joined the two lateral structures.

During normal operation of the orthosis, the air supply for the pneumatic muscles was provided by a pressure tank. To give an idea of its dimensions, a cylindrical tank with a volume of 0.002 m^3 provides pressurised air for about 6 operations (stored at 1.0 MPa), and has a diameter of approximately 120 mm, a length of 300 mm and a mass of about 4 kg. Figure 21.3 shows a photograph of the prototype.

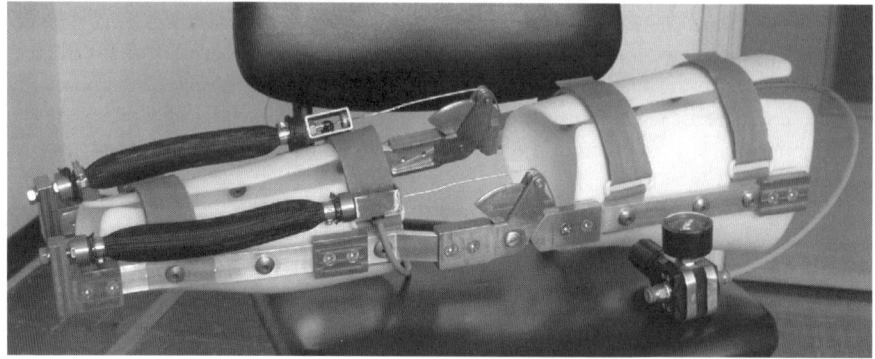

Figure 21.3. The realised prototype

21.3 The Control System

The control system has to meet the technical usability requirements. It has to permit natural movement, require minimal training, and utilise small, low weight components. The first idea was to use two buttons: one to drive the 'stand up' and the other the 'sit down' movement. Such a system was implemented for preliminary testing of the overall system. It assumed the hands were to be used to push the buttons. This was not the ideal situation since the hands could be useful to maintain equilibrium during movement. A device able to automatically recognise the user's intention would be better. To obtain this goal, a sensor that detected user intention by measuring the hardness of the femoral muscle was developed.

With regard to the control system, the basic idea was to consider the operator as the central control element. Often, a focus on disability regards only the motion capability of the limb, while the sensorial proprioceptive system is still able to detect the actual position and effort of the limb.

The idea was to give an active role to the user's vision and proprioceptive sensorial systems to control the orthosis. The user will control the real movements with reference to measures of force and velocity. The orthosis will have the task of providing the assisting force as requested from the user.

In such a way the orthosis will 'become' a part of the user, an 'extension' of him and the user will maintain the sensation of interacting with the environment in the same way as for healthy people, thus providing a good sense of control. For these reasons the system, constituted by the orthosis and the limb, can work like a human limb.

Since the user knows very well how to move their limbs, the use of the orthosis does not involve training. The idea described above is near to the so-called impedance control without the need to implement feedback sensors, resulting in a simple device.

The device is not separate from the user and this permits simplification of the overall system. It is the opinion of the authors that this type of strategy, by which the user assumes a central role in the control system, is preferable to others in which the device on its own completes the task. This is because the user has more motivation since he is more active and because the system is simpler and hence more reliable and cheaper (Raparelli et al., 2003).

With regard to the control system architecture, two strategies were developed, both making use of the signal from the developed sensor. The first made use of on/off logic while the other made use of proportional control.

21.3.1 The Electro-Pneumatic Sensor

An electro-pneumatic sensor was developed to detect the hardening of the femoral muscle. It consisted of a little bag made of silicon rubber connected to a pressure transducer. The lightly pressurised bag was placed on the femoral quadriceps and secured by a nylon inextensible belt.

During movement the muscle hardens in proportion to the requested effort and thus leads to an increase of pressure inside the bag. Figure 21.4 shows photographs of the sensor bag and its mounting arrangement.

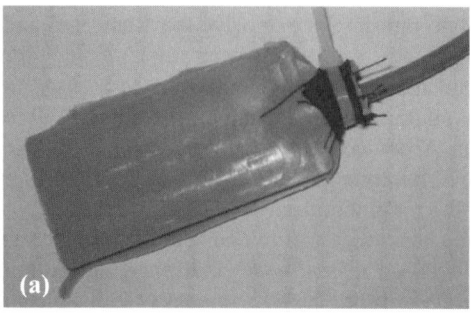 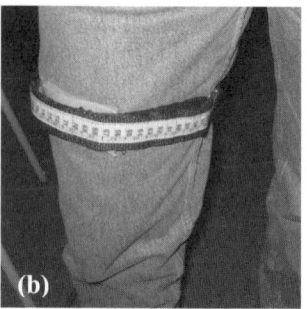

Figure 21.4. The sensor: (a) fitted to a tube; (b) mounted on the femoral muscle

The sensor was characterised experimentally. Preliminary tests indicated that the signal level provided by the sensor depends on many factors: initial pressure level, fastening force of the belt, bag dimensions and stiffness of the bag wall.

A procedure for mounting the bag was defined: with the leg stretched, the bag was placed on the quadriceps; the belt was placed around the leg and fastened in such a way that the length of the belt overlapped by a given percentage of the leg circumference.

Tests were carried out to determine the optimal values of these parameters to achieve a good level of output signal. Several sensors with different dimensions, made of pure silicon rubber and of silicon and a tissue inside (for stiffening purposes), with different belt fastening characteristics and with different initial pressure levels were carried out.

Tests were conducted on four people of different height and weight. The data were acquired using a pressure transducer (accuracy ± 0.5 % full scale of 0.5 MPa), a data acquisition board (National Instruments) and specially written C code. The best results, considering all the different users, were obtained for a stiffened bag, with dimensions 80 × 40 × 6 mm, a fastening overlap of 3.5 % and an initial pressure of 0.025 MPa. Figure 21.5 shows a typical output from the sensing system during stand up and sit down movements.

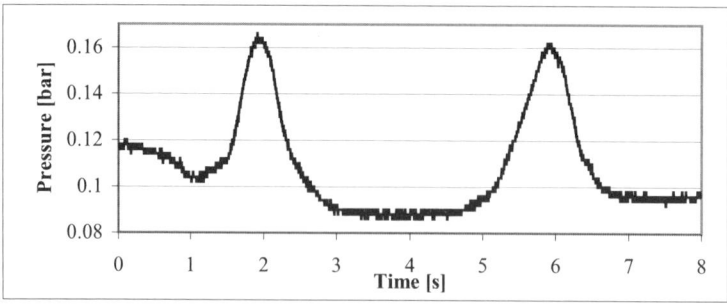

Figure 21.5. Typical behaviour of sensor system during stand up and sit down movements

21.3.2 The Control Strategies

Two control strategies were implemented to drive the orthosis: an on/off and a proportional one. Figure 21.2(b) shows that the force from the pneumatic muscle is similar to that required from the orthosis to provide movements in relation to the actual position.

The same goes for the torque, since this is related to the force by the pulley radius. This particular condition creates a stable system from the control perspective without the need to implement further hardware and software to improve stability.

The on/off control system has an architecture comprising: the sensor bag, a pressure transducer, a data acquisition board mounted on a personal computer, a home made photocoupler driver board and two pneumatic valves type SMC EVZ512 ($C = 1.62E\text{-}8$ m^3/s/Pa a.n.r, $b = 0.5$, catalog data) – see Figure 21.6(a).

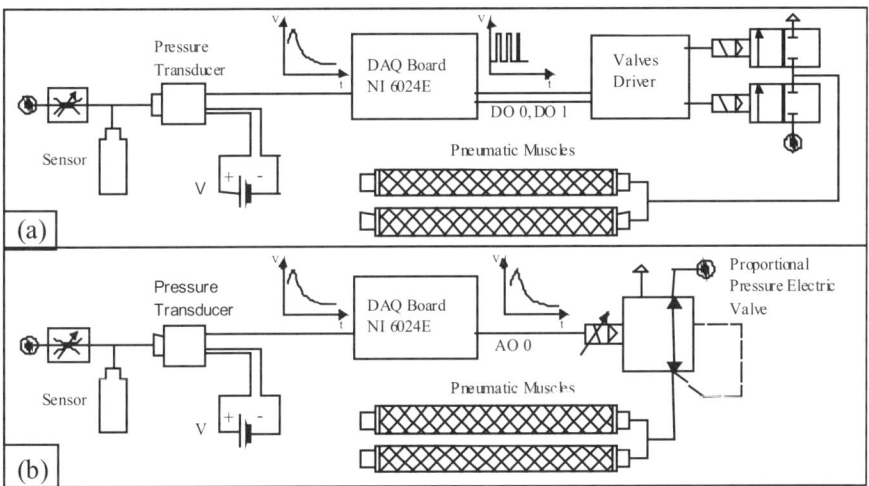

Figure 21.6. Scheme of the control system: (a) on/off; (b) proportional

With regard to the control algorithm, by considering the typical behaviour of the signal detected by the sensor during movement, two different level of signal were chosen to define three zones (Figure 21.7): the 1st zone ranges from zero to the first level, the 2nd from the first level to the second level, and the 3rd from the second to the maximum level.

When the detected signal falls within the 1st zone the exhaust valve is opened, thus decreasing the pressure in the actuators. If the signal falls into the 2nd zone, then both the valves are closed, holding the pressure in the actuators constant. Finally, if the signal falls into the 3rd zone the supply valve is opened, thus increasing the pressure in the actuators.

The supply pressure to the valves was set at 0.5 MPa, which was considered to be a safe level, since 0.65 MPa was the maximum pressure allowed to avoid failure.

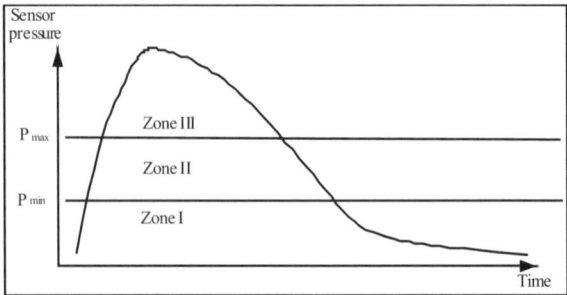

Figure 21.7. The three zones delimited by the two pressure levels to define the drive signals for the valves in the on/off control

With regard to the proportional control system, the architecture was the same as for the on/off control. The only difference was that the on/off valves were replaced by a proportional pressure valve, type SMC VY1200 output pressure $0.05 \div 0.88$ MPa. This system allows the actuator force to be controlled without use of a force feedback sensor. The control algorithm is also simple: the pressure inside the muscle (and so the force provided by the muscles) is proportional to the signal detected by the hardness sensor (see Figure 21.8). The gain constant was chosen such that the maximum sensor signal corresponded to a pressure reference of 0.5 MPa, which was the maximum permissible working pressure for the muscles.

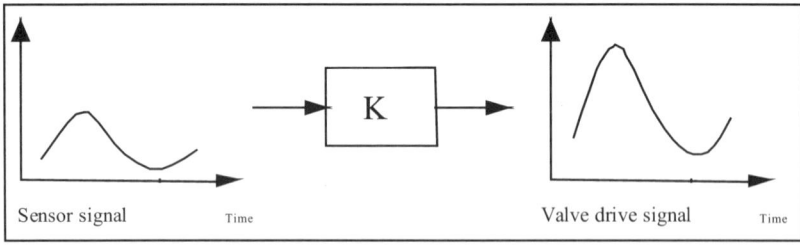

Figure 21.8. Transformation of the signal from the sensor to the valve drive signal in the proportional control

21.4 The Experimental Tests

Experimental tests on a healthy person were conducted using the on/off and proportional control architectures. The tests observed the performance of many stand up and sit down movements. The users' impressions were that the device provided substantial assistance. It was very easy to use since the user had to do nothing more than he was already able to do: just stand up and sit down. The system automatically detected the user intention and applied the assisting force. Figure 21.9 shows two frames of a sequence from a stand up movement. During the movements some noise due to the interaction with the structural part could arise, thus suggesting further improvements to the structural plastic interfaces.

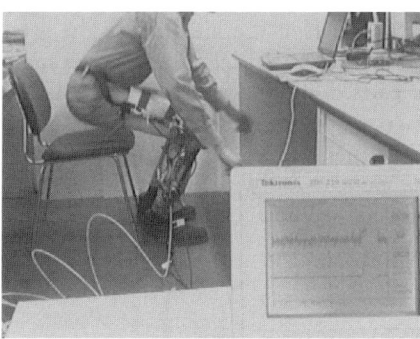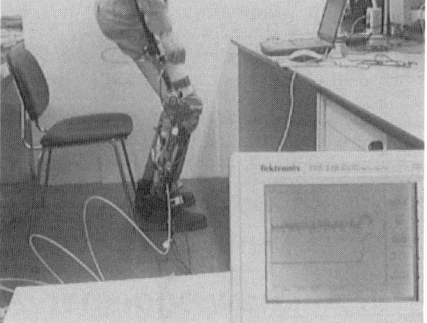

Figure 21.9. Two photos taken during a stand up movement

The main difference between the two control systems was that the proportional control exhibited smoother and quieter behaviour. The on/off control had to cycle the open and close valves to modulate the output signal while the proportional valve was moved in a continuous way to control the orifice. To provide a quantitative measure, the pressure inside the pneumatic muscle was monitored during the tests, thus determining the force provided by the pneumatic muscles and the torque applied at the knee.

The device provided, on average, approximately 55% of the torque necessary for movement with both control approaches. Figure 21.10(a) shows a comparison of the supplied torque versus angle (θ) for the on/off control while Figure 21.10(b) shows the same comparison for proportional control. Although 55% was a great help, it would be possible to increase the level of assistance by using more efficient pneumatic muscles to provide higher forces.

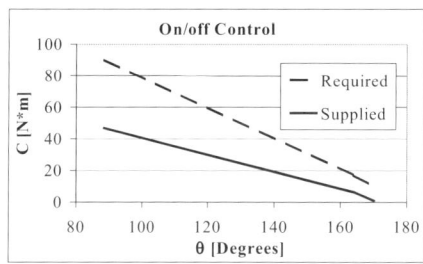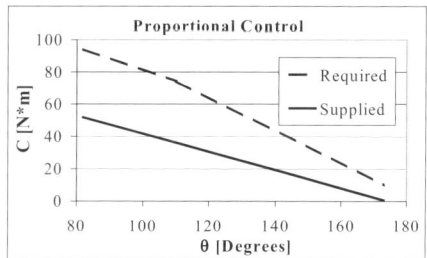

Figure 21.10. Supplied and required torque during stand up movement: (a) on/off control, (b) proportional control

21.5 Conclusions

In this chapter, the process of developing a powered lower limb orthosis is presented. The orthosis is designed to assist older people and those with some types of disability with standing up and sitting down movements. The orthosis has one degree of freedom, with a joint at the knee, and is driven by pneumatic muscle actuators. A control system, which automatically detects the intention of the user, was developed and two control algorithms based on on/off and proportional logic were implemented. Experimental tests were carried out with a healthy person and the device demonstrated good performance, providing up to the 55% of the torque required to stand up. Further developments are planned to improve the structural interfaces, and to miniaturise the control components, in particular, the controller and valves. Finally, clinical trials with older users will be undertaken.

21.6 Acknowledgements

The authors wish to thank Dr. Adriano Ippati for his help in the experimental tests, SOM s.r.l. for providing the plastic mechanical interfaces of the orthosis, and MIUR for their financial support.

21.7 References

Sanada K (1999) A study on control techniques for power-assisted chair. In: 4th JHPS, Int. Symp. On Fluid Power, Tokyo, Japan

Raparelli T, Beomonte Zobel P, Durante F (2000) On the design of pneumatic muscle actuators. In: 2nd Internationales Fluidtechnisches Kolloquium, Dresden, Germany

Raparelli T, Beomonte Zobel P, Durante F (2002) Development of a pneumatic knee orthosis. 5th JFPS, International Symposium on Fluid Power, Nara, Japan

Raparelli T, Beomonte Zobel P, Durante F, Raparelli F (2003) Development of a powered upper limb orthosis. In: 5th ICORR, Daejeon, Korea

Chapter 22

Collaborative Control Aspects for Rehabilitation Robots

A.H.G. Versluis, B.J.F. Driessen, J.A. van Woerden and T.T. ten Kate

22.1 Introduction

22.1.1 The Manus

A Rehabilitation Robot (RR) as e.g. the Manus Manipulator is an assistive device for severely motor handicapped users. With it, users can perform daily tasks that would otherwise be impossible or very difficult. The appreciation of the Manus robotic manipulator is reflected in the following reactions:

> "I wouldn't want to be without the Manus, since it has given me a certain amount of independence that I didn't have before",

> Ms. Eva Almberg, Sweden, (Neveryd 1999).

> "I feel good because I am more independent through the robot arm".

> (Veronica 2003).

However, the control of a complex device like the Manus is cumbersome for persons with very limited rest functions. Manus has six degrees of freedom (DOFs), e.g. X, Y, Z, Yaw, Pitch and Roll. These DOFs cannot be controlled simultaneously, because the user input device often allows for no more than 2 DOF control input (e.g. the wheelchair joystick). Therefore, the user is able to map his 1 or 2 DOFs to several different gripper co-ordinates during the execution of a task. This can be done in different co-ordinate frames, such as Cartesian mode and cylindrical mode. The DOFs that aren't controlled by the user are kept constant. Unfortunately, because of this switching in mappings, execution of tasks can take quite some time, though the maximum velocity of the Manus is sufficient in itself.

We propose a solution in which a number of the remaining DOFs are controlled using information from extra sensors, such as cameras, force torque sensors and infrared distance sensors. This reduces the cognitive load on the user as well as the need for control and the number of mode switches. In this way, task execution can be sped up.

It is not the intention to build a fully autonomous Manus. On one hand, this is very difficult because of the unstructured environment in which Manus has to operate. On the other hand, the philosophy of Manus has always been that the user retains supervision and actively controls Manus.

The combination of user and semi-autonomous sensor control is known in literature as "collaborative control". In this chapter, we will apply this concept to Manus and extend it to incorporate more than one sensor. A scheme is provided which provides easy addition of extra sensors and flexible mapping of DOFs to sensors and user. Special consideration is given to the interaction between user and sensor control (object selection, active feedback) in order to provide an intuitive user interface.

22.1.2 Collaborative Control

As stated earlier, the addition of extra sensors, like a camera or force-torque sensors, might provide extra control, but they might not be suited to handle every situation. For instance, a camera might not recognise every object even when a priori knowledge is available.

Collaborative control, the concept of combining computer accuracy with user intelligence has been proposed as a solution to this problem, see e.g. (Fong *et al.*, 1999).

In Fong *et al.* (2000) this collaborative control takes the form of an active dialogue between the user and a mobile robot. By exchanging information they negotiate the next action. The application of collaborative control to Manus is a relatively new concept, first seen in Martens *et al.* (2001). In this work, the interaction also takes the form of a dialogue, employing speech recognition. Though the course of action is negotiated in both related studies, the actual manipulation is still a more or less autonomous action. As stated earlier, this is not desirable in our case.

In later work, the collaborative control is extended from only one sensor and one user to multiple identical sensors and one user (Fong *et al.*, 2000; Goldberg *et al.*, 2001). The emphasis in these papers is put on the enhanced robustness rather than improved versatility. Because versatility is also an important design issue, we have extended the collaborative control to incorporate multiple *non-identical* sensors. We propose a special scheme to facilitate this incorporation.

22.2 Manus Collaborative Control

22.2.1 Control Scheme

A Manus collaborative control system differs from standard solutions for collaborative control on the count that it incorporates the user into the control loop to a much further degree.

Unlike the work mentioned in Section 22.1.2, the role of the user is not limited to issuing prescribed high-level commands. Instead, the user actively engages in the control of a part of the number of DOFs. User control is augmented by the other sensors that control the remaining number of DOFs. The intention of the user is determined from his/her input in an intuitive way, bypassing tedious dialogue. Constant feedback is provided to the user so that he/she retains supervision.

As mentioned earlier, multiple sensors are combined in order to control Manus. The strength of each sensor, such as camera versatility and distance sensor accuracy, is used to compensate the weaknesses of the other sensors as well as possible. The control scheme is shown in Figure 22.1:

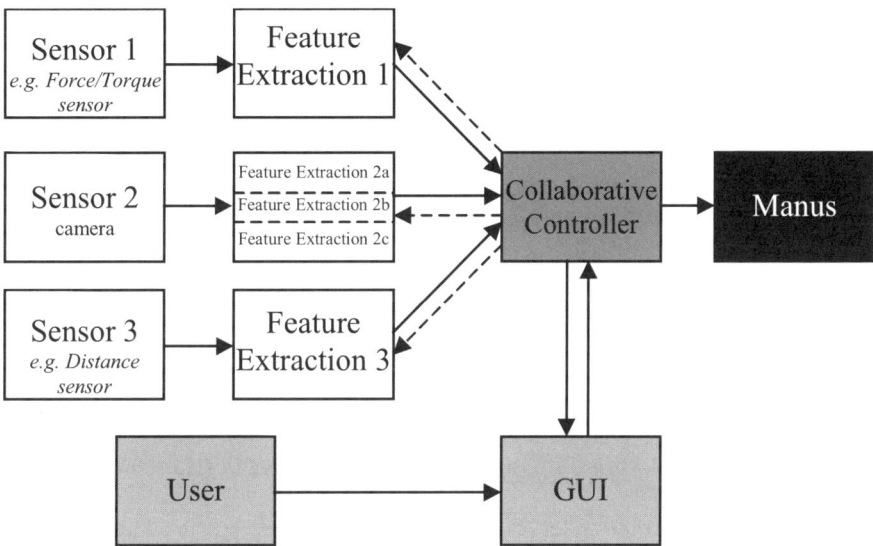

Figure 22.1. Control scheme. The collaborative controller combines the output of the sensors with the user input. Each sensor has its own algorithm to calculate control features. In the case of the camera, multiple algorithms are used.

In this scheme, the user is provides input, just like the sensors extract features, reflecting his incorporation in the loop (continuous arrows, indicate information). The collaborative controller communicates which features are to be calculated, and for which object (dashed arrows, indicate commands). This decision is made based on user input and sensory information. The present state of the controller, including the selected object is fed back to the user via the GUI. Finally, the controller combines the features from the sensors and the user input into a control signal for Manus. This is done by assigning DOFs to the user or certain sensors. Another possibility would be to add the signals together

An important sensor is the camera. Because it is the most versatile sensor, it plays an important role in not only the tracking of the object in order to provide control signals, but also in the initial selection of the object. To this end, the user is provided with the camera image, along with feedback on the selected object.

Because the camera provides by far the most data of all the sensors, the information obtained from it is often hard to process and therefore hard to interpret. This makes feature calculation more difficult and somewhat unreliable.

To aid in this interpretation, a similar solution to the combined control scheme is presented: The data from the camera is used by several image processing algorithms and the results of these algorithms are combined for a more reliable outcome in much the same way as the sensors are combined in the greater control scheme (see Figure 22.1).

In our research, the following sensors are available to Manus:

- user;
- camera;
- infrared distance sensor;
- force/torque sensor.

Our camera is a standard analogue camera, 1×1×2 cm, 768×576 resolution at 25 Hz and is mounted on the gripper. The distance sensor provides a single voltage, which is a measure for the distance to the nearest surface directly in front of the sensor. It has a range of 30 cm and an accuracy of about 0.2 cm.

22.2. 2 Visual Servoing

In this paragraph, a more in-depth description is given of how the robot is controlled using the camera.

Two widely used architectures for visual servoing are *image based visual servoing* (IBVS) and *position based visual servoing* (PBVS) (Hutschinson *et al.*, 1996; Corke *et al.*, 1993).

In PBVS a 3D world-model is constructed by the vision system. This 3D world model is used by a path-planner, which will guide the arm to the desired position. Calculating a 3D world model can be carried out using different techniques (stereovision, usage of a-priori knowledge about the objects, etc.). These techniques are not preferred, since they need extra cameras, or explicit a-priori information (which is in most cases not available in unstructured environments).

In IBVS, the required position of the manipulator is defined in terms of image features (e.g. required location of corners of a cube). The visual servo continuously calculates the actual values of these features, and calculates a correcting control action in feature space. Feature errors are translated to robot co-ordinates (defined in the frame set by the collaborative controller). This requires the calculation of the inverse of an image Jacobian (J_i), defined in the following equation:

$$\frac{df}{d^c x_o} = J_i(^c x_o) \tag{22.1}$$

where f represents the feature vector and $^c x_o$ the pose of the object with respect to the camera frame.

Of the two architectures, IBVS is incorporated into our control scheme, because the signals can more easily be combined with the signals of the user and the other sensors.

22.2.3 Co-ordinate Frames in the Collaborative Controller

As stated earlier, several co-ordinate frames are available to the user in order to control Manus. However, for each sensor, other co-ordinate frames might be preferable. For instance, a camera operates best in a Cartesian frame attached to the gripper, where the camera is placed. A force torque sensor might require a different frame, based on where it is placed on the Manus.

The collaborative controller facilitates this by using transformation matrices ^cTu to convert signals from each preferred co-ordinate frame into one single frame, which the collaborative controller uses to control Manus. An example of what the collaborative controller looks like for a user and a single camera is shown in Figure 22.2:

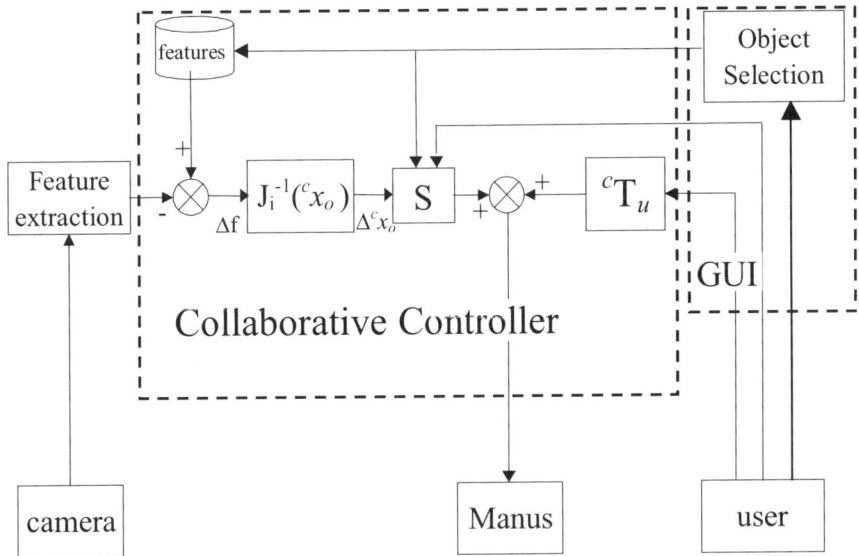

Figure 22.2. A scheme for a collaborative controller for a user and a single camera. The communication with the sensors has been excluded for simplicity's sake.

Whenever a user wants to execute a certain task, he/she selects an object and an appropriate set of desired (image) features are selected from a database. Different features may be selected during different stages of the task. The desired features are compared with the measured features, resulting in a feature error. The inverse image Jacobian J_i^{-1} translates feature errors to Cartesian errors (with respect to the camera frame). These errors are multiplied by a selection matrix S, which is a diagonal matrix of ones and zeros. A one in element S_{ii} implies that the ith Cartesian DOF is actively used for visual servoing.

In parallel, the end-user may drive the robot in his/her preferred co-ordinate system. The specified user input is transformed into the camera frame too, and added to the output of the visual controller. The controller uses the combined signals to control the robot. Note that when the entire selection matrix S is set to 0, the traditional MANUS controller is realised.

22.2.4 User Interface

In order to properly select an object, the user needs on-the-fly feedback about the object that has been segmented by the camera. To this end, a display is available, in which the selected object is constantly highlighted in a real-time video stream. In this manner, the user is able to check whether the camera information is still being processed correctly (hasn't gone off track).

22.3 Case Study

22.3.1 System Set-up

In order to test our theories, we have selected the following "sensors": user and camera. In the near future we plan to also incorporate the distance sensor. The set-up of the collaborative controller is the same as in the previous paragraphs, see Figure 22.2. The commands to the robot are given in a Cartesian frame attached to the gripper. The DOFs are therefore X, Y, Z, Yaw, Pitch and Roll.

For the camera, wide-angle lenses were used, preventing failure of feature calculation at close proximity. For segmentation of the object, normalised colour information is used, providing brightness independent colour segmentation. From the segmented image, several features are calculated.

To increase robustness, a second algorithm calculates Hu moments, which are a measure for the shape of the object. If the shape changes too much, the features are considered unreliable. A third algorithm measures the pixels on the border in order to detect whether the object is out of view.

For servoing in the $^c x$ and $^c y$ directions, the centre of mass of the pixels belonging to the object is calculated by taking the median of the pixel co-ordinates. This is more robust than the mean of the co-ordinates, as can be seen in Figure 22.3.

A feature for the Roll is obtained by calculating the centre of mass for both the upper and lower half of the object. The angle of these two points with the y-axis is used as a measure of the Roll. This way, the system tends towards a symmetric image in which long objects are aligned with the y-axis.

More than one possibility exists to use the features for visual servoing. For example, the centre of mass can be used for controlling the $^c x$ and $^c y$ of the gripper, or for controlling the yaw and pitch orientation angles. The user determines this using the selection matrix.

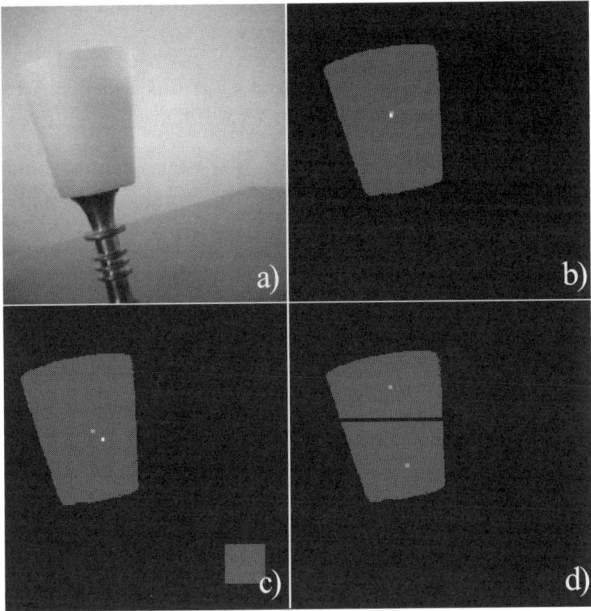

Figure 22.3. Calculated features: *a)* The cup. *b)* Centres of mass using median (light grey, more robust) and mean(white). *c)* Centres of mass in case of segmentation error (grey square). Roll feature, cup divided in two halves.

22.3.2 Stability

Our set-up has some special consequences for the stability of the system. Although the relationship between the position of the object with respect to the camera and the features in the image is linearised through the Jacobian, the Jacobian itself is dependent on $^c x_o$.

This means that the 'gain' between one pose parameter and its feature is influenced by other pose parameters. For instance, the centre of mass appears to be moving faster in the camera image when an object is close. This is caused by the perspective of the camera. The Jacobian has large diagonal values for smaller values of $^c z_o$, which may result in instability. This effect is called cross coupling.

Whilst this is a problem in all IBVS set-ups, here it cannot be compensated, because not all pose parameters, like $^c z_o$, are known from the camera. We solved this problem by considering possible cases of cross coupling and tuning the gain to a stable system in the worst case of this cross coupling. The system should then be stable in all other cases.

Additionally, some constraint may be imposed on a DOF to pose a limit on this worst case. For the aforementioned example of the centre of mass, this means that the movement is constrained to a minimum Z and the gain is tuned to a stable system for this Z_{min}. With the future addition of a distance sensor, the gain might be tuned dynamically.

22.3.3 Experiments

The system was tested with several different DOFs assigned to user and camera. The task was to pick up a coloured cup. The experiments served two goals:

- to investigate the stability of the proposed visual control architecture;
- to investigate the usability issues of the combined visual / user control system.

In all cases we were successful in picking up the cup. The roll feature performed adequately, as did the centre of mass. The computer was able to steer the gripper towards the cup in a stable way. Additionally, assigning X and Y to the user and Yaw and Pitch to the computer resulted in a situation in which the user was able to have the gripper 'circle around' the cup in a natural way.

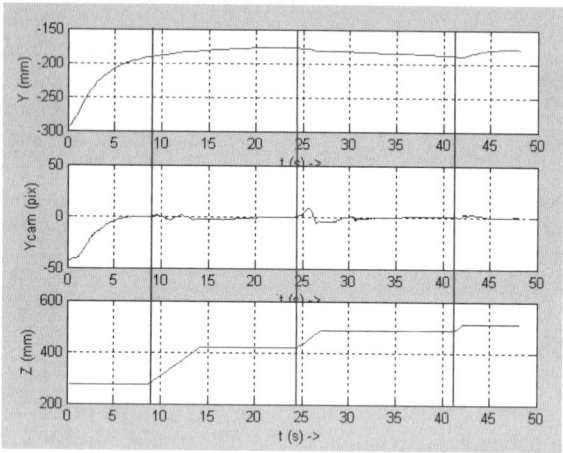

Figure 22.4. Position of the gripper in X, Y and Z. The user has given three inputs in the Z direction, indicated by the ramps.

The stable combination of control signals is illustrated in Figure 22.4. In this experiment, the user controlled the Z-direction (i.e. the distance between the gripper and the cup) manually, whilst the visual servo controlled the X, Y and roll DOFs. Yaw and pitch angles remained constant.

22.4 Conclusions

By combining the user and multiple sensors we have shown that a stable, robust and versatile system can be created to aid severely handicapped people in execution of daily tasks at reduced cognitive load. The future work comprises of developing more tracking algorithms, adding more sensors and providing a better user interface. To this end, several experiments will be done, including important constant user trials. These will be presented at the workshop.

22.5 References

Corke P, Hashimoto K (ed.) (1993) Visual control of robot manipulators – A review. World Scientific, Singapore

Fong T, Thorpe C, Baur C (1999) Collaborative control: A robot-centric model for vehicle teleoperation. In: AAAI 1999 Spring Symposium: Agents with Adjustable Autonomy, Stanford, CA. Available at: http://vrai-group.epfl.ch/projects/ati/

Fong T, Thorpe C, Baur C (2000) Advanced interfaces for vehicle teleoperation: Collaborative control, sensor fusion displays, and remote driving tools. Autonomous Robots 11(1) Available at: http://vrai-group.epfl.ch/papers/AR01-ATI-TF.pdf

Goldberg K, Chen B (2001) Collaborative control of robot motion: Robustness to error. In: IEEE/RSJ International Conference on Robots and Systems, October 2001. Available at: http://www.ieor.berkeley.edu/~goldberg/pubs/robust-iros01.pdf

Hutchinson S, Hager G, Corke P (1996) A tutorial on visual servo control. IEEE Transactions on Robotic and Automation 12(5): 661-670

Martens C, Graser A et al. (2001) The semiautonomous robotic system "FRIEND" consists of an electric wheelchair with a robotic arm and utilises a speech interface. IEEE Robotics & Automation Magazine. Available at: http://icat.snu.ac.kr/robotics/PDF/16_30/FRIEND.pdf

Neveryd H, Eftring H, Bolmsjö G (1999) The Swedish experience of rehabilitation robotics. In: Proceedings of Workshop Rehabilitation Robotics, Hoensbroek, The Netherlands

Veronica (2003) Manus the robotarm. Available at: http://members.lycos.nl/veronicasclubhuis/ manus_de_robotarm.html

Chapter 23

Effects of Repeated Exposure to a Humanoid Robot on Children with Autism

B. Robins, K. Dautenhahn, R. te Boekhorst and
A. Billard

23.1 Introduction

This work is part of the Aurora project which investigates the possible use of robots in therapy and education of children with autism (Aurora, 2003), based on findings that people with autism enjoy interacting with computers, e.g. (Powell, 1996). In most of our trials we have been using mobile robots, e.g. (Dautenhahn and Werry, 2002). More recently we tested the use of a humanoid robotic doll. In (Dautenhahn and Billard, 2002) we reported on a first set of trials with 14 autistic subjects interacting with this doll. In this chapter we discuss lessons learnt from our previous study, and introduce a new approach, heavily inspired by therapeutic issues. A longitudinal study with four children with autism is presented. The children were repeatedly exposed to the humanoid robot over a period of several months. Our aim was to encourage imitation and social interaction skills. Different behavioural criteria (including Eye Gaze, Touch, and Imitation) were evaluated based on the video data of the interactions. The chapter exemplifies the results that clearly demonstrate the crucial need for long-term studies in order to reveal the full potential of robots in therapy and education of children with autism.

23.1.1 Autism

Autism here refers to the term Autistic Spectrum Disorders with a range of manifestations of a disorder that can occur to different degrees and in a variety of forms (Jordan, 1999). The exact cause or causes of autism is/are still unknown. Autism is a lifelong developmental disability that affects the way a person communicates and relates to people around them. People with autism often have accompanied learning disabilities. According to the National Autistic Society (NAS, 2003) people with autism have impaired social interaction, social communication and imagination. This can show itself in difficulties in social relationships, the inability to relate to others in meaningful ways, difficulty with verbal and non-verbal communication and in the development of play and imagination. Usually people with autism show little reciprocal use of eye-contact and do rarely get engaged in interactive games. Autism affects more males than females (NAS, 2003).

23.1.2 Imitation and the Case of Autism

Imitation plays an important part in social learning both in children and adults. From birth, imitation plays a critical role in the development of social cognition and communication skills, helping an infant in forging links with other people (Nadel *et al.*, 1999). Imitation and turn taking games are used in therapy to promote better body awareness and sense of self, creativity, leadership and the taking of initiative both in children and adults (as used in Dance Therapy by Kalish 1968; Levy 1988; Payne, 1990). There are currently contradictory findings in respect of imitative deficits in autism. Some researchers suggest autism-specific impairments in imitation (Rogers and Pennington, 1991; Meltzof and Gopnik, 1993) whilst others show that autistic children are able to engage in immediate imitation of familiar actions (Hammes and Langdel, 1981).

Nadel explored the use of imitation as a communicative means in infant with autism (Nadel *et al.*, 1999) and found significant correlation between imitation and positive social behaviour. Her findings indicate that imitation is a good predictor of social capacities in children with autism. In addition, it was also found that autistic children improve their social responsiveness when they are being imitated (Dawson and Adams 1984; Tiegerman and Primavera, 1981; Nadel *et al.*, 1999). In therapy too, imitation, reflection and synchronous movement work has been used with autistic children to develop social interactions (Costonis, 1974; Adler, 1968).

23.1.3 The Aurora Project

In most of the trials conducted within the Aurora project we have been using mobile robots (e.g. Dautenhahn and Werry, 2002). More recently we tested the use of a humanoid robotic doll, called Robota (Billard, 2003). In (Dautenhahn and Billard, 2002) we reported on a first set of trials with 14 autistic subjects. The central theme of these trials was imitation games between the robot and the children. A camera system analysed gross arm movements of the children that in turn could trigger the robot to imitate the child. Also, Robota performed movements on its own in order to encourage the children to mirror the robot's movements. It was thus hoped to initiate imitative interaction games between Robota and the children. However, the results were inconclusive, and we identified a number of drawbacks of the original set-up.

Firstly, the set up required the children to sit still at a table, facing the robot, and moving their arms in a very distinct manner, due to limitations of state of the art vision systems that cannot identify subtle movements. Secondly, the children's participation in the interaction games substantially depended on explicit encouragement by a teacher who sat next to them. Overall, our experiences showed that the particular set up did not seem to facilitate the emergence of spontaneous, proactive, and playful interaction games. Lastly, in these previous trials each child was only exposed once to the robot, a situation were accidental parameters can potentially have a significant effect on the interactions observed. A small number of exposures to the robot is also not likely to give any indications with regards to any therapeutic or educational effects.

For the purpose of the present study we therefore decided a) to use a much more unconstrained set up, posing only very little constraint on the children's behaviours and postures that are allowed during the interactions, b) to pursue a longitudinal study and expose each child a number of times to the robot, and c) to reduce the intervention of carers so as to focus on spontaneous and self-initiated behaviour of the children.

23.2 The Research Questions

The primary aim of this chapter is to investigate to what extent repeated exposure to a humanoid robot, over a long period of time, can help to increase basic social interaction skills in children with autism. Also, varieties of interactions that can be observed will be documented.

23.2.1 Longitudinal Research

As mentioned above, the longitudinal repeated measure design reduces the influence of variables that could lead to 'accidental outcomes', because the same subjects are used. For example, we noticed that unplanned changes in the schedule of activities prior to a trial, such as cancelling the school's assembly, can significantly affect the children's behaviour because of the change to their routine. Also in longitudinal studies there are fewer cases of random variation to obscure the effects of the experimental conditions.

It is very common in therapy to design programmes of intervention/treatment to take place over a period of a year or longer, where, for example, 50 or more sessions of Art Therapy are not unusual (Evans and Dubowski, 2001), or in Dance Movement therapy (Seigel, 1984; Adler, 1968) where case studies show that it might take six months or more for the first breakthrough in the interaction between the therapist and an autistic child to occur.

Similarly, in education there is increasing use of the Qualification and Curriculum Authority's (QCA's) P-scales assessment method (QCA, 2003) to assess pupils' performance and to support monitoring of progression and target setting for pupils with learning difficulties. This is usually done once a year and although in many cases the pupils move up a level at the end of a year, often pupils show very slow progress in some developmental areas and stay at the same level for more than a year, simply covering more ground at that level.

A common approach in therapy involves the therapist to gradually attune to the client. This slow process reduces anxiety and distress levels and allows the gradual development of the therapeutic relationship. For these reasons, and because of the long-term projection that is used in education, we designed our trials to take place over a longer period of time. On the one hand we wanted to minimise the anxiety and distress the autistic children might find themselves in, caused by a change of routine, being in a novel situation with a new and unusual toy (the robot), and a new person (the investigator). On the other hand we wanted to allow enough time for the children to use any interaction skills they might have (e.g. eye-contact, turn-taking, imitation), in a reassuring environment, where the predictability and repetitive behaviour of the robot is a comforting factor. Furthermore, we intended to allow enough time and opportunity for the children to improve their social interaction skills by attempting imitation and turn-taking games with the robot while slowly increasing the unpredictability of the robot's actions. We also wanted to be able to monitor the children's reaction to different appearances of the robot, (cf. Ferrara and Hill 1980) study where children with autism play with different non-robotic toys. In our study this involved two different appearances of the robot, namely a 'pretty girl doll' as opposed to plain clothing with a featureless head (the comparison of these two experimental conditions is beyond the scope of this chapter and will be discussed in a separate publication).

Overall, this approach has been designed to allow the children to have unconstrained interaction with the robot with a high degree of freedom, on their terms to begin with (providing it is safe for the child and safe for the robot), and to build a foundation for further possible interactions with peers and adults using the robot as a mediator (Werry et al., 2001).

23.3 The Trials

The trials took place in Bentfield Primary School in Essex, UK, a mainstream school with approximately 220 typically developing pupils. The school also has an Enhanced Provision unit to cater for nine pupils with various learning difficulties and physical disabilities. These pupils, each accompanied by a carer, pursue their own unique curriculum and are integrated in the mainstream classes, according to their age group. They participate in any class activity that they are able to.

23.3.1 The Set-Up

The trials were conducted in the Light & Sound room at the school. This is a familiar room for the children, as they often use it for various activities. The Light and Sound area, which is an extended part of the room, was closed off by a curtain leaving a large empty area of approximately 5.5 m × 4.5 m, with a carpeted floor. The room had one door and several windows overlooking the school playgrounds.

The robot was connected to a laptop and placed on a table against the wall at one side of the room. Two stationary video cameras were placed in the room, one at the side to capture the area in front of the robot and the children when approaching the robot, and the other camera placed behind the robot to try and capture the facial expressions of the children as they interacted with the robot in close proximity. We felt that having manned cameras (with yet more adult strangers in the room) would be too intrusive and would cause additional stress to the children. However, despite having two cameras in most of the trials, there were periods of time when the children moved outside the range of the cameras, as the nature of the trials gave them the freedom to move around in the large room.

23.3.2 The Robot

The robot used in these trials is Robota – a 45 cm high, humanoid robotic doll (Billard, 2003). The main body of the doll contains the electronic boards (PIC16F870, 4 MHz and 16F84, 16 MHz) and the motors that drive the arms, legs and head giving 1 DOF to each. The robot has also the capability of being connected to various sensors such as infrared emitters/ receivers, light detectors and more, which were not used in these trials. The arms, legs and head of the robot are plastic components of a commercially available doll. The robot can react to touch by detecting passive motion of its limbs and head through its potentiometers. For a complete description of Robota's hardware see (Billard, 2003).

Robota is connected through a serial link to a PC and can use speech synthesis, speech processing and video processing of data from a quick-cam camera. Using its motion tracking system, Robota can copy upward movements of the user's arms, and sideways movements of the user's head when the user sits very still and close to the robot, looking straight at it, engaging in turn-taking and imitation games with the robot. Machine learning algorithms allow Robota to be taught e.g. a sequence of actions as well as a vocabulary.

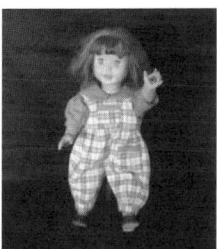 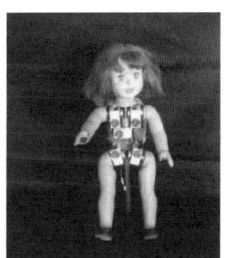 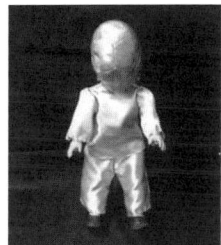

Figure 23.1. The robot in its two different appearances (the centre figure shows the 'undressed' version revealing the robotic parts that control its movement)

Robota has originally been developed as a robotic toy that supports a rich spectrum of multi-modal interactions with typically developing children, involving speech, music and movements. However, all of the behavioural qualities required in situations of social interaction are less natural to children with autism. Such qualities would include: being still, having a long enough focus of attention, and maintaining gaze on another's face. These are advanced tasks for these children to perform as it lies directly in one of the main areas of their impairment –

communication and social interaction. Therefore, in the current trials, Robota's features of speech processing, motion tracking, and learning were not used. As explained above the trials are designed to be unconstrained, with minimal structure, to allow the children to have the greatest degree of freedom. Possibly other features of Robota could be used in future experiments where we will slowly introduce more structure and complexity into the trials, allowing the children time to build their confidence and increase their social interaction skills according to their abilities.

In the current set of trials, the robot has been programmed to operate in two basic modes:

1. as a 'dancing toy' where it moved its arms, legs and head to the beat of pre-recorded music. We used three types of music – children's rhymes, pop music and classical music, following the teacher's advice as to the children's liking;
2. as a puppet, whereby the investigator is the puppeteer and moves the robot's arms, legs or head by a simple press of buttons on his laptop.

23.3.3 The Children

Four autistic children age 5-10 from the Enhanced Provision unit at Bentfield Primary School were selected by their teacher to participate in the trials. Each child participated in as many trials as was possible for him during that period (nine trials each on average). The children are:

*   E.M. – age 5, in the Reception class. E.M. uses only two or three words but is beginning to communicate using the Picture Exchange Communication System (PECS);
*   B.B. – age 6, in year one. B.B. has some limited verbal expression, which he uses to express some needs, likes and dislikes. He understands simple directions associated with routines;
*   B.S. – age 10 , in year 5. B.S. has autism combined with severe learning difficulties. He has no verbal language and uses symbols and signs to make choices and to express basic needs. He will generally have a go at whatever task he is presented with unless he is feeling unwell when his behaviour deteriorates;
*   T.M. – age 10 , in year 5. He has verbal language, which he may use to express needs but often elects not to do so. He can be very difficult to motivate and it is sometimes very difficult to channel his attention towards a particular task.

Once a year the school assesses the pupils' performance using the QCA's P-scale method. It is important to view the children's behaviour during the trials in the context of their personal development level, which was assessed by their teacher six months prior to the trials.

According to the assessment of their personal and social development level, in the subject of attention, E.M. and B.B. have been assessed at a level where they pay rigid attention to their own choice of activity, and are highly distractible in activities or tasks led by others. B.S. and T.M. have been assessed at a level where they can attend to an adult directed activity but require one to one support to maintain their attention. In the area of interacting and working with others, E.M. was assessed at a level where he engages in solitary play or work and shows little interest in the activities of those around him. B.B., B.S. and T.M. were assessed at level where they might take part in work/play with one other person and take turns in simple activities with adult support.

23.3.4 Trial Procedures

Before each trial, the robot was placed on a table ready to start with a click of a button from the laptop. The investigator was sitting next to this table operating the laptop when necessary. The cameras, operated by a remote control, were set to 'standby' mode ready to record.

The children were brought to the room by their carer, one at a time. Each trial lasted as long as the child was comfortable with staying in the room. The trials stopped when the child indicated that he wanted to leave the room or if he became bored after spending 3 minutes already in the room. The average duration of trials was approximately three minutes. A few of the trials lasted up to five minutes, a few others were just under three minutes, and two ended very shortly after they started when the children left the room after 40 and 60 seconds.

The trials were designed to progressively move from very simple exposure to the robot to more complex opportunities for interaction. There were three phases to this:

Set-up A: during the first three trials, the robot was placed inside a large open box painted black inside, similar to a puppet-show setting (see Figure 23.2). At this stage in the trials the robot was operating in its 'dancing' mode moving its limbs and head to the rhythm of pre-recorded music. This was simply intended to attract the children's attention to the robot. The children mostly watched while sitting on the floor or on a chair but occasionally left the chair to interact with the robot more closely, (watching closely, touching etc). This section of the trials was designed mainly for the children to familiarise themselves with the robot (a new toy) and so the carer gave no instructions or tasks for the children to do, simply minimal verbal encouragement if and when this was needed (e.g. "look , there, what is it?" etc.). The children were left to do what they chose to do. The carer and the investigator were generally only observing, intervening only if the child was about to harm the robot (i.e. pushing /pulling the robot's limb using excessive force). The investigator did not initiate communication or interaction with the child, but did respond when addressed by the child.

Set-up B: in later trials, the box was removed, the robot was placed openly on the table and the children were actively encouraged to interact with the robot. In this stage the carer introduced physical encouragement, standing with the child near the robot and moving the child's limbs to show him how the robot could imitate his movement (see Figure 23.2). The children could then continue the interaction with the robot on their own. In this situation the robot was operating in its 'puppet mode', where the investigator as puppeteer caused the robot to accurately respond to the child's arm, leg and head movements (even when the child was not facing the robot directly or was not in close proximity to the robot). Note that the investigator's control of the robot was hidden from the children.

Set-up C: in the last couple of trials, whenever possible, the children were not given any instructions or encouragement to interact with the robot, and were left to interact and play imitation games on their own initiative if they chose to do so. On these occasions the robot was operated as a puppet by the investigator again. The investigator was able to recognise even subtle expressions of the child and to quickly respond to the child's movements, and also to introduce further complexity of turn-taking and role-switch into the simple imitation game.

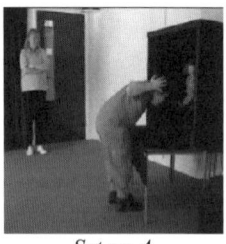   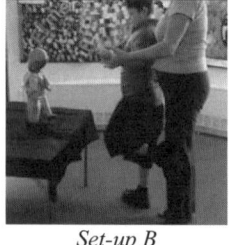   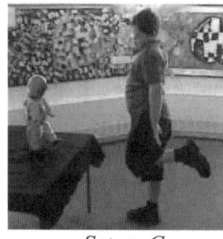

Set-up A   *Set-up B*   *Set-up C*

Figure 23.2. The three phases of the trials

23.4 Data Processing and Analysis

In our trials we defined four elementary behaviour criteria that we evaluated throughout the period of trials, based on the video footage. These behaviours were:

- eye gaze (when directed at the robot);
- touch (when the child touched any part of the robot);
- imitation (this included direct imitation of the robot's movements, delayed imitation and response to the robot's movement, and attempted imitation of the robot's movement);
- near (this included the child approaching the robot and staying in close proximity to the robot regardless of the child's other behaviours).

23.4.1 Quantitative Analysis

The video data from each and every trial for a given child was segmented into one second intervals. The trials were coded by scoring the above defined elementary behaviours every second of the trial (*cf.* Tardiff *et al.*, 1999; Dautenhahn and Werry, 2002). The scores for each trial were then summed up and yielded the total number of occurrences of each behaviour during a specific trial and the total duration the child was engaged in each behaviour during that trial. The trials varied in duration, therefore the duration of a behaviour was standardised by expressing it as a proportion of the trial duration.

This data analysis produced various graphs showing changes in the children's behaviour (during the child robot interaction) over a period of time. For each child we followed the trend of each of their behavioural criteria from day one, when the first trial took place, to day 101 when the last trial was conducted.

The graphs in Figure 23.3 give samples of the results. Figure 23.3 (left) shows that the values for the behaviours of Touch, Imitation and Near all increase considerably towards the later trials, i.e. from day 92 onward.

For Eye Gaze highest scores occur during the first two trials on day 1 and day 8. This could be attributed to the novelty of the situation and due to the fact that the child was given a chair to sit in front of the robot to watch this new toy. Naturally the high score for Eye Gaze can be expected in this situation. However if we disregard these first two trials, we see that the trend for Eye Gaze, too, increases from the third trial onwards, resulting in a relatively high score on the last trial on day 101.

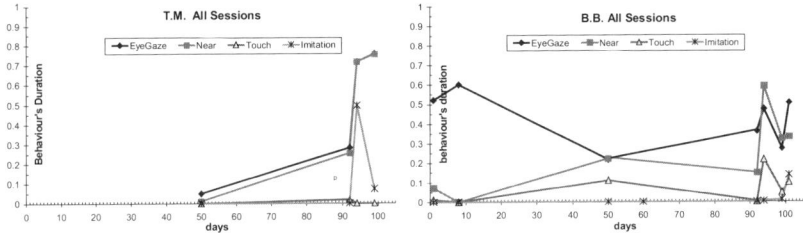

Figure 23.3. The graph shows the scores for the four behavioural criteria during all the trials that B.B. (left) and T.M. (right) participated in

Figure 23.3 (right), which shows the behaviour criteria of T.M. during the trials, demonstrates a considerable increase of the scores for Near, Eye Gaze and Imitation toward days 92 and 94. Touch, although with a very low score, also occurred only on day 92. The data that we have processed also allowed us to monitor each behaviour criteria separately, over the whole period of the trials, across all the children. The graphs in figure 23.4 show samples of these results.

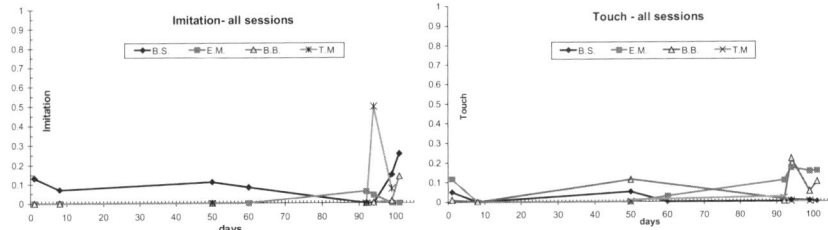

Figure 23.4. The trends of scores for Imitation (left) and Touch (right) throughout the investigation period

Figure 23.4 (left) shows a trend of Imitation scores as it appeared in all children throughout all the trials with a visible increase at the end of the trial period – from day 92 onwards. In Figure 23.4 (right) the Touch scores increase for some of the children in the last trials, days 92 – 101.

23.4.2 Qualitative Analysis

As stated earlier, one of the overall questions that we are investigating within this project is whether exposure to and interaction with the robot help increase the autistic child's social interaction skills using imitation and turn-taking games for this purpose. During the analysis of the video recordings of this set of trials we noticed several occasions when the children also interacted with the adults in the room (i.e. their carer, or the investigator). Sometimes this occurred in relation to the robot, when the robot acted as a mediator or an object of shared attention, but at other times these interactions were not robot related. To understand the events that take place in such interactions requires attention to the autistic child's activities in their interactional context. The quantitative analysis alone, based on the frequency and duration of the basic behaviours, cannot reveal some important aspects of social interaction skills (imitation, turn-taking, role-switch) and the communicative competence that the autistic children showed during the trials.

A comprehensive qualitative analysis of some of those segments of the trials where the children showed such interaction skills and communicative competence is beyond the scope of this chapter and will be discussed in a separate publication. However, Table 23.1 gives a description of a very short segment (duration of 32 seconds) taken from one child's trial, which reveals such interaction skills.

Table 23.1. A sample of one child's trial

Action	Response
1. Robot raises left arm	Child mirrors and raises right arm
2. Robot raises left arm	Child mirrors and raises right arm
3. Robot raises left arm	Child mirrors and raises right arm
4. Robot raises right arm	Child mirrors and raises left arm
5. Robot raises right arm	Child mirrors and raises left arm
6. *pause (under 1 sec)*	
7. Child raises right arm	Robot mirrors and raises left arm
8. Robot raises left arm	Child starts to raise left arm, quickly drops it and raises right arm
9. Child raises left arm	Robot mirrors and raises right arm
10. Robot turns head to the right	Child mirrors and turns head to left
11. Robot turns head to the right	Child mirrors and turns head to left
12. Child shakes head up and down	Robot turns head to left.
13. *child pauses*	
14. Robot raises right arm	Child starts to raise right arm, quickly drops it and raises left arm

We can see that during this segment the child showed the following social interaction skills: a) straightforward imitation of various body parts' movements (lines 1-5, 9-11,14), b) the child realised when he made a mistake in imitation and corrected himself (lines 8, 14), c) the child initiated interaction as part of the imitation and turn-taking game without any pre-determined cue thus causing a role-switch (lines 7,9), and d) the child tried to initiate interaction using a new movement – shaking the head up and down. The child indicated a comprehension that this movement is beyond the robot's capability and so moved on without insisting on that movement (line 13). As stated earlier, those skills shown here would not be revealed in a purely quantitative analysis.

23.5 Conclusion

This chapter presented a novel study of longitudinal research on the exposure of a humanoid robot to children with autism. Relatively little work has been done on using autonomous robots in autism therapy, cf. (Dautenhahn and Werry, 2002) for a comprehensive overview on related work where usually the same children are only exposed once, or a few times to a robot. In contrast, our current approach of repeated trials over a long period of time allowed the children time to explore the interaction space of robot-human, as well as human-human interaction. In some cases the children started to use the robot as a mediator, an object of shared attention, for their interaction with their teachers (*cf.* Werry *et al.*, 2001). Furthermore, once they have got accustomed to the robot, in their own time and on their own initiative, they all opened themselves up to include the investigator in their world, interacting with him, and actively seeking to share their experience with him as well as with their carer. We believe that this is an important aspect of the work, since this human contact gives significance and (emotional, intersubjective) meaning to the experiences with the robot. Future work will, for example, address the statistical analysis of the video data, verify the interrater reliability of the method used, as well as continue the development of new interaction games with Robota and other robots we are using.

23.6 Acknowledgements

We are grateful to the teaching staff, parents, and children at Bentfield Primary school. Our special thanks go to the Head-teacher Mr. Draper for his continued support.

23.7 References

Adler, J. (1968) The study of an autistic child. In: Proceeding of the 3rd annual conference of the American Dance Therapy Association 1968, Madison, Wisconsin, USA

Aurora (2003) The aurora project. Available at: http://www.aurora-project.com

Billard A (2003) Robota: Clever toy and educational tool. Robotics & Autonomous Systems 42: 259-269

Costonis M (ed.) (1978) Therapy in motion. University of Illinois Press, Urbana

Dawson G, Adams A (1984) Imitation and social responsiveness in autistic children. Journal of Abnormal Child Psychology 12: 209-26

Dautenhahn K, Billard A (2002) Games children with autism can play with robota, a humanoid robotic doll. In: CUWAAT'02, Springer-Verlag London, UK

Dautenhahn K, Werry I, Rae J, Dickerson P, Stribling P, Ogden B (2002) Robotic playmates: analysing interactive competencies of children with autism playing with a mobile robot. In: Socially Intelligent Agents. Kluwer Academic Publishers

Evans K, Dubowski J (2001) Art therapy with children on the autistic spectrum: Beyond words. Jessica Kingsley Publishers, Philadelphia, PA

Ferrara C, Hill S D (1980) The responsiveness of autistic children to the predictability of social and non-social toys. Journal of Autism and Developmental Disorders 10(1): 51-57

Hames J G, Langdell T (1981) Precursors of symbol formation in childhood autism. Journal of Autism and Developmental Disorders 11: 331-44

Jordan R (1999) Autistic spectrum disorders - An introductory handbook for practitioners. David Fulton Publishers, London, UK

Kalish B (1968) Body movement therapy for autistic children. In: Proceeding of the 3rd Annual Conference of the American Dance Therapy Association 1968, Madison, Wisconsin, USA

Levy F (1988) Dance movement therapy – A healing art. The American Alliance for Health, Physical Education, Recreation and Dance, Reston, VI

Meltzoff A, Gopnik A (1993) The role of imitation in understanding persons and developing a theory of mind. In: Perspectives from autism. Oxford University Press, UK

NAS (2003) National Autistic Society UK. Available at: http://www.nas.org.uk

Nadel J, Guerini C, Peze A, Rivet C (1999) The evolving nature of imitation as a format of communication. In: Imitation in Infancy, Cambridge University Press, UK

Payne H (1990) Creative movement and dance. Winslow Press, Oxfordshire, UK

Powell S (1996) The use of computers in teaching people with autism. In: Autism on the agenda: papers from a National Autistic Society Conference. London, UK

QCA (2003) The Qualifications and Curriculum Authority. Available at: http://www.qca.org.uk/ca/foundation/profiles.asp23p_scales

Rogers S J, Pennington B F (1991) A theoretical approach to the deficits in infantile autism. Development and Psychopathology 3: 137-162

Siegel E V (1984) Dance-movement therapy: mirror of our selves - the psychoanalytic approach. Human Sciences

Tardiff C, Plumet M-H, Beaudichon J, Waller D, Bouvard M, Leboyer M (1995) Micro-analysis of social interactions between autistic children and normal adults in semi-structured play situations. International Journal of Behavioural Development 18(4): 727–747

Tiegerman E, Primavera L (1981) Object manipulation: An interactional strategy with autistic children. Journal of Autism and Developmental Disorders 11: 427-38

Werry I, Dautenhahn K, Ogden B, Harwin W (2001) Can social interaction skills be taught by a social agent? The role of a robotic mediator in autism therapy. In: CT2001, Springer Verlag, London, UK

Chapter 24

The Gloucester Smart House for People with Dementia – User-Interface Aspects

R. Orpwood, C. Gibbs, T. Adlam, R. Faulkner and
D. Meegahawatte

24.1 Introduction

This chapter describes the development of support devices to be used within a smart home for people with dementia, and in particular the way end users were involved in this design process. At first sight it might seem that the reasonably sophisticated technology used in smart homes was completely inappropriate for use with people with dementia. The severe memory loss that is the hallmark of dementia and the inability to learn new tasks would make it seem that people with dementia would not be able to interact with the technology and would probably become extremely anxious and upset by its introduction.

However the vision that lay behind the project was that it should be possible to design new support devices that would be completely invisible to the user and not require them to interact with them directly. Such equipment could monitor the behaviour of the user and their interaction with household appliances, and only intervene to provide prompts and reminders, or to turn household devices on or off in appropriate circumstances.

In other words the house should be able to act in a similar manner to a live-in carer, only providing care for 24 hours a day without becoming tired or frustrated. Of course such technology could never replace human care and support, but it could augment such caring and hopefully also provide some respite for personal carers. This chapter describes the work undertaken, with a focus on how the complex user interface was dealt with.

24.2 User Survey

From the design team's background in assistive technology it was standard practice to use a user-led approach to design, and with this project the first exercise carried out was an information gathering one. Many discussions were held with professional carers of people with dementia to listen to their understanding and anecdotes about the problems faced by their clients.

A comprehensive user survey was carried out through the use of a questionnaire sent to personal carers of people with dementia. The aim of the questionnaire was to ask the carers to relate the difficulties they encountered as they went through a typical day spent looking after their relative. The questionnaire led to a whole series of problem areas to be listed, and to a quantified appraisal of the importance of each of the problems. The survey provided an ideal starting point for the design work and the results were published as a reference for other workers (Jepson and Orpwood, 2000).

24.3 Design Philosophy and Approach

Most design teams working within assistive technology follow a user-led design methodology (Poulson et al., 1996) and the Institute had long followed its own version of such methodologies (Orpwood, 1990) which has been very effective. The methodology incorporates a stage of recognising that most of the difficulties and unknowns occur with the user-interface aspects of the design, and tries to evolve solutions for these aspects by working on them in isolation with typical end users in an iterative fashion.

Users try out early prototypes of the user interface aspects of the design, accepting that the design will require modifications to deal with the problems that become highlighted during simple tests. Implicit in this process is the need for users to become involved as part of the design team. For devices for people with dementia this introduces many ethical concerns about whether it is appropriate to expose such users to devices at an early stage when there will inevitably be problems. An alternative design methodology has been followed that has evolved from the dementia design work carried out at the Bath Institute of Medical Engineering (Orpwood et al., 2003). The methodology relies heavily on the involvement of personal carers of people with dementia and on their intimate understanding of the problems faced by them. A close working relationship has to be developed with many personal carers for this process to be effective. This was done in several ways with the current project.

- designers were involved in a number of discussion sessions with carers through the help of day clubs organised by the Alzheimer's Disease Society;
- professional care staff from a number of local authorities organised informal gatherings of carers so that we could discuss problems and designs with them;
- more formal focus groups were run with both personal and professional carers with the same end in mind.

All these meetings were used to explore the problems the carers faced, to present design ideas for feedback and comment, to present early prototypes for their reactions, and to set up simple user tests of early prototypes.

24.4 Carer Emulation

A key requirement for the design team was to adopt a design philosophy that would enable them to generate design solutions that hopefully would be effective, without too much involvement of people with dementia until fairly mature products were available. The key approach used was to listen to the solutions adopted by personal cares in their dealing with the various problems they confronted. It was argued that carers had the greatest intimate understanding of the problems involved and if they had found effective strategies, then these ought to form a good starting point for any design work. A design approach of trying to emulate carers has proved to be very effective.

An illustration of the power of this approach is the design used for a tap monitor system for use in the bathroom or kitchen. We had several anecdotes related to us where people with dementia had started to run a bath, but then walked off and flooded the bathroom. A straightforward engineering solution would be to use a level sensor in the bath such that when the water reached that level the water supply could be turned off using a solenoid valve. However if this was done, although the flood would have been prevented, it could cause a lot of confusion on the part of the user. If they came back to the bathroom and tried to run some more hot water into the bath because it had cooled they would find the taps no longer worked. It was this sense of the house taking control that we were particularly keen to avoid. In contrast to this approach the support provided by a personal carer would be quite different. In many situations like this one where there was an inappropriate use of equipment, carers tended to employ a three-stage response.

- firstly they would provide a reminder ("Don't forget you've left the bath running");
- secondly, if the user didn't respond to the reminder, they would intervene to turn off the tap;
- thirdly they would let the user know what they had done ("Your bath is ready. I've turned the water off").

The end result of these actions would be that the situation had been dealt with without taking control away from the user. They could still run some more water in if they wanted. They would not be made anxious and confused because they had been told about the interventions carried out.

The above approach implies a need for communication and this will be dealt with below. It also requires a tap water control that acted like the carer and didn't take control away from the user. To do this a tap design was evolved that is shown in Figure 24.1. The tap itself didn't control the water flow directly but was simply connected to an encoder which provided an electric valve with information about how far the tap had been turned, and water was supplied through the valve appropriately. If the water level sensor indicated the bath was full enough the water supply could be turned off, but at the same time a brake could be applied to the tap shaft to make the tap feel like it was turned off. The encoder on the shaft could then be reset to zero. Consequently as far as the user was concerned the tap was turned off but they could still interact with it and use it in a normal way. The tap design is quite novel but the important point is that it wasn't just a good idea thought up by the designer. It was the result of a lot of consideration of user responses and designed to meet a specific user need. This user-led approach is felt to be crucial to work of this kind.

Tap

Water control
valve

Encoder

Brake

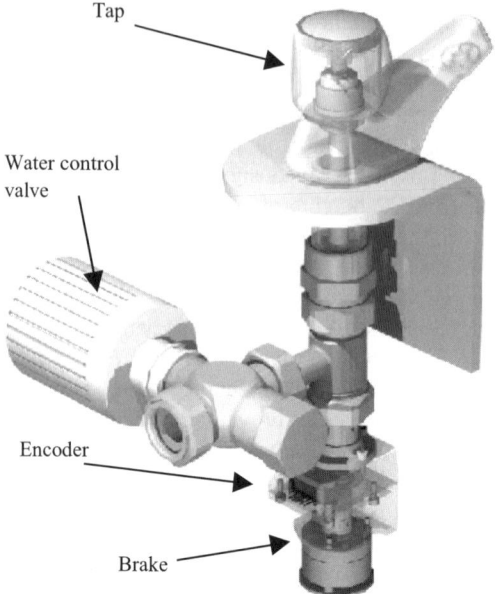

Figure 24.1. Replacement tap for water control

24.5 The Need for "Normal" Appearance

People with dementia find learning new tasks very difficult if not impossible in the short term. If they are presented with such a task they are likely to become very anxious and are more than likely to just reject it. This reaction has important implications for the design of assistive technology. Any appliance that the user has to interact with has to look, feel and work just like the kind of appliance they have always been used to. The tap described above was successful because it just felt and operated like taps always had. The cooker monitor described below had to be an add-on to the user's normal cooker rather than an introduction of a replacement high-tech device that incorporated all the safety features felt to be necessary. Pans used on the cooker had to be ones that had always been used. Simple devices such as light switches had to be standard fittings rather than some of the excellent but inappropriate versions available as part of commercial smart home fittings. Any monitoring sensors had to be hidden away or they would cause alarm, so the level sensor used for the bath for example could not rely on something stuck onto the inside of the bath like a thermistor. The sensor used for the bath was a capacitance sensor stuck to the outside of the bath that used the bath water as a dielectric, and gave a good enough indication of when the limiting water level had been reached.

24.6 Dealing with the Complexity of Human Behaviour

24.6.1 Monitoring Behaviour

It became quite clear during the project that the major difficulty in using sensors to monitor human behaviour was that human behaviour is actually very complicated and variable. The information from the sensors had to be used in a way which provided a judgement about what the user was doing despite this variability. A good example of this was the use of sensors to detect dangerous use of a gas cooker. This monitor was a crucial part of the smart home system being explored because it is a major cause of people having to go into residential care.

The cooker monitor had to be able to detect three sources of danger. First of all it had to detect if the gas had been turned on but not lit. Secondly it had to be able to detect when food was becoming burnt or fat was getting a little too hot. And thirdly it had to detect when pans had been allowed to boil dry or overheat. Raw gas detection was fairly straightforward using commercial sensors. Burning food and hot fat could very easily be detected with commercial smoke detectors, with variable sensitivity ones being particularly helpful. These smoke sensors are particularly sensitive to hot fat which emits an aerosol of fat droplets to which they are very sensitive.

For detecting hot pans and pans that had boiled dry many different systems were explored but the one finally used incorporated single point infrared sensors. Thermograms of pans boiling dry had shown how effective infrared imaging was for this situation. The emissivity of the pans was very variable but we were looking at trends rather than measuring actual temperatures so the information was very useful.

As can be seen from Figure 24.2 the output from the IR sensor showed a gradual increase until the boiling point was reached where it stayed fairly constant until the water boiled dry. Thereafter, and within a few seconds, there was a rapid increase in temperature. It was felt that it should be easy to detect this sudden rise. However this simple temperature/time curve was complicated by the behaviour of users. A similar pattern could be obtained for example if the user turned the heat of the gas up and down.

It could also be obtained if the pan was moved from one ring to another. These likely behavioural actions complicated what was superficially quite a straightforward response. Algorithms were eventually derived which enabled the boiling dry situation to be detected but this could only be done after much monitoring of different situations during the real use of the cooker. The algorithm was effective about 80% of the time, with the emphasis on false positives for the failures.

The difficulty of detecting certain behavioural traits has been evident in many problem situations, from detecting wandering to detecting when someone has got out of bed. Behaviour is often complicated, and a lot of measurement work in real life situations is required to derive effective algorithms that use the sensor data.

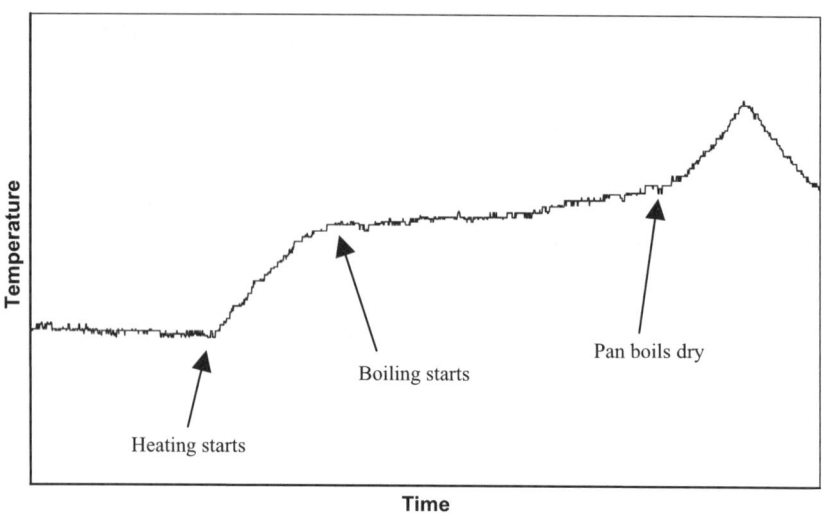

Figure 24.2. Temperature/time curve as pan boils dry

24.6.2 User Reaction to Interface Design

It proved to be very difficult to make judgements about how a user might respond to a given situation, even with the guidance provided by personal carers. For example a system was tested that would fade up a bedroom light if someone got out of bed at night, and then fade the light off once they got back into bed. Even this straightforward action was found to lead to complications. The original turning off facility waited until the user was back into bed.

However it was found in practice that the user might often sit on the bed to deal with slippers or dressing gown before getting back into bed. With the original system once the user sat on the bed it was assumed they were lying down and the lights would go off, causing some confusion. It was a fairly trivial exercise to put a delay in the lights before they faded off, but the experience illustrated how difficult it is to make assumptions about the way that people behave even in simple situations.

Some user reactions were quite subtle and yet the designs they were using could be profoundly affected by their reaction. One system designed provided a locator for objects that were mislaid. A small panel had a series of buttons on its face to depict objects that might be mislaid, such as keys, purse, walking stick, etc. When the user pressed the button next to a picture of the object a tag attached to the object bleeped until it was picked up. People with dementia found the panel confusing and so it was modified so that just a touch panel was presented with pictures of the objects that had to be touched in order to find them. This proved to be even less easy to use. When the panel was touched there was no movement and no click, and the user had no sense of their having done anything. A moving membrane panel was needed to solve the difficulty.

Another lesson learnt about user behaviour concerned their tendency to fiddle with support devices. We had been warned from our user meetings that people with dementia will tend to fiddle with things in their environment if they were unusual. The first test of the night light system described above fell victim to this trait. The user was clearly concerned about the box of electronics next to their bedside lamp, and fiddled with the wires so much they became detached. Making support device fiddle proof is quite an important feature for assistive technology for people with dementia.

24.7 Evaluations

A key part of development work for assistive technology is the need for thorough user evaluation to assess effectiveness and to carry out any further development. For the smart house system there were many complicated factors to be explored and several ways in which different support devices could interact. Consequently it was decided quite early in the project that the evaluations would be carried out in two stages. The individual systems would first of all be tested with users and refined in their own right as stand-alone systems. Once we were happy with their performance the second phase would be to integrate them into complete smart home systems to explore their use and whether further complications arose from the way that the devices interacted. Consequently for all the support devices developed, stand-alone versions were constructed for initial assessment, firstly by personal carers, and then by people with dementia themselves. This procedure has been very effective and a whole raft of support devices has now been the subject of testing, and most have completed further development to correct any problems that arose. Some of this work overlapped with a European Commission funded project called ENABLE which aimed to evaluate a series of items of support equipment for people with dementia. At the time of writing complete smart home systems are being planned to be installed in a couple of apartments in sheltered accommodation run by Housing 21, the housing association that has been supporting the project.

24.8 Exploring Communication Devices

As would be apparent from the discussion above a key part of the new developments for people with dementia is the need to be able to communicate with them in order to provide prompts and reminders. At the start of the project many of the professional carers were very sceptical about how effective such communication might be. The most flexible and "normal" communication is through the use of voice. However we were reminded that people with dementia might be very confused by voices not coming from people. In addition if they recognised the voice they may well start to look around the house for the person they think must be there. However work on voice communication was felt to be important to explore. Another commonly relayed anecdote was that people with dementia often respond to voice on the radio or television as though they were being spoken to directly themselves. Sometime users had been found to be quite upset, for example, by items on the news because of their personal reaction and a sense of guilt.

It was felt that using this observation it might be possible to provide voice communication without alarming the user by ensuring the voice came out of the radio or TV, or possibly the telephone. The initial tests have all been done with voices coming from the radio. A radio has been developed which will interrupt its programme by relaying a message at an appropriate time, or if it is turned off, by temporarily turning on to provide the message.

It has been found to be very complicated to test these ideas for communication. Simple tests with users to see if they understand can provide some indication of comprehension and have some value. But the aim of the communicator is to affect the user's behaviour and in order to do that the communicator has to be used as part of a complete support system.

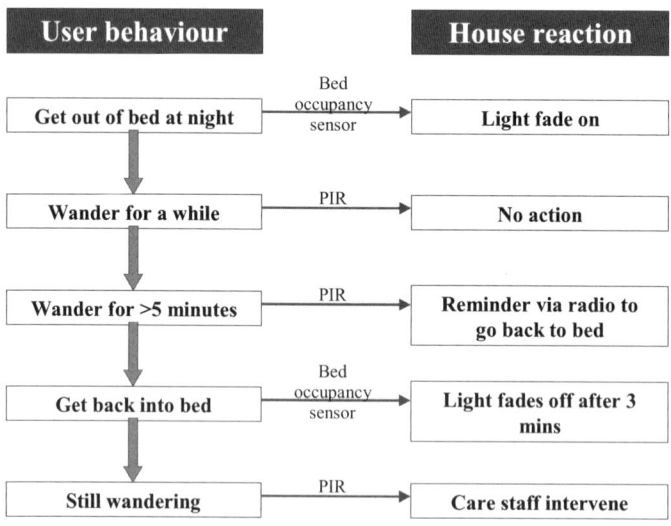

Figure 24.3. Sequence of house reactions in response to user behaviour

To illustrate these difficulties consider Figure 24.3, which depicts the sequence of events that had to be set up to test a simple radio communicator. It was set up in conjunction with a bedside night light that had the automatic fade up and down capability discussed above. First of all the night light had to be set up in a care home so that the user had good professional support. If they got out of bed the light would fade up. If they then got back into bed within a few minutes the light would wait a while and then fade down again. If they didn't get back into bed within a few minutes the voice communicator would provide a message such as, "It is still night time Mrs Brown. I should go back to bed". If they went back to bed that was fine and the light would fade down again. If they didn't the system would wait a little longer and then call the support staff through their alarm pagers so that they could go in and provide some support.

All this system had to be set up to explore how well someone would react to a message and allow us to explore such things as the voice used and the content of the message. There is no doubt that there is a lot of potential for using voice messaging with people with dementia but it is a complicated exercise to explore the important variables involved. It is also important that the actions of the user and the support device are electronically logged so that the sequence of events can be monitored, This has proved to be particularly important for verbal reminders tested as part of a system to discourage night-time wandering. Without logging you have no idea whether the person has been deterred from leaving the house in the middle of the night by your system or whether they simply haven't wandered at all for a while.

24.9 Conclusions

The interaction between someone with dementia and assistive technology designed to support them is quite complex. If new designs are to be effective then a lot of work has to be undertaken to ensure the user interface aspects of the design are carefully considered. This project has shown a lot of guidance can be obtained from close working with personal carers of people with dementia, but that the designer must expect many unpre-edited responses to occur once devices start to be tested and these responses must be carefully taken into account.

24.10 Acknowledgements

We would like to acknowledge support for the work presented from the EPSRC under their EQUAL programme, and from the European Commission for a 5th framework supported project called ENABLE.

24.11 References

Jepson J, Orpwood R (2000) The use of SMART home technology in dementia care. In: Proceedings of Annual Conference of College of OTS, Keele, Slovenia

Orpwood R (1990) Design methodology for the disabled. Journal of Medical Engineering and Technology 14: 2-10

Orpwood R, Faulkner R, Gibbs C, Adlam T (2003) A design methodology for assitive technology for people with dementia. In: Assistive technology – shaping the future. IOS Press, Amsterdam

Poulson D, Ashby M, Richardson S (1996) A practical handbook on user-centred design for assitive technology. ECSC-EC-EABC, Brussels

Chapter 25

Standards and the Dependability of Electronic Assistive Technology

G.D. Baxter, A.F. Monk, K. Doughty, M. Blythe and G. Dewsbury

25.1 Introduction

Electronic Assistive Technology (AT) includes both technology to help people with their daily activities, such as a door entry, and sensors that can raise alarms on detecting a fall or some other incident in the home i.e. home tele-healthcare (usually abbreviated to Telecare).

Electronic AT is of great economic and social value as it allows people to remain in normal homes when otherwise they would be forced to move to some sort of institutional setting.

25.2 Electronic Assistive Technologies As Critical Systems

Electronic ATs are critical systems in the sense that if they fail there may be resulting injury or distress.

A door entry system that locks an older person into their home, or opens the door at random times when interfering radio signals are received will cause considerable distress. A social alarm system that leads someone who has had a fall to believe help is on the way, when it is not, is a danger to life.

Given the critical nature of these systems one would expect them to be covered by extensive legislation to enforce high standards of design and manufacture.

This chapter examines the measures that can be taken in this respect. It can be viewed as preparatory to a survey of current practice which has yet to be carried out and as the beginning of a campaign to encourage more visible evaluation of the dependability – essentially, the trustworthiness – of electronic ATs, particularly within Europe.

25.3 Legislation, Standards, Codes of Practice and Guidelines

It is well-established practice in engineering to record guidelines and standard procedures to ensure good design practice and in most companies these are formalised as part of the product quality assurance process. Where this is true, staff are expected to be able to demonstrate that they comply with these procedures. A company that invests significantly in developing the required knowledge and procedures to ensure dependability of their products will want to demonstrate this to their customers. It is thus in their interest to join with other companies and professional bodies to develop public standards that they can sign up to. Eventually, these standards may become legal requirements upon all manufacturers. EC directives, for example, are implemented as national legislation by individual member countries of the EC. Manufacturers can show compliance with the legislation (where required) by conforming to the appropriate standards which have been developed as a way of promoting perceived wisdom and best practice. Compliant equipment carries a CE marking.

The process of developing and publishing a standard is the business of a standards agency. There are specialist standards organisations, which are national or international such as the British Standards Institute (BSI), and the International Standards Organisation (ISO). Within individual industries, professional organisations also develop their own standards, such as the Institution of Electrical Engineers (IEE) in the UK and the Institute of Electrical and Electronic Engineers (IEEE) in the USA. Trade organisations also exist, such as the Association of Social Alarm Providers (ASAP), who have developed their own code of practice for the operation of a call centre, with which all of its members should comply. However, these codes of practice tend to be very much less formal in their definition and in measures of compliance. Also, membership of professional and trade organisations is generally not mandatory.

Some standards have been very influential. The ISO 9000 series, for example, are very widely used to demonstrate a systematic quality assurance process. The US military standards (DEF STAN) set the gold standard for risk analysis

In this chapter two approaches to providing standards in the area of electronic AT are examined. One is to develop an overarching standard specifically for this purpose and the next section examines medical devices legislation as a way of doing this. The alternative is to use a variety of standards as they apply to different components of the system. This is examined in section 25.4.

25.4 Medical Devices Legislation and Electronic AT

The Medical Devices Agency (MDA) in the UK was recently made part of the Medicines and Healthcare Products Regulatory Agency. The MDA is largely responsible for implementing the three medical devices directives (The Active

Implantable Devices Directive (90/385/EEC), The Medical Devices Directive (93/42/EEC), and The In Vitro Diagnostic Medical Devices Directive (98/79/EC)) under the auspices of the Secretary of State for Health. These were recently implemented in the UK by the Medical Devices Regulations 2002 (SI 2002 No. 618). One of the latest updates (EN60601-1-2:2002) provides an international standard for EMC testing of Medical Electrical Equipment. This is important both because medical devices need to operate correctly in hospital environments that can be quite hostile in terms of interference from other equipment, and because they need to provide very limited electronic 'noise' so that other sensitive equipment may not be disturbed.

If a *manufacturer* makes a *medical device* and intends *placing (it) on the market*, then the Medical Devices Regulations apply. Each of the italicised terms are defined by the regulations.

Manufacturers are defined in a fairly broad sense. The term includes people who build systems from existing components, with the intention of placing the resultant system on the market. There is one key exception, which is the person who assembles or adapts devices already on the market to their intended purpose for an individual person.

A *Medical Device* is defined as "an instrument, apparatus, appliance, material or other article, whether used alone or in combination, including software necessary for its proper application , which –

a. is intended by the manufacturer to be used for human beings for the purpose of:
    i diagnosis, prevention, monitoring, treatment or alleviation of disease,
    ii diagnosis, monitoring, treatment, alleviation of or compensation for an injury or handicap,
    iii investigation, replacement or modification of the anatomy or of a physiological process, or
    iv control of conception; and
b. does not achieve its principal intended action in or on the human body by pharmacological, immunological or metabolic means, even if it is assisted in its function by such means."

This is a very broad-based definition. In its literature the MDA provides an incomplete list of examples of medical devices that includes walking aids, prescribable footwear and "equipment for disabled people". The latter term would seem to embody what many people would describe as assistive technology.

Medical devices are divided into three classes by the Directive. These classes directly relate to the level of risk associated with the device, so Class I devices are those generally regarded as low risk, and Class III devices are those generally regarded as high risk; medium risk devices are divided into two subclasses of Class II. Classification of the devices is determined using a set of rules that form part of the regulations, and there may be a fee for obtaining compliance. Of course, this fee is but a small part of the cost of employing an engineer to perform a risk analysis, document the risk management applied and submit the application for compliance. There are interesting differences between Europe and the USA where the Food and Drug Administration (FDA) enforces the equivalent legislation, however, in both cases obtaining compliance with this standard is expensive and can be a problem for small start-ups with a single product or large companies with families of devices to register (Mackenzie, 2002). For these reasons companies will look for exceptions that allow them to bypass this legislation. There are also some problems with the associated standard, ISO 14971 – Application of risk management to medical devices. These include a lack of definition of risk management as part of the system quality assurance process, and uncertainties in the ways that risk scoring is performed (Mackenzie, 2002).

As noted above, a person "who assembles or adapts devices already on the market to their intended purpose for an individual person" is exempt. This excludes individual installations that may differ from home to home. Devices that are developed within one organisation for use within that same organisation are also considered to be exempt, because they are not placed on the market. This means, for example, that systems developed by the medical physics department in a NHS trust hospital for use on patients elsewhere in the hospital, are exempt. In addition to the explicit exemptions, there are grey areas in the regulations. If a person buys a device of their own volition as an aid to daily living, for example, then it is not normally considered as a medical device. Similarly, there are some devices that can be considered as having a medical role when they are used by disabled people, but can also be used by able-bodied people. Such devices are not considered as medical devices. A door entry system, for example, which allows the person in the home to see who is at the door, and remotely open it is obviously very useful for someone with mobility problems. Such systems are also sold to people without mobility problems, so it would not normally be considered as a medical device. More generally, one can claim that if the technology is sometimes used by people without disease, injury or handicap then it is not primarily intended for "diagnosis, prevention, monitoring, treatment or alleviation" of those afflictions and so the regulations do not apply.

Given the major grey areas and exceptions that are embodied within the legislation, the meaning of a CE marking on electronic AT is not at all clear. If the relevant legislation and standards are not easily defined, what does it mean to say that the device meets all relevant European legislation? It is thus very difficult for the standards to do their job and demonstrate to customers that a product meets high standards of dependability.

25.5 Alternative Standards for Electronic AT

In trying to identify the current standards that apply to electronic AT, the MDA was contacted directly. They indicated that they do not keep a list of the relevant standards. A similar response was also received from the Health and Safety Executive: they do not have any ongoing work relating to the use of electronic AT in the home. There are, however, a number of standards that could be applied to different system components.

Figure 25.1 is a block diagram representation of a typical telecare system. The sensors and the client are shown in a box that represents the home. In addition to the client, the system will normally have at least one other type of user: the person who monitors the client's status through a computer system in a call centre, and may interact with the carer network (social worker, informal carer, GP and so on).

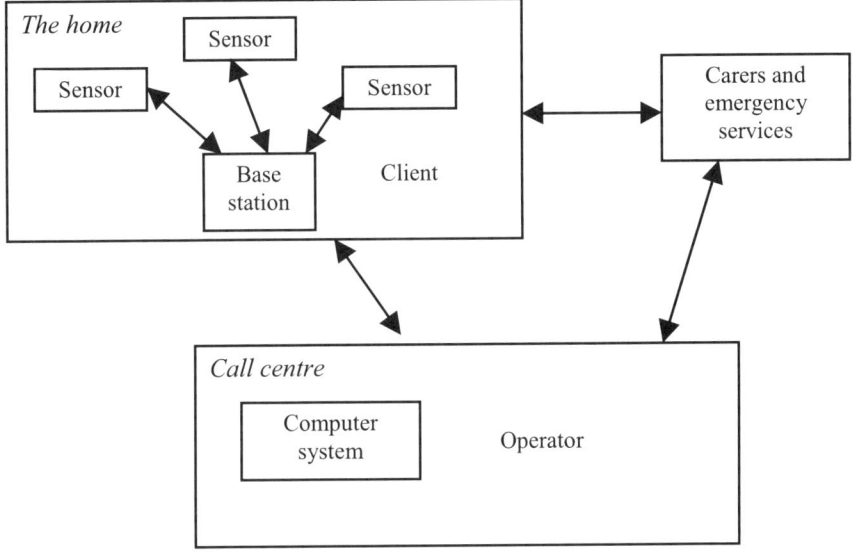

Figure 25.1. Typical telecare system, see text for explanation

Based on Figure 25.1, there are three obvious areas where standards exist that could be useful in assessing how good an electronic AT system is: computer systems (the base station in the home, and the computer system in the call centre); people (operator, professional carers and emergency services), and infrastructure.

There is a plethora of standards available that apply to systems development. The situation has been described as "The Frameworks Quagmire" (Sheard, 2001), since there are at least seven identifiable frameworks, each of which has several associated standards.

Fortunately, there does seem to be a gradual evolution towards new frameworks which encompass the best bits from the old frameworks. Sheard's assessment of the situation only addresses systems development in the most general sense. In other words, Sheard does not consider the particular standards associated with the development of safety critical systems.

Given the impetus for a move towards more care being carried out in the home, and the use of various monitoring technologies for medical purposes, it is fairly easy to see that electronic AT systems will take on an increasingly critical role in individual health care.

There are some natural parallels here with existing industrial safety critical systems where a culture has evolved which has identified the unique features of such systems, and standards have been introduced to help to assure the quality of such systems (Hone *et al.*, submitted). There are costs associated with the development of critical systems to ensure that they meet the extra, more stringent requirements, although these can normally be justified by a cost-benefit analysis.

The clients will normally be the main users of the system however they are not open to regulation (Dewsbury *et al.*, 2003). There are other identifiable users, however. In some electronic AT systems, there is a monitoring station that allows a carer, for example, to monitor multiple clients. The interface required for the carer will be different to that required by the user. There are existing standards that apply to the selection of people who work as carers. These are beyond the scope of this chapter. Similarly, although there are various building standards, these are not discussed here. Neither are the available network cabling and communication standards.

Table 25.1 shows the relationship between the attributes of dependability and the system components in Figure 25.1, and where the various standards fit in. It is not intended to be exhaustive, but does give a reasonable picture. A longer list of standards that are (potentially) applicable to the development of an electronic AT system is given in Table 25.2. Note that the issue of network communication standards has not been addressed, and basic electrical standards (wiring regulations, radio interference, and so on) are assumed.

It may be apparent, that some components of a telecare system such as the pendant trigger or an automatic sensor (e.g. a bed occupancy device) that has been built on the infra-structure of a social alarm system might also be used in an Environmental Control System used by a disabled and, hence, vulnerable person. Different standards will apply in the two cases.

On the one hand, environmental control systems, which are used by little over 4000 people in the UK, must comply with MDA regulations. Social alarms, and extended systems based on them (i.e. 1st generation telecare) need to comply only with the relevant sections of EN50134 which are far less stringent but extremely pertinent to the industry in which they are used.

It follows that a manufacturer of components of Assistive Technology devices may need to apply different standards according to the end application. This would be practically impossible and would give manufacturers of the lowest cost elements of AT an administrative burden that cannot be justified. The responsibility for ensuring compliance with the relevant standards should therefore lie with the system integrators, commissioners and installers.

The attributes of dependability that are important in home technologies in general, and electronic AT in particular, have been enumerated by Dewsbury *et al.* (2003). A selection of these attributes that are particularly relevant to Telecare are given below, expressed from the end user's point of view:

- safety: Can I injure myself when using it?
- reliability and availability: Will it always work when I need it?
- adaptability: Can it be changed when my needs change without introducing new faults?
- confidentiality and integrity: Will it make my data publicly available?
- usability and learnability: Will I be able to work it?
- fitness for purpose: Does it meet my real needs?

Table 25.1. Dependability-related standards as they apply to Telecare Monitoring System. Italics indicate where an existing standard could potentially be used.

Physical systems	Safety	Reliability and availability	Adaptability	Confidentiality and integrity	Usability and learnability	Fitness for purpose
Component devices (e.g., sensors such as a fall detector, the base station, call centre software and computer)	ISO 13485 ISO 13488 ISO 14971 *IEC 61508?*			IEC 61508 Data Protection Act	ISO 9241 ISO 13407	Not applicable to single device
Communicating components	*IEC 61508?*			IEC 61508 Data Protection Act	ISO 9241 ISO 13407	Not applicable to single device
Socio-technical systems						
Home system + call centre (incl. Operators and Procedures)	BSI EN 50134 *IEC 61508?* ASAP COP Part 1	*BSI EN 50134?* ASAP COP Part 1	ASAP COP Part 1	IEC 61508 Data Protection Act ASAP COP Part 1	ISO 9241 ISO 13407	
Home system + call centre + care support network	BSI EN 50134 ASAP COP Part 1 BS 5979 *IEC 61508?*	BSI EN 50134 ASAP COP Part 1		IEC 61508 Data Protection Act ASAP COP Part 1	ISO 9241 *ISO 13407?*	

The categories of systems shown above the thick line in Table 25.1 can be considered as physical systems, in that they can all exist independently of any users and an environmental context. Those systems below the line are socio-technical systems, in which there is at least one set of users, and the systems are all embedded into some context. These systems are essentially the result of installing a physical system into a particular setting. What is clear from the table is that adaptability and fitness for purpose are not catered for at all.

Adaptability, being able to modify components or the system as a whole as the client's abilities and needs change, is partly covered in the ASAP code of practice but the advice given is very informal. Similarly, fitness for purpose – whether the system is appropriate to the real needs of the user – is not covered. Consumer protection law will ensure that a device performs the function specified, but is this really the function that the client needs?

There is no real advice on how one assesses the real needs of a client in these engineering standards. While there are duties of care for health professionals there is little agreement as to how this should work more generally, and little concern with the detailed specification of the equipment prescribed. In general, assessment of clients for electronic AT has been criticised as having a very narrow notion of client need (Hone *et al.*, submitted).

The future will undoubtedly see the introduction of more advanced telecare systems, many of which will include physiological alarm sensors such as hypoglycaemia detectors and epileptic fit detectors. These will need to be approved medical devices. Will the remainder of the telecare system, i.e. the care phone, the call centre and the telecoms arrangement, also need to be MDA approved in order to provide the same level of quality throughout? Second generation telecare involves the data mining of lifestyle information gathered through a variety of sensors, most of which will have been designed and manufactured for security applications rather than for care purposes. This will mean that the entirety of the data set will not be reliable. Should this limit the use of, and belief in the outputs of the system? Clearly, a new set of standards will be needed to ensure that errors in measurement do not result in wrong assessments which, in turn, lead to inappropriate levels of care provision being offered.

25.6 Conclusions

As things currently stand, there is no simple way for a system purchaser to easily determine the dependability of an electronic AT system, as there is no appropriate single standard it may demonstrate compliance with. One solution would be to modify the Medical Devices Regulations to make them more applicable, by creating either a subcategory within it or a completely new standard. Such a standard has to close the various loop holes by which manufacturers currently avoid providing a full risk analysis, but at the same time, reduce the costs and practical difficulties that make them seek these loop holes in the first place. For some suggestions about alternative risk analysis procedures see Williams et al. (2000) and Hone *et al.* (submitted).

Another way round the problem would be for the people who purchase the electronic AT to insist on compliance with multiple standards. This document has shown that, even though coverage is patchy, there are existing standards that can be applied to electronic AT. The drawback with this approach, however, is that unless a manufacturer is already working to some of these standards, there may be a high cost involved in attaining compliance. It is likely that at least some of this extra cost will be passed on by the manufacturer to the people who purchase the systems or that valuable ideas will not come to market. There may, again, also be problems of clearly defining which standards are applicable.

Whatever route is taken, the need to report failures to a central authority is an important requirement. This authority can then record and track these problems and, where appropriate, issue safety bulletins as the MDA does for other devices at the moment. This probably means establishing a similar reporting scheme for electronic AT, outside of the MDA. Such systems exist in other domains, although there are obvious logistical problems – such as who would run the system, and who would pay for it – none of which appear insurmountable. Such a system would provide another useful source of data for the designers of electronic AT systems and for those updating the standard.

Table 25.2. Standards (potentially) applicable to the development of electronic AT systems

Year	Reference	Title
2001	ISO 13485	Quality systems -- Medical devices -- Particular requirements for the application of ISO 9001
1996	ISO 13488	Quality systems -- Medical devices -- Particular requirements for the application of ISO 9002
2001	ISO 14971	Medical Devices: Application of Risk Management
2002	BS EN 50134-1	Alarm systems. Social alarm systems. System requirements
2000	BS EN 50134-2	Alarm systems. Social alarm systems. Trigger devices
2001	BS EN 50134-3	Alarm systems. Social alarm systems. Local unit and controller
1996	BS EN 50134-7	Alarm systems. Social alarm systems. Application guidelines
2002	ASAP COP	Association of Social Alarm Providers Code of Practice: A Management framework for best practice. Part 1 – Call handling operations
2000	BS 5979	Code of practice for remote centres receiving signals from security systems
1997	DEF-STAN 00-42	Software reliability. Reliability and maintainability (R&M) assurance guides. Part 2: Software
1997	DEF STAN 00-55	Requirements for safety related software in defence equipment
1997	DEF STAN 00-56	Safety management requirements for defence systems
2000	DEF STAN 00-58	Hazop studies on systems containing programmable electronics
2000	ISO 9001	Quality Management Systems – Requirements
1995	ISO/IEC 12207	Software Life Cycle Processes
1998	ISO 15504	Software Process Assessment (9 parts)
2001	ISO/IEC 9126-1	Software Engineering – Product Quality. Part 1: Quality Model
1999	IEC 61508	Functional safety of electrical/electronic/programmable electronic safety related systems
1995	AECL CE-1001-STD	Standard for software engineering of safety critical software
1992	RTCA DO-178B/ED-12B	Software considerations in airborne systems and equipment certification
1996-2000	ISO 9241	Ergonomics requirements for office work with visual display terminals (VDTs)
1999	ISO 13407	Human centred design process for interactive systems
1998	DPA	Data Protection Act

25.7 Acknowledgements

Baxter, Monk, Blythe and Dewsbury were supported by the Dependability Interdisciplinary Research Collaboration ("DIRC") funded by the UK EPSRC (grant number GR/N13999).

25.8 References

Dewsbury G, Sommerville I, Clarke K, Rouncefield M (2003) A dependability model for domestic systems. In: Proceedings of Safecomp 2003, Springer Verlag, Berlin, Germany

Hone K, Monk AF, Lines L, Dowdall A, Baxter G, Blythe M, Wright P (submitted) Risk analysis in the home: enabling people with disabilities and the elderly to live independently

MacKenzie DM. (2002). Medical device risk management. In: Proceedings of the 20th International System Safety Conference. The System Safety Society, Unionville, VA, USA

Sheard SA (2001) Evolution of the frameworks quagmire. IEEE Computer 34(7): 96-98

Williams G, Doughty K, Bradley DA (2000) Safety and risk issues in using telecare. Journal of telemedicine and telecare 6: 249-262

Chapter 26

If I had a Robot at Home…
Peoples' Representation of Domestic Robots

M. Scopelliti, M.V. Giuliani, A.M. D'Amico and
F. Fornara

26.1 Introduction

The decrease in childbirth and the great increase in life expectancy represent typical demographic trends in industrialised countries. These tendencies make more concrete the issue regarding elderly people: the more they grow old, the more they are likely to need medical, social and personal care services. Nursing home care services are probably the most important example in terms of social costs, not only because they are extremely expensive from an economic point of view, but also because they determine a forced relocation of elderly people. To be compelled to live in a new place, completely depending on other people's assistance, has unquestionably a deep psychological impact (Hormuth, 1990): probably more difficult to assess than the economic expenditures, but definitely not less significant. Elderly people undoubtedly prefer living independently in a familiar domestic and residential setting. Anyway, a new series of problems arises, due to the shortage of residential infrastructures and facilities and the lack of home service workers compared to the large number of people who need assistance. As for domestic settings, in addition, the psychological impact of a long term home care assistance is still far from well understood: assistance provided by other people can generate a stronger negative influence upon final users, in that they may perceive a loss of control in their living space, and they may look at home service caregivers as privacy intruders. This condition may represent a menace to self-esteem and to the integrity of personal identity.

26.1.1 Assistive Technology

An alternative solution to human home care assistance may be represented by assistive technology. The term "assistive technology" refers to a broad array of devices which can accomplish several tasks at home. First of all, they can be used in treatment and rehabilitation of debilitated people who suffer from accidents and diseases which temporarily impair their normal functioning. Second, they can be used as assistive devices in long term care for people with chronic illness. Electronic devices give the possibility of checking a variety of health conditions. There are monitoring machines capable of detecting common health indicators, ranging from blood pressure to temperature and weight, as well as more advanced technology which can recognise severe breathing or heart problems and prevent respiratory and cardiac arrest by immediately warning a caregiver (Stewart and Kaufman, 1993); similarly, in the event of a fall, detectors that "sense acceleration, change of position and impact could automatically report to a caregiver" (ibid., p. 4). Finally, they can be used to help ageing people with near-normal functioning levels to manage everyday tasks at home. Smart sensors and intelligent units in telecare systems are non-intrusive devices which can provide for a wide range of domestic warnings, preventing different risks such as overflowing in bathroom and kitchen, gas escape, extreme room temperature and so on (Doughty, 1999).

Despite advances in technology and robotics that make available innovative devices for the care of elderly people, the practical advantage of their use (e.g. reducing economic costs) is far from being the only issue. Assistive technology often fails to be adopted or used because of inadequate training on how to use it; because all the potential benefits to people's independence are not understood; because their design appears cumbersome (Elliot, 1991). In addition, the psychological implications of either having a human caregiver or a technological device supporting one's daily life and activities at home are undoubtedly different.

Theoretical and empirical evidence is available to support this statement. Doughty (1999) argues that technological devices can provide continuous care, they are objective in their analysis, and they never get stressed or tired. They can foster elderly people's independence and improve their quality of life. Nonetheless, they are not able to "substitute for the tender loving care that can be given thanklessly by dedicated individuals". Stewart and Kaufman (1993) claim that activities such as eating and personal hygiene represent areas in which technological assistance is preferred to human aid, because perceived control over life is enhanced. Monk and Baxter (2002) underline that one of the advantages of the smart home can be the opportunity to socialise for people experiencing loneliness, through video conferencing facilities. The care of elderly people is a complex experience in which social, emotional and environmental factors play a central role (Hirsch et al., 2000). Beyond the impact of design on usability (too small buttons, printed letters hard to read, etc.), an important task is to understand what are the real needs of final users. Ignoring this aspect would pose serious difficulties for the adoption of potentially useful devices. Gitlin (1995) tried to deepen the user's perspective, shedding light on the reasons why elderly people may accept or reject the use of assistive technology. Depending on personal factors, helping devices may be viewed either as mechanisms by which to regain independence or as threats to self-identity and social life. Independence, however, is not only a matter of personal ability, but must be considered as the result of person-environment fit (Steinfeld and Shea, 1993). Houses are often full of physical barriers, which are frequently underestimated by elderly people. Home modification may improve people's independence, but elderly people often consider difficulties as conditions they have to live with, hardly seeing good reasons for change. From a psychological point of view, continuity in place experience is a key factor in preserving personal identity (Breakwell, 1986).

26.1.2 Interactive Robots

Beyond technology related to domestic risk prevention and aimed at increasing home suitability, a greater challenge consists in the implementation of a new generation of technological devices, which can interact with people, providing personal assistance in common everyday activities. Mahoney (1997) reviewed the market of rehabilitation robot products, paying particular attention to a device designed to help people to eat; Baltus *et al.* (2000) developed a project aimed at the implementation of a mobile robot which can accomplish various personal-aid tasks in many primary functions. It goes beyond health care (data collection, health indicators detection, tele-medicine, etc.) to safeguarding the elderly person and monitoring the environment and other people inside the home. It is also a useful device to remind health-related activities (e.g. to take a medicine) and, in general, things to do. Although its vocabulary is not very large, it can provide information related to different daily activities, such as the television programs and the weather forecast. Furthermore, it is able to interact with people through a real-time speech interface consisting of a speech recognition and a speech synthesis system.

The possibility of using such a device is definitely a further step in evolution compared to the smart home technology. However, it probably implies a different kind of psychological reaction in people, mainly because robots cannot be simply considered as assistive devices but also as entities to interact with in a more or less humanlike relationship. Today, robotic agents can engage in a variety of peer-to-peer relations, reacting to human behaviour or actively encouraging social interaction (Fong and Nourbakhsh, 2003). The interaction can also consist of a continuous human-robot dialogue, called "collaborative control" (Nass and Moon, 2000), through which the robot asks questions to the human being in order to get assistance and to solve problems.

Regardless of which activities robots can actually perform, another important psychological question is how people would react to them. It has been shown recently through a series of experimental studies (Nass and Moon, 2000) that people may unconsciously attribute social rules and gender stereotypes to computers, and may engage in a humanlike interaction, which implies politeness, reciprocity and self-disclosure. Duffy (2003) argues that humans sometimes tend to anthropomorphise inanimate entities, by attributing cognitive/emotional states to them and by interpreting their behaviour as if it were governed by rational choices and consideration of their desires (Dennett, 1996). It is suggested that robots can be more acceptable if they resemble human beings in some way.

Science fiction is probably a source of influence for people's representation of humanlike robots: it gives a twofold image of robots as helping assistants or, on the other hand, as more frightening potential competitors – or, even worse, overwhelming entities! However, a *domestic* robot is probably difficult to conceive, because it can hardly be associated with any kind of real experience.

Nonetheless, the aim of exploring people's ideas about such advanced devices would allow the designers to adjust its features to what people need and expect. Khan (1998) developed a questionnaire to assess people's attitude towards getting help from a domestic robot in Sweden. Respondents were shown to be rather positive towards having a robot performing domestic tasks. In addition, they felt safe about it and did not feel that it would intrude their privacy. Speech was found to be the preferred way of communicating, showing again the tendency to favour a humanlike interaction with the robot. The results of the study can be a useful agenda for robot producers, who aim to fulfil the user's needs and expectations in terms of design and functionality (Oestreicher et al., 1999).

26.2 The Research

The aim of this study is to investigate people's representation of domestic robots by using a psychological approach. Particular attention is focused on age-related, gender and educational level differences.

In a pilot study (Cesta et al., 2003), we interviewed the members of six families, including three different generations, asking them questions partially extracted from Kahn's tool (1998). We found that elderly people generally care about a harmonious integration of robots in the socio-physical environment of the home, asking for requirements such as "the robot must not frighten the pets" or "it should not be a cumbersome obstacle". The robot's shape is described in a wide array of different ways, ranging from a minimum to a maximum degree of anthropomorphism (from "cylinder to parallelepiped, with no reference to human beings" to "it should be like a child, so that I will not see it as a stranger"). Respondents often imagine the potential interaction with the robot by referring to social dynamics which are typical of human beings ("I would like it to mind its own business" or "I would speak to it as if it were a person, I would never give it an order like a dictator would"). These data were used to develop a questionnaire, in order to collect quantitative data and to compare the representations of people at different stages of their life.

26.2.1 Method

Sample. We contacted a sample of 120 subjects, balanced by gender and age group (18-25, 40-50, 65-75). People were all urban residents, living in different neighbourhoods in Rome, and as heterogeneous as possible with respect to educational level and familiarity with technology.

Tool. The questionnaire centred on several topics which emerged as highly important in the pilot study. In addition to collecting socio-demographic data, the questionnaire addresses the following topics:

- Section one – Attitudes towards technology.
  13 5-point Likert-type items asking people to what extent they agreed/disagreed with sentences (from 0 = "I completely disagree" to 4 = "I completely agree") regarding features, advantages and disadvantages of modern technology;
- Section two – Robot capabilities.
  16 items focusing on the perceived capability for a robot to perform different everyday activities at home. Participants were asked to check each activity as "impossible", "probably available in the future", or "currently performed";
- Section three – Emotional response to robots.
  16 5-point Likert-type items focusing on emotional response to domestic robots. People were asked to check each adjective from 0 = "not at all" to 4 = "very much";
- Section four – Image of robots.
  9 categorical items focusing on people's preferences and expectancies about robot's shape, size, colour, cover material, speed, etc.;
- Section five – Human-robot interaction.
  15 categorical items focusing on people's preferences and expectancies about robot's personification (given name, etc.) and modalities of human-robot communication and interaction.

Analyses. Multivariate statistical procedures were applied to the data in order to unify and condense into a single comprehensive framework the several relationships underlying the observed data.

A two-phase strategy was adopted. First, two separate Factor Analyses were performed in order to identify the dimensions underlying a) people's attitudes towards technological devices, and b) emotional response to domestic robots. The factors extracted were used as dependent variables in a one-way ANOVA, in order to assess differences related to socio-demographic variables. In addition, an index of "trust in robotics achievements" was constructed by using the scores of "robot capabilities" items.

Secondly, Multiple Correspondence Analysis and Cluster Analysis were carried out in order to detect both the main patterns describing different preferences about the robot's aspect and interactive modality, and the main features of the various types of robot. Factorial scores obtained by subjects on the previous analyses and socio-demographic data were used as illustrative variables in order to show the relationships with the types of robot.

26.2.2 Results

Attitudes Towards Technology. The general attitude towards new technologies showed to be quite positive (mean score: 3.11), with no significant differences between age groups. By contrast, they use different strategies when learning how to use a new machine: young people use a "trial and error" strategy, adults read the instruction and elderly people ask more expert persons for help (χ^2= 32.06, df= 4, p< .001).

A Factor Analysis performed on 13 items yielded three different dimensions explaining a large proportion of variance (46.9%). The first dimension (labelled "Benefits of Technology": 23.6% of total variance) summarises the advantages provided by technology: they help people not to get tired and not to waste time, they allow them to perform different tasks and to be independent of others, etc. The second dimension ("Disadvantages of Technology": 13.1 of total variance) synthesise practical negative aspects: electronic devices break down too often, they are not easy to use and instructions are hard to understand. The third dimension ("Mistrust": 10.2% of total variance) emphasises a general negative feeling towards technology, in that sophisticated devices are not perceived as stimulating objects and people don't trust in them.

The ANOVA performed on attitude factors showed no significant effect of age group on the first two dimensions; on the opposite, the effect on "Mistrust" ($F_{(2, 115)}$ = 5.90, p<.01) was significant. The Bonferroni test (p< .05) showed that older people perceive mistrust towards technology significantly more than adults and young people. Also the effect of gender was significant on "Mistrust" ($F_{(1, 116)}$= 8.58, p< .01): females revealed a stronger diffidence towards technology than males.

Assessment of Robots Capability. We found that people's representation of robot capabilities is somewhat distorted. On the one hand, activities that imply object manipulation (such as dusting, cleaning windows, making beds, laying and clearing the table, using the washing-machine and finding objects) are perceived as much easier to implement by robotic technology than they are in fact. On the other hand, people underestimate the actual implementation of such activities as entertainment and home safety control, which imply cognitive tasks and are indeed already available. Nonetheless, they accurately recognise the current availability of robotic devices that are able to remind of engagements and prompt things to do. They are also realistic about the difficulties of implementing robots that can help people cook and cut their nails. The total score obtained on the 16 items was transformed in a categorical variable with three modalities: "optimistic" towards advances in robotics, "pessimistic" and "realistic".

Emotional Reactions to a Domestic Robot. A Factor Analysis performed on 16 items yielded two different dimensions, explaining a large proportion of variance (57.9%). The first dimension, labelled "Positive Feelings", explains 38.7% of total variance. It describes a positive reaction, which implies the representation of robots as lively, dynamic, interesting, stimulating, etc. entities. The second dimension, labelled "Negative Feelings", explains 19.2% of total variance. It describes a negative reaction, in that robots are perceived as dangerous, scary, potentially out of control, cumbersome, etc.

The ANOVA on the emotional response factors revealed a significant effect of age group on both "Positive Feelings" ($F_{(2, 111)}$= 3.47, p< .05) and "Negative Feelings" ($F_{(2, 111)}$= 4.97, p<.01). Post hoc analysis showed that young people express a more positive emotional response than older people; older people showed a more negative emotional response than both adults and young people (Bonferroni, p< .05). The effect of the educational level was significant on the variable "Negative Feelings" ($F_{(2, 111)}$= 8.82, p< .01): people with lower educational level expressed more negative feelings than people who attended high-school and people who have a degree (Bonferroni, p< .05).

Preferences about Robot's Aspect and Interaction Modalities. In order to obtain a global description of the set of associations among variables, Multiple Correspondence Analysis was performed on 19 variables describing the preferences. In this application the study focused on the first three axes which reproduced 76% of the total information (Benzécri's correction).

The first three factorial axes were interpreted using the absolute contributions together with two-dimensional graphical representations. The first axis opposes a lack of preferences as to the physical aspect of the robot and a preference for a not speaking device, controlled by a keyboard, to the specificity of expressed preferences. The second axis opposes a preference for a device executing fixed tasks, made by plastic material, moving slowly, and communicating by acoustic signals, to an autonomous and human-like robot. The third axis opposes an amusing pet-like object, with low autonomy, to a serious device, with a name given by the producer and communicating through luminous signals. The first two axes are significantly associated to the age groups, the first opposing adults to young and elderly people; the second opposing the elderly to young people and adults.

Table 26.2.1. Robots' representations in the 5 groups

N. of ss. x group	Significant associations in each cluster (p <.01)
Group 1: N=37	Human and amusing aspect (skin-like cover), male name/voice, free to move and to autonomously act, humanlike mode of interaction, introduced by given name, personalised aspect, not disturbing privacy
Group 2: N=37	Female name/voice, not free to move, not called by given name
Group 3: N=15	Pet-like size/name, moving slowly, standard aspect, tasks executor, disturbing privacy
Group 4: N=20	No voice, (communicates through luminous signals), called by remote control/keyboard, market name, introduced as a device, not free to move
Group 5: N=11	No preferences as to aspect, size, colour, cover material, name, human-robot interaction

Different types of robots emerged as a result of a hierarchical cluster analysis carried out in the factorial space of the first three axes. A 5-group partition was found at a level of 71% for the Inertia inter/Total Inertia ratio. The active variables significantly associated to each cluster are summarised in Table 26.2.1.

As regards the age groups, the young are mainly oriented towards the types represented in clusters 1 and 2, the adults towards types 1 and 5, and the elderly towards type 2 and 3. The large majority of people who choose type 5 are adults, and the preferences towards type 4 are nearly equally distributed among the groups.

The barycentre of the five clusters was projected on the factorial space of the first two axes together with the illustrative variables, in order to graphically represent the association between the robots' representation and the other characteristics of the respondents (Fig. 26.2.1).

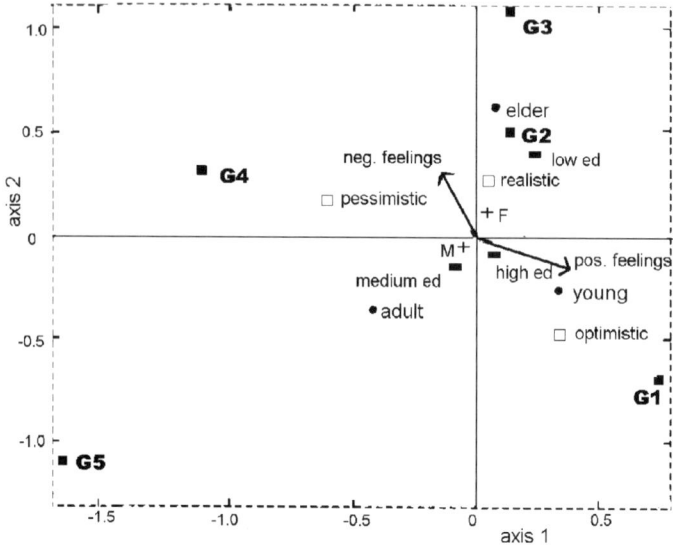

Figure 26.2.1. Two dimensional representation (axis 1 and 2) of cluster barycentres (G1-G5) and illustrative variables

As shown in the figure, the continuous variable representing the affective reaction is significantly related to the clusters, in particular regarding positive feelings, which are positively related to G1 and negatively related to G5. Negative feelings are negatively related to G1. The educational level and the representation of robot capabilities do not have any significant association with the clusters.

26.2.3 Discussion

Results show that the general idea on technology is rather positive in our sample. However, when speaking about a domestic robot, which is a more specific device, the global evaluation becomes much more multi-faceted. A strong coherence between robot aspect and modality of human-robot interaction emerged; in addition, variables related to preferred interaction highly characterise the different representations.

On the one hand, young people have a strong familiarity with technology and a friendly idea of robots: in fact, young people score higher on "positive feelings" than the other groups. In their representation domestic robots are not useful devices, but humanlike entities to interact with in leisure situations; almost all of them would like to have a speaking robot, mainly with a young voice, and the possibility to personalise its aspect, which would be in general amusing.

On the other hand, elderly people are the most frightened at the prospect of having a robot at home, and they try to ward off their anxiety by attributing to the robot features able to reduce the impact with the machine: small size, slow motion, feminine voice, and executing collaborative tasks. Although technology can be useful, older people show a slight mistrust towards machines that are likely to be unsafe to some extent.

Adults seem to be by far the least homogeneous group in expressing ideas, preferences, attitudes and emotional responses to the possibility of having a robot at home. A substantial percentage of them is highly characterised in terms of "absence of preferences" as to their physical features and type of human-robot interaction. In addition, they show mid-point scores on attitude and emotional dimensions extrapolated from Factor Analyses. It could depend on a sort of disenchantment with technology, in that adults probably undervalue both the stimulating/exciting (appreciated by young people) and the practical/functional side (appreciated by elderly people) of having such innovative devices. They probably consider a domestic robot as a device which is too futuristic to spend time in thinking about. However, part of them share with young people a more friendly view of such a device, even if the majority of them would prefer to have complete control over it.

Gender and educational level differences were shown to be far less important.

26.3 Conclusion

This study represents an attempt to understand the potential impact of the introduction of domestic robots in people's everyday life. The analysis of the general attitudes towards technology and the specific representations of such futuristic devices seemed to be a good starting point to identify some basic acceptability requirements, which would provide robot designers and producers with useful guidelines for further innovation. A deeper knowledge on this topic could be achieved by using a larger sample and by comparing representations of people from different cultures. Despite the huge advances in technology and robotics, the psychological implications of human-robot interactions still remain a scarcely explored field. An inquiry into people's representations of domestic robots appears to be a suitable way for bridging the gap between the possibilities granted by new technologies and the users' needs.

26.4 Acknowledgements

This research is partially supported by MIUR (Italian Ministry of Education, University and Research) under project RoboCare (A Multi-Agent System with Intelligent Fixed and Mobile Robotic Components).

26.5 References

Baltus G, Fox D, Gemperl F, Goetz J, Hirsch T, Magaritis D et al. Toward personal service robots for the elderly. In: WIRE' 00. Available at: http://www.cs.cmu.ed/~nursebot/web/papers.html

Breakwell G (1986) Coping with threatened identity. London: Methuen

Cesta A, Bahadori S, Cortellessa G, Grisetti G, Giuliani MV, Iocchi L, et al. (2003) The RoboCare project. Cognitive systems for the care of the elderly. In: Conference on Aging, Disability and Independence. Washington DC, USA

Dennett DC (1996) Kinds of minds. New York: Basic Books

Doughty K (1999) Can a computer be a carer? In: 9th Alzheimer Europe Meeting & Alzheimer's Disease Society Conference, London, UK

Duffy BR (2003) Anthropomorphism and the social robot. Robotics and Autonomous Systems 42: 177-190

Elliot R (1991) Assistive technology for the frail elderly: An introduction and overview. Washington: U.S. Department of Health and Human Services

Fong T, Nourbakhsh I (2003) Socially interactive robots. Robotics and Autonomous Systems 42: 139-141

Gitlin LN (1995) Why older people accept or reject assistive technology. Generations, Journal of the American Society on Aging 19: 41-46

Hirsch T, Forlizzi J, Hyder E, Goetz J, Stroback J, Kurtz C (2000) The ELDer Project: Social and emotional factors in the design of eldercare technologies. In: Conference on Universal Usability. Arlington, Virginia, USA

Hormuth SE (1990) The ecology of self: Relocation and self-concept change. Cambridge: Cambridge University Press

Khan Z (1998) Attitude towards intelligent service robots. Technical Report No. TRITA-NA-P9821. Stockholm: NADA, KTH

Mahoney RM (1997) Robotic products for rehabilitation: Status and strategy. In: Proceedings of ICORR '97 - International Conference on Rehabilitation Robotics. Bath, UK. Available at: (http://www.bath.ac.uk/bime/icorrproc/mahoney1.pdf)

Monk AF, Baxter G (2002) Would you trust a computer to run your home? Dependability issues in smart homes for older adults. In: A New Research Agenda for Older Adults, Workshop at BCS HCI 2002, London, UK

Nass C, Moon Y (2000) Machines and mindlessness: Social response to computers. Journal of Social Issues 56: 81-103

Oestreicher L, Hüttenrauch H, Severinsson-Eklund K (1999) Where are you going little robot? CHI 99 Basic Research Symposium, In: ACM CHI'99. Available at: http://www.nada.kth.se/iplab/hri/publications/chi99/

Steinfeld E, Shea S (1993) Enabling home environment: Identifying barriers to independence. Technology and Disability 2(4): 69-79

Stewart LM, Kaufman SB (1993) High-Tech home care: Electronic devices with implications for the design of living environments. In: Life-span Design of Residential Environments for an Aging Populations. AARP: Washington DC, USA

Index of Contributors